PRACTICAL CLINICAL BIOCHEMISTRY
Volume 2

PRACTICAL CLINICAL BIOCHEMISTRY

VOLUME 2
HORMONES, VITAMINS, DRUGS AND POISONS

BY

HAROLD VARLEY
MSc, FRIC

Honorary Consultant Biochemist, Manchester Royal Infirmary.
Formerly Head of the Biochemistry Department, Manchester Royal Infirmary
and Lecturer in Clinical Pathology, University of Manchester.

ALAN H. GOWENLOCK
MSc, MB ChB, PhD, FRIC, FRCPath

Consultant Chemical Pathologist, Manchester Royal Infirmary and Associated Hospitals,
Reader in Chemical Pathology, University of Manchester.

MAURICE BELL
MSc, FRIC

Chief Biochemist, Manchester Royal Infirmary and Associated Hospitals.

FIFTH EDITION

WILLIAM HEINEMANN MEDICAL BOOKS LTD
LONDON

First published.	.	1954
Second Edition	.	1958
Reprinted	. .	1960
Third Edition .	.	1962
Reprinted	. .	1963
Reprinted	. .	1964
Reprinted	. .	1965
Reprinted	. .	1966
Fourth Edition reset.		1967
Fifth Edition reset	.	1976
Reprinted	. .	1981

ISBN 0 433 33803 2

© Harold Varley 1976

All rights reserved

Printed in Great Britain by
The Whitefriars Press Ltd, London and Tonbridge

PREFACE TO THE FIRST EDITION

THE rapid development of clinical biochemistry has been an outstanding feature of medicine during the past twenty to thirty years. The present book is a survey of the whole field of this subject from the standpoint of workers in hospital laboratories. It is hoped that it will appeal particularly to registrars training in clinical pathology, to hospital biochemists, and to laboratory technicians. The book should be especially useful to technicians studying for the examination in Chemical Pathological Technique of the Institute of Medical Laboratory Technology. As the tests described are also used in many laboratories not directly concerned with diagnosis and treatment, so far as possible the needs of workers in medical research laboratories have also been borne in mind.

While the purpose of the book is essentially practical, it was felt that summaries of the findings in health and disease would add considerably to its value. Although these are necessarily brief they are provided to obviate frequent reference to larger works on the interpretation of biochemical tests. No claim is made that these replace entirely such books a few examples of which are given in the short bibliography on p. 764.

My debts to other authors are many. In a rapidly developing subject such as this much is owed to the various journals which publish papers on biochemical methods. Full references to these are given. Books on practical methods which I have found valuable are also listed in the bibliography already referred to.

I wish gratefully to acknowledge permission to use material by the following: *Acta medica Scandinavica,* for material from Supplement 128 (1942) by Dr. H. O. Lagerlöf; *American Journal of Physiology* for Table XVII; Bayer Products Ltd. for Fig. 4; British Drug Houses Ltd. for the list of primary standards on p. 756; Messrs. J. and A. Churchill Ltd. for normal values for haemoglobin from "Practical Haematology", by J. V. Dacie on p. 587; Evans Electroselenium for Figs. 81 and 82; Harvard University Press for Fig. 86 adapted from "Chemical Anatomy, Physiology and Pathology of Extracellular Fluid," by J. L. Gamble; Ilford Ltd. for Figs, 9 and 10; *The Journal of Clinical Endocrinology* and Dr. S. Soskin for Fig. 36; *The Lancet* for Fig. 26a; *The Lancet* and Dr. J. D. Robertson for Table XVIII; Messrs. H. K. Lewis and Co. Ltd. for material on p. 375 from the *British Journal of Experimental Pathology*; Messrs. E. S. Livingstone for the table of Standard Weights on p. 762 from "A Textbook of Dietetics," by L. S. P. Davidson and I. A. Anderson; Dr. G. Lusk for Table XX; The Josiah Macy Jr. Foundation for material from the booklet "Copper Sulphate Method for Measuring Specific Gravities of Whole Blood and Plasma," by Phillips *et al.*; Messrs. May and Baker Ltd. for material on pp. 744-747 from their booklet "The Estimation of Sulphonamides"; Dr. M. Somogyi for Table XI; Dr. J. H. van de Kamer for Fig. 76; Drs. D. D. van Slyke and G. E. Cullen for Table XIV; Messrs. Williams and Wilkins for material on Indicators and Buffers on pp. 758-760 from "The Determinavi _Preface_

tion of Hydrogen Ions," by W. M. Clark (published in Great Britain by Baillière, Tindall and Cox Ltd.).

I should like especially to express my thanks to my wife who did nearly all the diagrams and formulae, and to several of my friends and colleagues from whose help I have benefited considerably. Dr. J. E. Kench has read the whole of the proofs whilst Dr. H. T. Howat, Dr. S. W. Stanbury, Mr. M. Bell and Mr. J. E. Southall have each read sections. I have received constant encouragement and advice from Dr. R. W. Fairbrother. For any errors either of omission or commission which still remain the author must accept sole responsibility.

Finally, I should like to thank my publishers for their unfailing consideration and patience during the period in which the book was being written and published.

H. V.

October, 1953

PREFACE TO FIFTH EDITION, VOLUME 2

Shortly after the publication of the fourth edition of this book in 1967 its original author retired from his post at Manchester Royal Infirmary, which he had occupied for over forty years. When the time came to consider the preparation of a further edition, the need for some assistance was obvious. He therefore invited two colleagues with whom he had been associated for many years to collaborate with him in producing the fifth edition. These are Dr A. H. Gowenlock who had been appointed as Consultant Chemical Pathologist and Director of the Biochemistry Department of the Manchester Royal Infirmary and associated hospitals (now Manchester Area Health Authority (Teaching), Central District) and Mr Maurice Bell, Chief Biochemist in the same department.

It was early decided that although considerable changes had been made in successive editions resulting in an increase of about 50 per cent in the original length of the book, with the ever increasing rate of advance in the subject, a more detailed and complete revision was now required. This started in 1971. For a variety of departmental and personal reasons and because of the enormous amount of new work in practically all branches of the subject, progress was slower than anticipated. It became apparent that the resulting increased size of the book would produce a volume undesirably large and too unwieldy for a bench book. On reflection it was decided that the text should be divided into two volumes. The more highly specialised subjects of hormones, vitamins, drugs and poisons form the chapters in the second volume. The remaining topics which form the basis of the work of all clinical chemistry departments appear as the first volume of a size similar to the single volume of the last edition. As events have turned out the second volume is ready for publication first. We hope that this solution of our difficulties will be acceptable to the many users of this book and we would like to express our regret at the delay in publication.

We have introduced the use of SI units in both volumes but have retained equivalent values in traditional units in the majority of cases. Although this makes for increased length and some difficulty in reading the text, it was felt that at this stage, both sets of units were sufficiently widely used to make this dual approach justifiable. We have used the recommended abbreviations and have selected the litre as the unit of volume when expressing concentrations.

When making up reagents it is assumed that, unless stated specifically otherwise, the chemicals used are of analytical reagent grade and that they are dissolved either in distilled water or deionised water of high quality.

In this volume we have extended the sections on practical techniques to include newer methods within the scope of an average-sized laboratory. In addition there has been extra emphasis on background information to place these techniques in a proper context. This includes an abbreviated account of more specialised techniques. The sections on clinical interpretation have also been extended. It is hoped that the revised version will make this volume of use to several different grades of reader. It should be of help to the technician working at the bench and also preparing for qualifying examinations but it is also intended to assist more senior medical and scientific hospital staff in the understanding of these specialised aspects of clinical biochemistry and in the interpretation of the results of laboratory investigations.

We would like to acknowledge the aid we have received from many colleagues with whom we have had helpful discussions. In particular we thank Mr E. King, National Occupational Hygiene Service, Manchester, for permission to reproduce his method for the determination of lead. Dr A. T. Howarth and Mr D. A. Robertshaw, Bradford Royal Infirmary, allowed us to include their manual method for the fluorimetric determination of urinary oestrogens as did Mr G. Davies, Broadgreen Hospital, Liverpool for his method for methylmalonic acid. Mrs G. E. Price and Dr S. L. Ch'ng were responsible for extending the information on the colour reactions and absorption spectra of various drugs during investigations in our department. Some of the diagrams are the work of the Department of Medical Illustration, Manchester Royal Infirmary. We are grateful to Miss E. T. Cunningham and Miss C. M. Ratcliffe for their invaluable help in typing the manuscript. Finally, we would like to express our thanks to our publishers for their forebearance and for their help and advice, in preparing this edition. The responsibility for the choice of material, the opinions expressed and any residual errors in the text, however, rests with the authors.

H. VARLEY,
A. H. GOWENLOCK,
M. BELL.

CONTENTS

CHAPTER		PAGE
	Preface to the First Edition	v
	Preface to the Fifth Edition, Volume 2	vii
	Contents of Volume 1	x
	Abbreviations	xi
1.	THYROID FUNCTION TESTS	1
2.	STEROID HORMONES Introduction and Techniques for C_{19} and C_{21} Steroids	45
3.	STEROID HORMONES The Hypothalamic-Pituitary-Adrenal Axis	82
4.	OESTROGENS AND PROGESTOGENS TESTS OF GONADAL FUNCTION FETO-PLACENTAL FUNCTION TESTS IN PREGNANCY	105
5.	ADRENALINE, NORADRENALINE AND RELATED COMPOUNDS	193
6.	VITAMINS	215
7.	DRUGS AND POISONS	260
	Appendices	365
	Bibliography	377
	Index	379

CONTENTS OF VOLUME ONE

1. Hazards in the Biochemistry Laboratory.
2. Units.
3. Separative Procedures. Chromatography.
4. Separative Procedures. Electrophoresis.
5. Immunological Methods.
6. Instruments Using Measurements of Light Intensity.
7. Work Simplification. Automated Procedures.
8. Radio-isotopic Techniques.
9. Statistics.
10. The "Normal" Range. Reference Values.
11. Quality Control.
12. Collection of Specimens. Some General Techniques.
13. Blood Glucose and its Determination.
14. Glucose Tolerance. Tests for Investigating Hypoglycaemia.
15. Tests for Reducing Substances in Urine.
16. Diabetes Mellitus. Ketosis.
17. Non-Protein Nitrogen. Urea, Uric Acid, Creatine, Creatinine.
18. Amino Acids.
19. Plasma Proteins.
20. Urinary Proteins.
21. Lipoproteins and Lipids.
22. Enzymes.
23. Sodium, Potassium, Chloride.
24. Acid Base Regulation.
25. Calcium, Magnesium, Phosphorus, Phosphatases.
26. Iron, Copper, Zinc.
27. Porphyrins, Haemoglobin and Related Compounds.
28. Gastric Function Tests. Occult Blood.
29. Tests in Liver Disease. Jaundice.
30. Tests in Pancreatic Disease.
31. Tests in Diseases of the Small Intestine.
32. Renal Function Tests.
33. Urinary deposits. Calculi.
34. Urinary and Faecal Pigments.
35. Cerebrospinal Fluid. Milk.

ABBREVIATIONS

ACTH	Adrenocorticotrophic hormone
δ-ALA	Delta-aminolaevulinic acid
ALT	Alanine aminotransferase
AST	Aspartate aminotransferase
BDH	British Drug Houses Ltd.
BSA	Bovine serum albumin
CAH	Congenital adrenal hyperplasia
CPB	Competitive protein binding
CRH	Corticotrophin releasing hormone
DHA	Dehydroepiandrosterone
DIT	Di-iodotyrosine
DUH	Dysfunctional uterine haemorrhage
E1	Oestrone
E2	Oestradiol
E3	Oestriol
EDTA	Ethylenediamine-tetraacetic acid
EEL	Evans Electroselenium Ltd.
FAD	Flavin adenine dinucleotide
FIGLU	Formiminoglutamic acid
FMN	Flavin mononucleotide
FSH	Follicle stimulating hormone
FTI	Free thyroxine index
GLC	Gas-liquid chromatography
γ-GT	Gamma-glutamyl transpeptidase
HCG	Human chorionic gonadotrophin
5-HIAA	5-Hydroxyindoleacetic acid
HMG	Human menopausal gonadotrophin
HMMA	4-Hydroxy-3-methoxymandelic acid
HPA	Hypothalamic-anterior pituitary-adrenocortical axis
HPL	Human placental lactogen
HW	Hopkin and Williams Ltd.
IL	Instrumentation Laboratory Ltd.
2nd IRP,HMG	Second International Reference Preparation, HMG
LH	Luteinising hormone
MIMS	Monthly Index of Medical Specialities
MMA	Methylmalonic acid
MMPH	5-p-Methylphenyl-5-phenylhydantoin
MRC	Medical Research Council
NAD	Nicotinamide adenine dinucleotide
NADP	Nicotinamide adenine dinucleotide phosphate
NNDEA	N,N-Diethylaniline
NNED	N-Naphthylethylenediamine
NPGS	Neopentylglycol succinate
17-OGS	17-Oxogenic steroids
11-OHCS	11-Hydroxycorticosteroids
17-OHCS	17-Hydroxycorticosteroids
PBI	Protein-bound iodine
PGA	Pteroylglutamic acid
17-OS	17-Oxosteroids

xii

Abbreviations

RH	Releasing hormone
RIA	Radio-immunoassay
SD	Standard deviation
SE	Standard error
SHBG	Sex hormone binding globulin
T_3	Tri-iodothyronine
T_4	Thyroxine
TBG	Thyroxine binding globulin
TBPA	Thyroxine binding pre-albumin
THF	Tetrahydrofolic acid
TLC	Thin layer chromatography
TMS	Trimethylsilyl
TRH	Thyrotrophin releasing hormone
TSH	Thyroid stimulating hormone

CHAPTER 1

THYROID FUNCTION TESTS

THE THYROID gland contains two distinct endocrine systems which secrete different hormones.

1. The iodine-containing substances, *triiodothyronine* (3,5,3'-triiodo-L-thyronine) and *thyroxine* (3,5,3',5'-tetraiodothyronine), referred to as T_3 and T_4 respectively because of the number of iodine atoms in their molecules:

T_3 $\qquad$ $HO-\bigcirc-O-\bigcirc-CH_2 . CHNH_2 . COOH$

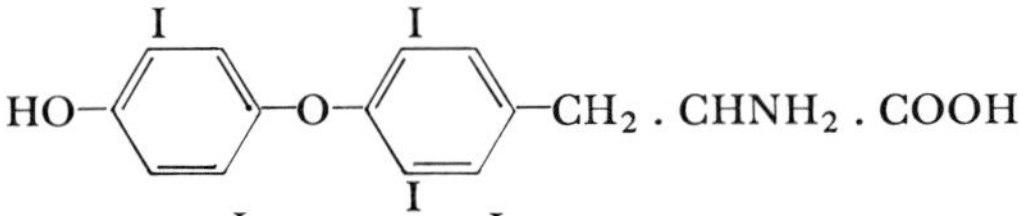

T_4 $\qquad$ $HO-\bigcirc-O-\bigcirc-CH_2 . CHNH_2 . COOH$

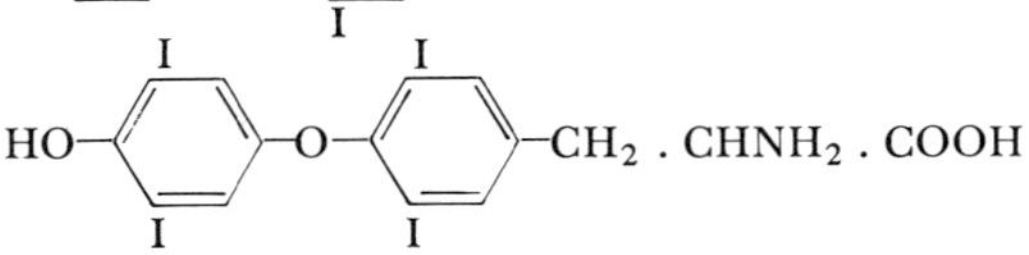

They are produced by the follicular cells of the thyroid (see Doniach, 1967), and act in a manner still imperfectly understood to increase the rate of metabolism of many metabolic processes in the body. There is increased metabolism of protein, carbohydrate and some lipids, with resulting overall increase in oxygen consumption. The production of these hormones is under the influence of thyrotrophin (thyroid stimulating hormone, TSH) secreted by the anterior pituitary. This glycoprotein is composed of two subunits, α and β. The α-subunit is also found in the gonadotrophins HCG, FSH, and LH (see Chapter 4). The secretion of TSH is partly directly controlled by a negative feed-back mechanism being stimulated by a low plasma concentration of the hormones and inhibited by a raised one. In addition, the thyrotrophin releasing hormone, TRH, produced in the hypothalamus, passes to the anterior pituitary and acts on the thyrotropic cells to produce a rapid release of TSH and probably increases TSH synthesis. It also causes the release of prolactin. It is now known that TRH is a tripeptide, L-pyroglutamyl-L-histidyl-L-proline amide.

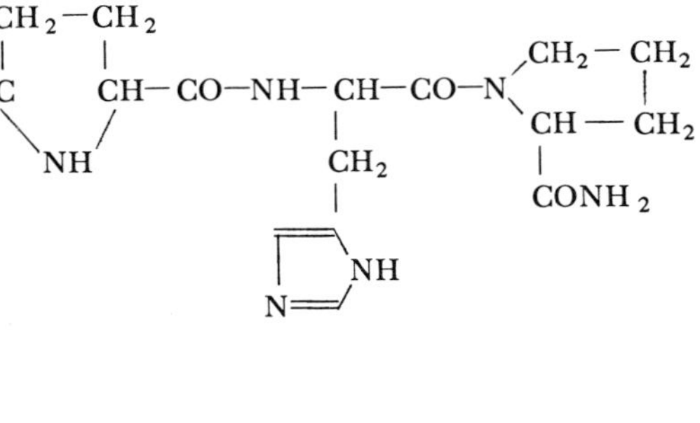

TRH

Its secretion is influenced by neural factors and its action on the anterior pituitary appears to be modulated by the level at which the feed-back action of thyroid hormones is set (see Reichlin, 1971).

2. *Calcitonin,* discovered much more recently (see McIntyre, 1967), is secreted by those cells in the thyroid known as C cells and acts to reduce the serum calcium by diminishing osteoclastic activity (see Chapter 25, Vol. 1).

These two activities are quite unrelated functionally. Thyroid function tests have been largely concerned either with the effect of disease on the production of the iodine-containing hormones and of the proteins which bind them or with the metabolic changes which result from increase or decrease in the amount of these hormones secreted.

The thyroid gland in mammals is characterised by its ability to concentrate iodide ions, a property shared with the salivary glands, gastric mucosa and mammary tissue. The conversion from inorganic iodide to the active hormones, T_3 and T_4, is a complex process not yet fully understood. The sequence of events is shown in Fig. 1,1. Inorganic iodide is concentrated into the cell in a process for which energy is required and is then oxidised to iodine by a peroxidase. The main iodinated product in the thyroid is the protein thyroglobulin, referred to histologically as colloid, which forms 70 to 80 per cent of the protein and contains nearly all the organic iodine in the normal thyroid. The intact molecule is a 19 S protein with mol. wt. about 640 000 which appears to consist of two types of tetramer made up of 8 S monomers of mol. wt. 160 000. The content of tyrosine residues in the thyroglobulin precursor, pre-thyroglobulin, amounts to about 3.1 per cent, equivalent to about 125 residues per molecule, some of which however are so placed that they cannot be iodinated. Iodination of the tyrosyl residues occurs within the pre-thyroglobulin molecule to give mono- and di-iodotyrosines (MIT, DIT). Coupling of these to form T_3 and T_4 follows. The hormones are then released by proteolytic degradation of the thyroglobulin molecule.

T_3 and T_4 are transported in the blood in relatively loose association with plasma proteins, not as peptides but in a form involving the free phenolic group of the hormones. These proteins must not be confused with thyroglobulin. The chief binding protein of human plasma is *thyroxine-binding globulin* (TBG) which migrates electrophoretically between the α_1 and α_2 globulins. It has a greater affinity for T_4 than for T_3, its capacity for T_4 being approximately 250 to 400 nmol/l (20 to 30 μg/100 ml) plasma and under normal physiological conditions carries 50 to 65 per cent of the plasma T_4. A second transport protein is *thyroxine-binding prealbumin* (TBPA) which carries 15 to 25 per cent of the T_4 and no T_3, having a total capacity of about 3 250 nmol/l (250 μg/100 ml). Albumin can also bind T_4 but with relatively low affinity and so plays little part in normal transport. Under normal physiological conditions about 75 per cent of the TBG sites and 99 per cent of the TBPA sites are unoccupied.

The reaction between T_4 and protein is reversible. In plasma there are always a certain number of free thyroxine molecules (FT_4) in constant

Thyroid Function Tests

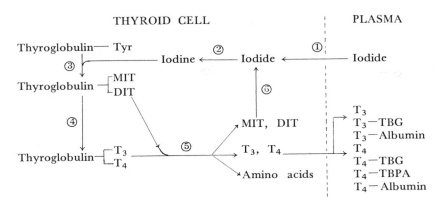

Where: 1 = iodide "carrier" or concentrating mechanism
(stimulated by TSH, inhibited by ClO_4^-, CNS^-)

2 = peroxidase
(stimulated by TSH, inhibited by thioureas)

3 = tyrosine iodinase

4 = "coupling" enzyme
(stimulated by TSH, inhibited by thioureas and sulphonamides)

5 = protease
(stimulated by TSH, inhibited by I^-)

6 = dehalogenase

Tyr = tyrosine residue in thyroglobulin molecule

MIT = monoiodotyrosine, $HO-\langle\bigcirc\rangle-CH_2-CH(NH_2)COOH$ (with I on ring)

DIT = diiodotyrosine, $HO-\langle\bigcirc\rangle-CH_2-CH(NH_2)COOH$ (with two I's on ring)

TBG = thyroxine-binding globulin

TBPA = thyroxine-binding pre-albumin

Fig. 1,1. Metabolism of Iodine in the Thyroid.

interchange with protein bound thyroxine molecules (PBT_4) while some protein binding sites have no T_4 bound to them (FP). The proportion of bound to unbound molecules in the case of a particular protein, is constant so long as the physical conditions of the medium do not change. This can be expressed as a dissociation constant

$$K = \frac{[FT_4][FP]}{[PBT_4]} \qquad \text{hence,} \qquad [FT_4] = K\frac{[PBT_4]}{[FP]}$$

There seems to be general agreement that FT_4, which has the higher diffusibility and is therefore better able to penetrate the extracellular space and reach the cells, is the biologically active fraction of the hormone. This, however, represents only 0.036 to 0.056 per cent of the total T_4 or from 35 to 74 pmol/l of serum (1.76 to 3.76 ng $T_4 I$ per 100 ml). Although methods have been devised for the determination of this fraction they are unlikely to be used for routine assessment of thyroid function. Similar remarks apply to serum T_3 for which values from 2.62 to 4.2 nmol/l (100 to 160 ng $T_3 I$/100 ml) have been obtained (Sterling, 1971). The free fraction is approximately 0.5 per cent of the total T_3 giving values for free T_3 of 13 to 21 pmol/l (500 to 800 pg $T_3 I$/100 ml). As T_3 possesses physiological activity approximately three times that of T_4 these figures suggest that the significance of T_3 in thyroid disease is greater than was previously thought. It has been estimated that about two-thirds of the total metabolic effect in human subjects may well be due to T_3 metabolism (Woeber *et al.*, 1970). Newer methods for investigating thyroid function based on the properties outlined here, such as the competitive protein binding (CPB) method for T_4, and the T_3 uptake test as a measure of the unsaturated TBG sites, will be discussed more fully later.

For further information concerning the synthesis and transport of the iodinated hormones see Pitt-Rivers (1967), Wolff (1970), Robbins and Rall (1967), Tong (1971), Oppenheimer and Surks (1971), and Reichlin (1971).

There are at present considerable technical difficulties in measuring free T_3 and T_4 in plasma, assays for TSH are insensitive at the lower end of the normal and in the subnormal range, and secreted TRH cannot be measured in plasma. Accordingly tests of thyroid function are rather less direct than theoretically desirable. These include the measurement of TSH over part of the whole range, the determination of total T_3 and T_4 or of protein-bound iodine in plasma, the extent of saturation of proteins binding T_3 and T_4, the indirect calculation of free T_3 and T_4, the uptake of iodine by the thyroid and the effect on various body systems of the biologically active free thyroid hormones.

These less direct procedures can be influenced by extra-thyroid factors including drugs, pregnancy, emotion, etc., and the normal ranges often vary appreciably between laboratories. Part of this problem arises from the lack of suitable standards. Certainly the degree of inter-laboratory variation with the commoner tests is considerable, that for the more complex tests is largely unknown.

TESTS OF THYROID FUNCTION INVESTIGATING CHANGES IN HORMONE PRODUCTION

I. In Vivo Tests of Iodine Uptake

These measure the ability of the thyroid to take up iodine. Following an oral dose of radioactive iodine in the form of inorganic iodide, the rate of

Thyroid Function Tests

accumulation of the isotope in the thyroid is measured using an external gamma-counter placed over the gland. [131] I with a half-life of about 8 days has been mostly used but the use of [132] I is increasing. This has a half-life of 2.6 h so that repeat determinations can be carried out after a relatively short period of time. The test is most useful for investigating hyperthyroid states in which uptake is high but is of less value in hypothyroid conditions.

II. Direct Methods for Determining the Amount of Circulating Hormone

Determination of Protein-bound Iodine (PBI)

In this still widely used method for the routine investigation of thyroid disorders, the proteins are precipitated and the iodine in the iodine-containing compounds carried down with them is converted into inorganic iodide by digestion or incineration. As precipitating agent Foss *et al.* (1960) used zinc hydroxide. Other agents used are trichloracetic or perchloric acids (Acland, 1958; Zak *et al.*, 1953; and Fischl, 1956). Drying of the washed protein has been in the presence of potassium hydroxide (Foss *et al.*), sodium carbonate (Barker *et al.*, 1951) or potassium carbonate (Widstrom and Bjorkman, 1958). Zak *et al.* (1952) used wet digestion with a mixture of chloric, perchloric and chromic acids. For modifications see Oneal and Simms (1953), Farrell and Richmond (1961) and Widdowson and Northam (1963) the last of whom used an aluminium block heater devised by Albert-Recht and Frazer (1961). Alternatively a strong anion exchange resin can be used to remove inorganic iodides before the digestion or incineration stages. Scott and Reilly (1954) used Dowex 2 and Zieve *et al.* (1956) Amberlite IRA 400.

The iodide is then measured by its catalytic action on the oxidation of arsenite by ceric sulphate in which the yellow Ce^{4+} ion is converted to the colourless Ce^{3+} ion. The final stage can be carried out manually as described below or using the AutoAnalyzer. The manual procedure was modified for use with the AutoAnalyzer by Welshman *et al.* (1966). Automation of the chloric acid digestion method was described by Widdowson and Northam (1964) and a fully automated technique after removing inorganic iodide by an ion exchange resin was developed for the AutoAnalyzer using a continuous digester by Riley and Gochman (1964).

Provided certain criteria are fulfilled the final colour reaction obeys first order kinetics and there is a logarithmic relation between extinction and iodine concentration so that a linear calibration curve is obtained when extinction is plotted against concentration on semi-logarithmic paper.

Protein-bound iodine includes T_3 and T_4 which are almost entirely protein bound, but also, depending on the protein precipitant used, variable amounts of MIT and DIT. Thus zinc hydroxide includes 90 per cent of any MIT and DIT present, trichloracetic acid less than 10 per cent. Also when present in large amounts inorganic iodide may interfere, but the most serious source of trouble is from organic iodine compounds much used as

6 *Practical Clinical Biochemistry*

contrast media in radiography most of which are included. Even using the fully automated technique with the AutoAnalyzer digester it is doubtful whether the time thus saved compensates for the trouble caused by these substances when assessing the relative merits of this technique and that for determining thyroxine iodine described below (p. 9).

The method for PBI determination given is that of Foss *et al.* (1960). For a discussion of the determination of PBI see Robbins and Rall (1967).

Reagents. 1. Zinc sulphate solution, 100 g $ZnSO_4, 7H_2O/l$.

2. Sodium hydroxide, 0.5 mol/l. Ten ml of the zinc sulphate diluted to about 60 ml with water should require 10.8 to 11.2 ml of this solution to give a faint permanent pink colour with phenolphthalein.

3. Potassium hydroxide, 2 mol/l.

4. Sodium arsenite solution, 6.50 g/l, or dissolve 4.95 g arsenious oxide in 50 ml 0.5 mol/l sodium hydroxide and make to a litre with water.

5. Sulphuric acid–hydrochloric acid mixture. Pour 98 ml concentrated sulphuric acid into about 350 ml distilled water, cool, add 27 ml concentrated hydrochloric acid and make to 500 ml with water.

6. Ceric ammonium sulphate solution. This should have an extinction of about 0.8 as the standard blank. Foss *et al.* used 12.65 g $Ce(SO_4)_2$, $2(NH_4)_2SO_4, 2H_2O/l$ in 1.6 mol/l sulphuric acid but the exact concentration may be a little different and should be determined.

7. Iodide standards. Dissolve either 120 mg sodium iodide or 132.8 mg potassium iodide in water and make to a litre. Use only highest purity reagents dried in a desiccator. These solutions contain 400 μmol I_2/l (10.16 mg I/100 ml). Prepare a more dilute stock standard by diluting 2 ml of this to a litre. This contains 800 nmol I_2/l (20.32 μg I/100 ml). For working standards dilute 20 ml of this dilute standard to 100 ml with water. This contains 160 nmol I_2/l (4.06 μg I/100 ml). All these solutions keep in the refrigerator.

Make all the above solutions with double distilled water. If too high a blank is still obtained it may be necessary to distil the water with substances such as alkali and permanganate. Acland (1958) used water purified by distilling from a metal still and passed through two columns of Amberlite Monobed MB-1 ion exchange resin, the second passage being made just before using. Use reagents of the highest purity with proven low blanks throughout.

Technique. Measure 1 ml serum into a Pyrex centrifuge tube (125 × 15 mm), dilute with 7 ml distilled water and add 1 ml zinc sulphate. Mix with a narrow glass rod (about 2 mm in diameter), add 1 ml sodium hydroxide and mix well. Remove any material adhering to the rod by rotating it against the wall of the tube. Allow to stand about 15 min, then centrifuge for 10 min at 2 000 r.p.m. Decant the supernatant fluid, add 10 ml distilled water and resuspend the protein precipitate with the stirring rod already used. Stir only sufficiently vigorously to give a uniform suspension. Centrifuge again and discard the supernatant. Carry out two further washings in the same way.

Thyroid Function Tests

After finally pouring off the supernatant fluid, add 1 ml potassium hydroxide and stir with the same stirring rod. Wash down the rod with 0.5 to 1.0 ml water added drop by drop down the rod. Place the tubes overnight in an oven at 100 to 105° C to drive off water. After thorough drying, ash in a muffle furnace. Place in the cold furnace, close the oven door to eliminate draught during heating. Vapour containing iodine forms during the later stages of heating up and conditions should aim to keep this in the tubes. Heat at 600° C. Bring to this temperature in 30 to 45 min. Heat for one hour. Open the door at 5, 25, 45 min after reaching 600° C. Then remove and allow to cool to room temperature. Add 10 ml water and stir well with the glass rod, removing any material from the walls of the tube. Centrifuge for 10 min.

Pipette duplicate 4 ml portions (= 0.4 ml serum) of the clear supernatant fluid into Pyrex test tubes. To each add 0.5 ml arsenite, then slowly add 1 ml sulphuric-hydrochloric acid. Mix and place the tubes in a constant temperature bath at $37 \pm 0.1°C$ for 10 min. Warm the ceric ammonium sulphate in the same way, then at 1 minute intervals add 1 ml of this to each of the tubes, mixing quickly by flicking with the fingers. At a fixed time which varies with the reagents but is in the period 15 to 20 min and which gives a fall in extinction from about 0.8 to 0.2 with the strongest standard, read the extinction at 420 nm in a spectrophotometer using a 10 mm path length. Run a reagent blank in duplicate with each set of tests, using 1 ml water instead of 1 ml serum put through the entire procedure. It is also useful to run a reagent blank with an internal standard, for example 1 ml of the standard containing 160 nmol I_2/l (4.06 µg I/100 ml).

Since the equivalent of 0.4 ml serum is used for the final stage, 1.0 ml of the standard containing 160 nmol I_2/l is equivalent to $320/0.4 = 400$ nmol

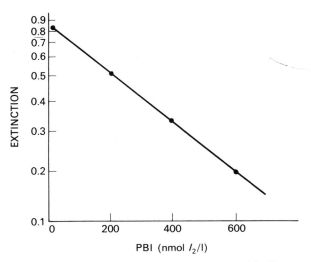

Fig. 1,2. Calibration Curve for Protein-Bound Iodine.

8 *Practical Clinical Biochemistry*

I_2/l or 10.15 μg I/100 ml. For a calibration curve (Fig. 1,2) put up a set of standards as follows:

Serum PBI (nmol I_2/l)	0	200	400	600
Serum PBI (μg I/100 ml)	0	5.08	10.15	15.23
Standard (ml)	0	0.5	1.0	1.5
Water (ml)	3.6	3.1	2.6	2.1

Add 0.4 ml potassium hydroxide and proceed with the addition of arsenite etc. as for the test.

Calculation. Read the iodine concentration for the test from the calibration curve and subtract from this the blank value found. This is usually of the order of 20 nmol I_2/l (0.5 μg I/100 ml). It should not exceed 40 nmol I_2/l. If it does, look for a source of possible contamination.

Notes. Glassware used must be scrupulously clean. After using the Pyrex tubes a few times they become badly etched and hence difficult to clean. Discard such tubes.

Tincture of iodine must not be allowed in contact with the skin and iodine-containing drugs (particularly Enterovioform) must not have been taken. Particular attention should be paid to whether iodine-containing substances used for X-ray procedures (cholecystograms, myelograms, bronchograms, angiograms) have been given to the patient. The effect of these can persist for months and give very high results immediately following their use. It is an advantage if a separate room can be used for the determination since when the test is carried out in the main laboratory the likelihood that a batch will be contaminated is considerably increased.

For useful additional information see Foss *et al.* (1960 and Foss (1963).

Zieve *et al.* (1956) absorbed inorganic iodide on to Amberlite IRA 400 resin in chloride form. To prepare the resin stir well with 1.0 mol/l hydrochloric acid and wash thoroughly with deionised water using suction and a Buchner funnel. After washing leave the suction on for an hour. Spread in 50 g quantities on Whatman 3 MM filter paper, dry at room temperature for 25-30 min and store in airtight polythene bottles. Shake 1.5 ml of serum with a little resin several times during 15 min, centrifuge, mix 1 ml supernatant with 1 ml of 2 mol/l potassium hydroxide solution and proceed as described on page 7.

Butanol Extractable Iodine (BEI)

One difficulty experienced with methods for PBI has been the inclusion of variable amounts of MIT and DIT. This was eliminated by preliminary extraction with butanol followed by back extraction with alkali. However, contamination with some contrast media still occurred and as the method cannot be automated it has fallen into disuse.

Thyroid Function Tests 9

Determination of Iodinated Hormones by Column Chromatography and Quantitation of Iodine

This has distinct advantages over the previous methods. The T_3 and T_4 are separated from inorganic iodide and other iodine-containing organic substances by the use of an anion-exchange resin as first described by Galton and Pitt-Rivers (1959). The hormones are adsorbed on the column and the other substances washed through. The T_4 can be eluted from the column. This column eluate is reacted with bromine in the non-incineration technique introduced by Pileggi and Kessler (1968) which liberates the organically-bound iodine as free iodine which is then determined by its catalytic effect on the decolourisation of ceric sulphate by arsenite as previously described for PBI. Inhibitors of this reaction which may be eluted from the column are eliminated by the bromine step. Alternatively, cation exchange resin methods have been used by Backer *et al.* (1967) and Miedema *et al.* (1971).

Semi-Automated Method for Determination of Serum Thyroxine

This technique is based on a combination of the methods of Kessler and Pileggi (1970) and Yee *et al.* (1971). The bromination and reduction stages are carried out using standard AutoAnalyzer modules. The technique is very much less subject to interference from contrast media and various drugs than the method for PBI and the rate of analysis compares favourably with the AutoAnalyzer digestion technique for PBI. It is recommended for routine use.

Reagents. 1. Ion exchange resin Bio-Rad AG 1-X2, 200-400 mesh, acetate form (Bio-Rad Laboratories Ltd., Porter's Wood, Valley Road, St. Albans, Herts). Wash the resin well by suspending in water and decanting until all fines have been removed. Three washes with settling for 15 to 20 min are usually sufficient. Store in this form, preferably in the refrigerator, ready for use. Check each batch for elution characteristics using standard thyroxine solutions and control sera. Slight alterations of elution volumes may be necessary from batch to batch. Collect the used resin from the columns for re-use after washing several times with 50 per cent acetic acid (reagent 8 below) and then with water until the excess of acid has been removed. This procedure tends to alter the flow characteristics slightly but recalibration is as for fresh resin.

2. Ammonium hydroxide, 0.8 mol/l, 53 ml 0.88 sp.gr. NH_4OH/l (BDH Aristar).

3. Acetic acid, 0.2 mol/l; dilute 11.6 ml glacial acetic acid (BDH Analar) to a litre with water.

4. Sodium acetate solution, 0.2 mol/l, 27.2 g $CH_3COONa,3H_2O$ per litre.

5. Acetate buffer, pH 5.6. Mix 1 volume 0.2 mol/l acetic acid with 10 volumes 0.2 mol/l sodium acetate. Adjust to pH 5.6 ± 0.2.

10 *Practical Clinical Biochemistry*

6. Acetate buffer, pH 4.0. Mix 4.2 volumes of 0.2 mol/l acetic acid with 1 volume of 0.2 mol/l sodium acetate. Adjust to pH 4.0 ± 0.2.

7. Acetic acid, pH 1.9. Mix 1 volume glacial acetic acid with 4.6 volumes water. Adjust to pH 1.9 ± 0.1.

8. Acetic acid, pH 1.3. Mix equal volumes water and glacial acetic acid. Adjust to pH 1.25 to 1.35. This is termed 50 per cent acetic acid below.

9. Stock arsenious acid reagent. Dissolve 49.5 g As_2O_3 and 20 g NaOH in about 800 ml hot water, cool and make to a litre.

10. Arsenious acid, working solution. To 100 ml stock solution add 26 ml concentrated sulphuric acid (BDH Aristar) and dilute to 1 litre with water.

11. Ceric ammonium sulphate, stock solution. Carefully add 52 ml concentrated sulphuric acid to 400 ml water, add 50 g ceric ammonium sulphate (BDH specially purified for PBI), cool and make to 1 litre with water.

12. Ceric ammonium sulphate, working solution. Dilute 100 ml stock solution to 1 litre with sulphuric acid containing 52 ml concentrated acid per litre. Depending on the purity of the other reagents this amount of ceric ammonium sulphate will need to be varied from time to time. The concentration chosen is such that the AutoAnalyzer recorder with all reagents pumping gives a baseline transmission of 15 to 17 per cent.

13. Stock bromine reagent. Dissolve 16.7 g $KBrO_3$ and 71.4 g KBr in water and make to a litre.

14. Bromine working solution. Dilute 25 ml stock reagent to 200 ml with water.

15. Sulphuric acid, 2 mol/l. Add 110 ml concentrated acid (BDH Aristar) carefully to 700 ml water, cool and make to a litre.

16. Stock standard thyroxine. The purity of commercially available L-thyroxine is variable. It can be obtained as the sodium salt pentahydrate or as free thyroxine. Gemmill (1955) found an extinction coefficient of 6.027 l cm^{-1} $mmol^{-1}$ in alkaline solution whereas Watson *et al.* (1974) investigating 8 samples from different suppliers found a range from 5.28 to 6.07. The higher the contamination with T_3 the lower the extinction coefficient. From this study Watson *et al.*, recommended the use of a figure of 6.1 for calibrating thyroxine standards. The T_4 obtained from Koch-Light has proved satisfactory. It was also acceptable for competitive protein binding methods (Watson and Lees, 1973).

Thyroxine has a mol. wt. of 777 but that of the sodium salt pentahydrate is 889. So 889 mg of the latter contains 1 mmol, equivalent to 777 mg free thyroxine and to 508 mg (2 mmol I_2) thyroxine iodine. Prepare a 1 mmol/l solution by dissolving 44.5 mg sodium L-thyroxine pentahydrate (Koch-Light) in 50 ml methanol-ammonia solution (99 volumes methanol to 1 volume 0.88 sp. gr. ammonia solution). Dilute this solution 1 in 20 with freshly prepared CO_2-free sodium hydroxide, 40 mmol/l, to give a solution containing 50 μmol/l. Read immediately in a 1 cm cell at 324 nm. The extinction should be 6.1/20 = 0.305. Therefore

Thyroid Function Tests

the actual concentration of standard in mmol/l is observed extinction/0.305. Take a suitable volume of the original standard and dilute to 50 ml with methanol solution to give a standard containing 200 μmol/l; approximately 10 ml is required. Dilute this standard 1 in 1 000 with 50 per cent acetic acid solution. Two stages can be used, 100 μl to 10 ml with acid, then 1 ml of this to 10 ml with acid. The final concentration is 200 nmol/l.

17. AutoAnalyzer working standards. To allow for the eluate volumes in the column chromatography stage the 200 nmol/l standard above needs a further 1 to 4.2 dilution which can be suitably made using 4.0 ml standard and 12.8 ml 50 per cent acetic acid which gives enough for the following standards. The equivalents/l serum assume the estimation is done using 1 ml serum.

Diluted standard (ml)	0.5	1.0	2.0	3.0	4.0	5.0
Acetic acid, 50% (ml)	4.5	4.0	3.0	2.0	1.0	0
Serum T_4 (nmol/l)	20	40	80	120	160	200
Serum T_4I (μg/100 ml)	1.02	2.03	4.06	6.10	8.13	10.16

Technique. *Column chromatography.* Suitable plastic columns are about 5 cm long, internal diameter 8 to 10 mm, with a built-in support for the resin. An additional extension funnel which can be added to the column during the washing stages is also necessary. The columns and funnels supplied with the Oxford T_4 kits are suitable; they can be washed and re-used quite easily. Transfer the prepared resin to the column to a depth of 2.5 to 3.0 cm, allow to drain and wash with 4 to 5 ml water. These columns are most conveniently prepared while the specimens are standing with ammonia. Pipette 1 ml of serum into suitable 10 × 1 cm plastic tubes and add 3 ml ammonia solution to each tube and leave to stand for 15 to 30 min. In the same way for each batch of analyses dilute a normal and a high control serum and a pipette 3 ml ammonia as a column blank. At the appropriate time transfer the diluted specimens successively to the columns collecting the eluate in the original tubes at this stage. When all the eluates have been collected transfer them once more to their respective columns and discard the final eluates. Wash each column successively with 4 ml of acetate buffer pH 5.6, acetate buffer pH 4.0 and acetic acid pH 1.9, allowing all the wash to pass through before applying the next one and directing the jet to the wall of the column so that the resin is disturbed as little as possible. The wash reagents can be quickly and efficiently dispensed from Zipettes. When the last wash has drained through wipe the tips of the columns with paper tissues, place the plastic elution tubes in position, and carefully add 0.2 ml glacial acetic acid (see also the note on standardisation of the ion exchange resin). When this has drained through add 4 ml of 50 per cent acetic acid to each column and collect in the same elution tube. This is the first eluate and contains the bulk of the T_4 the

12 *Practical Clinical Biochemistry*

exact proportion depending on the elution characteristics of the resin used. With new elution tubes in position add a second 4 ml of 50 per cent acetic acid and collect the second eluate. Stopper tubes and mix thoroughly. If not assayed immediately at this stage they can be stored in a refrigerator for a few days.

Automated ceric sulphate-arsenious acid reaction. The AutoAnalyzer flow diagram is shown in Fig. 1,3. The technique uses standard Auto-Analyzer equipment comprising the Mark II sampler operating at 60 samples/h with a 1 : 1 sample to wash ratio, pump, two-coil heating bath at $60° C$, colorimeter with 15 mm flow cell and recorder. Pump water through the manifold until a steady pattern is obtained, adjust the recorder to 98 per cent transmission with the 420 nm filters and suitable apertures in the colorimeter. Then transfer the pump tubes to the appropriate reagent bottles for 10 to 15 min before introducing the samples. Alternatively continue the base line pumping until the ceric sulphate solution appears at the colorimeter. However, this takes approximately 20 min with the double incubation coil causing unnecessary delay. With the optimal concentration of ceric sulphate a transmission of about 10 per cent is obtained when the ceric sulphate first appears; later when the sulphuric acid-bromine arrives this increases to 15 to 18 per cent, giving the most suitable conditions for the reagent background. Transfer the standards to the analyzer cups (protective gloves are desirable at this stage as 50 per cent acetic acid is corrosive) and start sampling. It is desirable to run two standard curves separated from each other by three cups of 50 per cent acetic acid. Also follow the second of these by three cups of acetic acid and then introduce the first eluates starting with the column blank followed by the normal control, the test solutions, and ending with the abnormal control. Separate this from the second eluates by three cups of acetic acid. After every tenth sample include an acetic acid wash for rapid identification of specimens.

The practice of first screening samples at 120/h to show the presence of any contaminated specimens as recommended by Kessler and Pileggi (1970) and by Yee *et al.* (1971) has not been found worth while, adding appreciably to the handling time (see p. 14). Dilute all eluates containing between 160 and 200 nmol T_4/l (8.0 to 10.0 μg I/100 ml) with an equal volume of 50 per cent acetic acid and re-run. Also re-run the eluates following such samples to check for possible carry-over. Re-run subnormal values in the same way with an acid wash preceding them.

Calculation. Plot the per cent transmission readings for the standards on linear graph paper to give curves similar to that shown in Fig. 1,2. The T_4 content for each eluate is obtained. Add these together and subtract the sum of the T_4 content of the column blanks to give the T_4 value for the test sera.

Notes. 1. *Standardisation of the ion exchange resin.* With an automated procedure where the second eluates can be estimated with little difficulty two approaches are possible. The fractions can be cut so that effectively all the sample comes in the first eluate, the second eluate being used only to

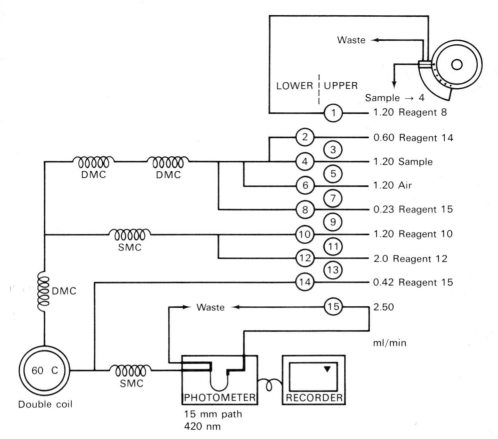

Fig. 1,3. AutoAnalyzer I Flow Diagram for Determination of Iodine. DMC, SMC - double and single mixing coils respectively.

check for any contamination. Alternatively, a fractionation with approximately 80 per cent in the first eluate can be used leaving an accurately determinable amount equivalent to 20 nmol T_4/l (1 μg I/100 ml) in the second eluate. In the latter case the T_4 contents of the two eluates are added to give the result. The relative proportions can be varied by changing the amount of glacial acetic acid used to prime the column. If a greater proportion comes out in the second eluate add 0.2 ml of acetic acid and run to waste before adding the second 0.2 ml which is collected as in the standard procedure. The use of a suitable control serum with each batch of analyses allows a continuous check on the performance and reproducibility of the method. There should be no difficulty in keeping within the quoted limits with the procedure described. With the manual procedures supplied in kit form by Bio-Rad and Oxford the characteristics of the bromination and ceric-arsenite reaction are such that standardisation must be carried out using standards or control sera carried through the full procedure. With the

14 *Practical Clinical Biochemistry*

present technique the inhibition due to materials from the resin column is completely overcome and calculations can be carried out using a standard curve as described. Kessler and Pileggi (1970) routinely include a KIO_3 standard in their Autoanalyzer runs and report greater than 95 per cent equivalent for the T_4I compared with the inorganic I whether in the form of KI, KIO_3, or KIO_4. This has not been used by us but continuity has been checked by routinely using assayed control sera.

2. *Screening for contaminated specimens.* Yee *et al.* (1971) described two procedures for screening for contaminated specimens and while this is undoubtedly necessary in the automated procedures for PBI it is not for T_4. Comparison of the method for T_4 with PBI results for the same sera has shown that gross contamination was usually completely removed in most instances and did not even show evidence of contamination in the second eluate. The results for T_4 were low or normal even when the PBI value was several hundred $\mu g/100$ ml. We have only encountered contamination three times in almost 3 000 consecutive estimations. In one, the specimen was collected shortly after a patient had received Biloptin for cholecystography; the apparent T_4 was approximately 2 800 nmol/l (140 μg I/100 ml) and the next three samples on the AutoAnalyzer were affected by carry-over. When the contaminated specimen was re-assayed using 1/10th of the sample, approximately 140 nmol/l (7.0 μg I/100 ml) appeared in *each* eluate showing that even at near normal values such contamination would still be apparent from the ratio between the two eluates. The need to screen all samples in the way suggested by Yee *et al.* would appear to be unnecessary. For detailed information concerning the type and extent of interference from various organic iodine sources see Cusick (1974).

3. A semi-automated version of this method using the prepacked columns supplied by Bio-Rad and Oxford has been fully investigated by Burnett *et al.* (1973). The introduction of a wire-wound 1 kΩ resistor as a range expander as described by Owen (1970) markedly increased the linearity and sensitivity of the method. This enabled the analyser to be run at 90 tests per hour. These workers still relied on the use of control sera as standards which is not necessary as the method can be standardised adequately against thyroxine when the semi-automated procedure is employed.

Determination of Thyroxine by Competitive Protein Binding Methods

Once established the test is extremely simple to perform and the problems due to iodine-containing contaminants are completely overcome. Complete sets of reagents are available from several manufacturers, but they are relatively costly and require equipment for counting [125] I. The principle of competitive protein binding (CPB) methods is described in Chapter 10, Volume 1.

Thyroid Function Tests 15

As an example the *Thyopac-4* test (Radiochemical Centre, Amersham) firstly involves separation of bound T_4 from serum proteins by ethanol precipitation. A proportion of the extract is added to a standardised amount of thyroxine-binding globulin (TBG) saturated with ^{125}I-labelled T_4 for the CPB assay proper. The assay mixture contains absorbent granules of unstated composition which take up unbound T_4 reversibly. After 30 min equilibration the granules are allowed to settle and the count rate of the supernatant fluid containing TBG-T_4 is determined. A standard serum of stated T_4 content and a serum free from T_4 are carried through the whole procedure at the same time. There is a linear relationship between the reciprocal count rate and T_4 concentration. The variable efficiency of ethanol extraction is compensated for by simultaneous processing of standards and the deterioration due to alcohol evaporation is avoided. The reversible nature of T_4 binding to the absorbent granules avoids the complications introduced by irreversible binding.

The *Res-O-Mat* kit (Malinckrodt-UK Ltd., Norman House, Long Lane, Stanwell, Middlesex) is similar in many respects. The differences lie in the removal of free T_4 on to a resin strip under controlled conditions, and in the method of calibration. For the two standard sera of zero and known high T_4 concentration the ratio of count rate after resin removal to the original total count rate is plotted linearly against concentration.

Ethanol extraction is avoided and Sephadex is used to remove unbound T_4 in the *Tetralute* kit (Ames Company, Slough, Bucks). T_4 is unbound from serum proteins in alkaline solution and a standard amount of ^{125}I-T_4 is added. On passing through a Sephadex G25 column all the T_4 is retained. After washing, a fixed amount of TBG (diluted pooled pregnancy serum) is added to the column and washed through. This elutes a fixed quantity of T_4 and the radioactive component is measured by counting. The method is calibrated by using known quantities of T_4 in albumin solution carried through the whole procedure.

The *Tetrasorb* kit (Abbott Laboratories, Queensborough, Kent) involves ethanol extraction followed by evaporation of the solvent. After equilibration with TBG saturated with ^{125}I-T_4, free T_4 is adsorbed at 0° C on to a resin sponge. After determination of the total count rate, the supernatant is removed, the sponge washed and then counted. The percentage absorbed on to the resin is related to the T_4 concentration in the original serum. One or more calibration sera are used to define which of a family of curves supplied by the manufacturers is appropriate for the current assay.

See Watson and Lees (1973) for an assessment of kit methods, and Seth (1973) for studies of a work simplified CPB method using Amberlite IRA 400 to remove the free T_4.

It has been possible to devise a radioimmunoassay method for T_3 (Chopra *et al.*, 1972) but suitable antisera are rare and interference by other factors is not reliably excluded.

Normal Ranges for Circulating Thyroid Hormone Concentrations

There is some confusion concerning the units used in reporting thyroxine concentrations. When determined as iodine by PBI methods the results could be unequivocally expressed in μg I/100 ml serum. When alternative methods became available, in order to give a similar normal range the results were usually expressed as T_4 iodine but confusion arose when results were given as T_4 without clear indication whether iodine was implied or not. Conversion to SI units adds further complications particularly in the case of PBI. The atomic weight of iodine is 127, the molecule is I_2 and one molecule of T_4 contains 2 molecules or 4 atoms of iodine. The use of SI units to describe T_4 concentrations requires a clear indication as to whether the mole refers to T_4, I_2 or I. With standardisation of T_4 by spectrophotometry in alkaline solution as given on p. 10 there is no need to quote T_4 results other than in nmol T_4/l however the determination is carried out. We have therefore quoted results in nmol T_4/l followed in brackets by the iodine equivalent in μg I/100 ml to give some continuity with the established usage in the past. Results for PBI expressed in nmol/l use the conversion involving I_2 with a molecular weight of 254.

Whichever method is employed each laboratory should determine its own normal range. As with any method the standard is important and spectrophotometric calibration given earlier should be used to correct for impurities in the T_4 standard. Some kit methods lend themselves to such external standardisation but others use control sera as standards which is less satisfactory. The recovery of added T_4 and its reproducibility is important in assessing the performance of the method. Workers in different laboratories vary in whether they correct for recovery before calculating the results.

PBI. Many normal ranges have been quoted but the most acceptable is 140 to 320 nmol I_2/l (3.5 to 8.0 μg I/100 ml). The PBI is raised in the first few days of life and may be as high as 640 nmol I_2/l (16 μg I/100 ml) in the first week falling to about 450 nmol I_2/l (11 μg I/100 ml) by the end of the second week and ranging from 160 to 420 nmol I_2/l (4 to 10.5 μg I/100 ml) from 3 weeks to 3 months of age (see also Acland, 1971). For conversion to nmol T_4/l divide by 2.

T_4 by column chromatography. The normal range for the T_4 method described above has been derived by us from over 6 000 consecutive routine analyses on hospital patients. The 95 per cent limits calculated using probability paper are 50 to 130 nmol/l (2.5 to 6.5 μg I/100 ml) agreeing closely with the alkaline CPB methods. Burnett et al. (1973) using a similar procedure found 95 per cent limits of 64 to 130 nmol/l (3.2 to 6.4 μg I/100 ml) assuming a Gaussian distribution but preferred the observed 95 per cent range of 60 to 133 nmol/l (3.0 to 6.6 μg I/100 ml). Using cation exchange methods Backer et al. (1967) and Miedema et al. (1971) both report a normal range of 60 to 120 nmol/l (3.0 to 6.0 μg I/100 ml).

Thyroid Function Tests 17

T$_4$ by competitive protein binding. All values (Table 1,1) have been expressed as nmol/l, with the equivalent iodine content in μg/100 ml in parenthesis. The latter figure is convenient for direct comparison with the PBI figures in the same units. Some methods give results which are higher than the PBI range although when direct comparisons are carried out the PBI is up to 1 μg I/100 ml higher in uncontaminated specimens. This is due to the presence of iodinated amino acids and other iodinated compounds. Few PBI methods correct for recovery which could also explain some of the discrepancy. Furthermore some CPB methods may be less specific than originally thought, particularly those using ethanol extraction.

TABLE 1,1

Normal Ranges for T$_4$ by Competitive Protein Binding Methods

Method	Range		Remarks
	T$_4$ (nmol/l)	(μg I/100 ml)	
Ethanol extraction techniques			
Murphy *et al.*, 1966	54-142	2.6-7.1	Uncorrected for recovery of 77%
	64-185	3.4-9.2	Corrected
Tetrasorb (Watson and Lees, 1973)	55-162	2.8-8.1	Corrected
Res-O-Mat	66-180	3.3-8.9	Corrected
Thyopac-4	57-170	2.9-8.5	Corrected
Alkali extraction methods			
Tetralute:			
Braverman *et al.*, 1971	58-138	2.9-6.9	
Seligson and Seligson, 1972	60-130	3.0-6.2	

The alkali extraction methods give lower results and are uncorrected for recovery which was reported to be virtually complete by Watson and Lees (1973). They also found that serum allowed to stand at room temperature develops material which mimics T$_4$ and so gives high results in the methods using ethanol extraction but not in the more specific Tetralute procedure.

Radioimmunoassay. This procedure for T$_3$ gives a normal range of 1.4 to 2.8 nmol/l (90 to 180 ng T$_3$/100 ml) (Chopra *et al.*, 1972).

III. Indirect Methods for Assessing Thyroid Function

T$_3$ Uptake Tests

These give a measure of the proportion of sites on TBG unoccupied by T$_4$ (and T$_3$). Again commercial kits are available for this test and have similar advantages and disadvantages to those for CPB methods.

There is a dynamic equilibrium between free T$_4$ and bound T$_4$ in serum. Usually some 75 per cent of the TBG sites remain free. In patients with normal TBG levels, the higher the T_4, the lower the proportion of free TBG sites which is estimated in the various T_3 uptake methods. T_3 is usually used because it is not bound by TBPA and very little by albumin, so its uptake should be more specific for the TBG sites. It also does not displace bound T_4. When ^{125}I-T_3 is mixed with serum an amount equivalent to the free binding sites is bound to the TBG. Separation of the free and bound ^{125}I-T_3 by red cells, ion exchange resin or Sephadex affords a means of assessing the relative proportion of these free sites. Two methods have been used in the final measurement: (1) determination of the percentage radioactivity bound to the secondary binder and therefore inversely proportional to the free binding sites, and (2) the proportion of the activity remaining with the serum and so directly proportional to the unbound sites.

The original observations on the distribution of T_3 between plasma and red cells were made by Hamolsky *et al.* (1957) by determining the percentage of the T_3 bound to the red cells after incubation and washing. Red cells lack uniformity and results are dependent on the haematocrit and absence of haemolysis. The result depends on the ability of the secondary binder to complex T_3. The binder was made more uniform by the introduction of anion exchange resin by Mitchell (1958). This allows the use of serum instead of whole blood so the results are no longer dependent on the haematocrit, the resin binding firmly any labelled iodide ions. Variations in the degree of radioiodide contamination will therefore lead to variations in the percentage uptake of the label by the resin. The presence of heparin can cause low results so that either serum or heparinised plasma should be used consistently. Abbott Laboratories (Queensborough, Kent) introduced the *Triosorb* ^{TM} *T-3* diagnostic kit using Triosorb resin sponge, a polyurethane resin-embedded sponge, which is of more uniform nature than red cells and can be washed more reliably and quickly. Another method relying on the counting of the secondary binder is the *Trilute* kit (Ames Company, Slough, Bucks.) where Sephadex G-25 is used. The *Res-O-Mat* T_3 test (Malinckrodt—UK Ltd., Norman House, Long Lane, Stanwell, Middlesex) uses a resin-impregnated wafer to remove the free T_3 but differs from the preceding methods in that the supernatant is counted making the method a direct assessment of the unsaturated binding sites. In addition a single count is required as the result is expressed as a ratio to that of the manufacturer's reference serum similarly treated. As each reference serum varies it carries a normalising factor to allow comparison with the mid-point of the normal range. This is given an arbitrary index value of 1.00. The ^{125}I-T_3 is supplied in vials to which serum is added followed by the resin wafer. After a suitable mixing time the wafer is removed and the residual activity in the whole vial counted. Thus there is one pipetting of serum only. Scholes (1962) introduced another variant of the T_3 uptake test using an absorbent binding T_3 reversibly; this is utilised in the *Thyopac-3* procedure (Radio-Chemical Centre, Amersham). ^{125}I-T_3 and a granular absorbent of unstated composition are supplied in vials to

TABLE 1,2

Comparison of Various T_3 Uptake Tests

Method	Isotope	Adsorbent	Preparation of material counted	Calculation
Red cell uptake	^{131}I	Red cell	Wash cells	$\% \text{ Uptake} = \dfrac{\text{Count rate, washed cells}}{\text{Total count rate}} \times \dfrac{10^4}{\text{haematocrit}}$
Triosorb	^{125}I	Resin sponge	Wash sponge	$\% \text{ Uptake} = \dfrac{\text{Count rate, washed sponge}}{\text{Total count rate}} \times 100$
Trilute	^{125}I	Sephadex G-25	Wash column	$\% \text{ Uptake} = \dfrac{\text{Count rate, washed column}}{\text{Total count rate}} \times 100$
Res-O-Mat	^{125}I	Resin impregnated wafer	Remove wafer	$\text{TBC index} = \dfrac{\text{Count rate, patient's serum}}{\text{Count rate, reference serum}} \times \text{normalising factor}$
Thyopac 3	^{125}I	Granular resin	Allow granules to settle	$\text{Thyopac-3 index} = \dfrac{\text{Count rate, patient's serum}}{\text{Count rate, reference serum}} \times \text{normalising factor}$

Total count rate = count rate of whole sample after adding T_3

20 *Practical Clinical Biochemistry*

which serum is added. On mixing, an amount of active T_3 proportional to the free binding sites is removed from the adsorbent and equilibrium is attained. The vials are allowed to stand until the adsorbent settles and an aliquot of the supernatant is removed for counting. Again only one count is required as the results are expressed in terms of a similarly treated manufacturer's reference serum, and different batches of serum carry a factor to allow comparison with the midpoint of the normal range. This is given an arbitrary index value of 100.

Table 1,2 illustrates the main points about the T_3 uptake methods quoted. Particular note should be taken of the normal values (Table 1,3)

TABLE 1,3

Summary of Diagnostic Ranges in T_3 Uptake Tests

	Normal value	Hypothyroid	Hyperthyroid
Red cell uptake	15-30%	< 10%	> 35%
Triosorb	25-35%	< 25%	> 35%
Trilute	40-60%	< 40%	> 60%
Res-O-Mat	0.87-1.13	> 1.13	< 0.87
Thyopac-3	90-110	> 110	< 90

for the methods where a reference serum is not used. For most methods used in investigating thyroid function it is advisable to determine the normal range for the local population as regional variations are known to occur. When calculating the free thyroxine index (see later) results for the Res-O-Mat and Thyopac-3 tests can be inserted directly in the mass action equation being a measure of the unsaturated binding sites. An alternative form of the equation has to be used for the calculation when red cell uptake, Triosorb or Trilute tests are used.

It must be emphasised that T_3 uptake tests do not give a measure of T_3 in serum. They are a means of assessing the relative amount of free TBG binding sites present compared with a normal population.

The Free Thyroxine Index

Difficulty in interpreting PBI and T_4 values may arise when the serum concentration of TBG alters. If this is raised, see p. 22, the protein bound T_4 fraction (TBG-T_4) will increase in order to maintain a normal free T_4 (FT_4) level. Thus patients in the euthyroid state will show increased values for circulating hormone as measured by the methods given above. Conversely, patients whose TBG is decreased will show a decrease as the protein bound fraction will also decrease in order to keep the FT_4 constant.

Thyroid Function Tests 21

By using a combination of T_4 and T_3 uptake results the free thyroxine index (FTI) proportional to the concentration of FT_4 can be obtained.

$$[FT_4] = K \cdot \frac{[TBG\text{-}T_4]}{[FTBG]} \simeq \frac{K'[PBI \text{ or } T_4]}{T_3 \text{ uptake}}$$

where FTBG is the part of the TBG unbound to T_4. This type of FTI involving two separate determinations has been called the "two-stage FTI" by McGowan (1975).

In persons without thyroid dysfunction the FT_4 and hence the FTI is kept constant as both factors in the above ratio move up or down together. In patients with thyroid hyperfunction the major change is an increase in FT_4 and FTI without a change in the binding protein concentration. The T_4 is increased with consequent reduction in T_3 uptake. The converse occurs in hypothyroid states. Again possible confusion between current and previous methods for T_3 uptake must be emphasised. In the original FTI method of Clark and Horn (1965) the Triosorb resin sponge method was used and the index calculated as PBI $\times T_3$ resin uptake. As previously explained the latter is reciprocally related in later T_3 uptake tests. In all cases the FTI is not equal to the free T_4 but proportional to it. The proportionality constant varies with the technique and mode of expressing the T_3 index.

The newest techniques for the investigation of thyroid function attempt to combine the T_4 competitive binding and T_3 uptake methods in a single test and have been referred to as "FTI (single stage) tests" by McGowan (1975). Where the method lends itself to a measurement of T_4 as a first step, the index finally determined may be called the "sequential FTI" (McGowan). Test kits which are examples of the first type are the: *Quantisorb T_4N* (Abbott Laboratories) and *Res-O-Mat ETR* (Mallinckrodt-Nuclear). Both work on the same principle. The T_4 is separated from the patient's serum by alcohol extraction and an aliquot corresponding to 100 μl serum added to TBG saturated with $^{125}I\text{-}T_4$ as in the usual CPB methods. Then a further volume of the patient's own serum is added to the mixture, 10 μl for the Quantisorb and 5 μl for the Res-O-Mat. Some of the T_4 including radio-T_4, binds to unoccupied sites on the patient's TBG. Tests of the "sequential FTI" type are the *Thyrolute* kit (Ames) and *Thyopac-5* kit (Radiochemical Centre). In the former the T_4 content of 100 μl of the patient's serum is determined as in the Tetralute (Ames) procedure (p. 15) using a Sephadex column. Then a further 20 μl of the same serum is passed through the column and the radioactivity finally remaining on the Sephadex is determined. In the second test the T_4 content of approximately 170 μl of the patient's serum is determined as in the Thyopac-4 (Radiochemical Centre) procedure (p. 15) using a resin. Then 5 μl of the same serum is added to the remaining fluid and resin. After equilibration an aliquot of the supernatant fluid is counted. In both

P.C.B.(II)–2

22 *Practical Clinical Biochemistry*

cases the patient's TBG removes a part of the T_4 held on the column or resin.

The tests differ in the final radioactive measurements. The unbound T_4 in the Quantisorb is adsorbed on to a resin sponge which is counted after washing and compared with the total radioactivity as a percentage uptake. In the Res-O-Mat system, the unbound T_4 is adsorbed on to a resin strip. After removing the strip, the bound T_4 is counted. Both methods require one or more reference sera to be run alongside the unknowns but differ in the final expression of the result. The Quantisorb test gives a ratio for each specimen. Similar ratios are obtained for two reference sera with stated "normalised" T_4 concentrations, above and below the normal range. Owing to variable extraction, losses on evaporation and other operating variables, the two reference serum ratios have to be fitted to one of a family of calibration curves provided by the manufacturer for that particular batch. The patient's result can then be read off directly as the concentration of T_4. In the Res-O-Mat variant, the manufacturer's reference serum is run alongside the unknown and the results are expressed as the ratio of the count rate using the reference serum to that using the patient's serum. This is referred to as the effective T_4 ratio, hence the test name—Res-O-Mat ETR. For the Thyrolute and Thyopac-5 procedures the results are expressed as a ratio of the result of the test serum to that of a reference serum. The midpoint of the normal range corresponds to a ratio of 1.00 for the last three tests.

In all cases the claim is that adding the patient's serum offsets variations in TBG content. Thus in pregnancy, TBG, TBG-T_4 and FTBG are increased. The second liberates more radio-T_4 during the CPB step but the extra FTBG in the added native serum binds this leaving a normal amount free. In hyperthyroidism TBG is near normal, TBG-T_4 increased and FTBG reduced. The final effect is an increase in unbound T_4. In hypothyroidism the converse holds.

The validity depends on the relative volumes of serum extracted and later added as native serum. The optimum ratio is found from the "normalising" effect on, for example, serum from pregnant euthyroid subjects. It is thus of interest that Ashkar and Bezjean (1972) added only $2\ \mu l$ patient's serum in their Quantisorb assessment, while Howorth *et al.* (1975) used only $10\ \mu l$ when evaluating the Thyrolute test.

The results for the two-stage FTI and the Res-O-Mat ETR test show rather poor correlation (Jørgensen, 1974; Wellby *et al.*, 1973) as is also the case for the Thyrolute test in patients with a raised TBG (Howorth *et al.*, 1975) although good correlation was found for hypothyroid, hyperthyroid, and other euthyroid patients. Hamada *et al.* (1975) also report a good correlation between the Thyopac-5 test and the two-stage FTI. It is not yet certain that the single-stage or sequential FTI tests offer any advantage other than speed and convenience over conventional two-stage tests. Indeed Howorth *et al.* (1975) consider they might have rather poorer discriminating power.

Thyroid Function Tests 23

Urinary T_3 and T_4 Excretion

As the biologically active non-protein bound fraction of T_3 and T_4 is filtered at the renal glomerulus, the excretion of these two hormones in the urine might also give an indirect assessment of free T_3 and free T_4. This involves collection of a 24 h specimen of urine and determination of either T_3 (Chan *et al.,* 1972) or T_4 (Chan & Landon, 1972). Initial results are encouraging but the place of this investigation has to be established.

Plasma Thyroid Stimulating Hormone Measurements

Determination of Thyroid Stimulating Hormone. TSH can be measured by radioimmunoassay and several available methods are reviewed by Hall (1972). There are still problems in that the antisera show cross reactivity with HCG, LH and FSH with which they share common antigens. The assays also lack sensitivity and this with the specificity problems leads to difficulties in separating pathologically low values from those in the lower normal range. The assays usually require incubation for several days thus reducing their value for the early reporting of abnormalities.

The normal ranges vary between different laboratories owing to these factors but figures ranging from "undetectable" or 0.4 mU/l up to 4 mU/l with a mean of about 1.6 mU/l are representative. The results are similar for both sexes and for children over 1 year old. They show a circadian rhythm being greatest at 02.00 to 04.00 h and least at 18.00 to 20.00 h.

In the absence of pituitary disease, hypothyroidism would be expected to lead to increased levels of TSH and hyperthyroidism to decreased levels. For the reasons just described the latter situation is not usually demonstrable and the investigation is not helpful for diagnosis. In the rare cases of primary pituitary or hypothalamic dysfunction leading to hyperthyroidism there is an increase in circulating TSH. The investigation is, however, most helpful in the investigation of hypothyroidism due to primary thyroid failure. Whereas hypothyroidism secondary to pituitary and hypothalamic disease is associated with low or normal TSH figures, primary thyroid failure is almost always accompanied by an increased TSH concentration up to 40 mU/l or more. The change is very sensitive to minor degrees of thyroid hypofunction. Evered and Hall (1972) classified patients into three groups. In those with myxoedema or overt hypothyroidism, the TSH increase is associated with other definitely abnormal thyroid function tests and is usually obvious clinically. In mild hypothyroidism routine thyroid function tests may give equivocal results and clinical diagnosis is uncertain. Also the TRF test (below) may be normal in many cases. Such patients usually benefit from replacement therapy. In subclinical hypothyroidism, the increase in TSH is the only abnormal finding. This leads to difficulties in defining the upper end of the normal range for TSH. The clinical progress of such patients is not established. In some cases a trial of thyroxine therapy may be warranted.

24   *Practical Clinical Biochemistry*

Many patients with non-toxic goitre have normal TSH levels but increases have been seen in auto-immune thyroid disease, iodine deficiency, in congenital enzyme defects and after ingestion of natural goitrogens.

Thyrotrophin Releasing Hormone Stimulation Test. The availability of TRH allows direct stimulation of the anterior pituitary to secrete TSH to be carried out. The response is modified by the existence of pituitary disease and by the negative feed-back arising from the level of circulating thyroid hormones. The latter may be altered by thyroid disease. When given intravenously TRH causes a rapid increase in plasma TSH which is maximal at about 20 min. In some cases a delayed response occurs, peaking at 60 min. The response increases with the dose of TRH up to 400 μg. The test conditions usually used require a dose of 200 μg TRH intravenously with determination of TSH in plasma collected 20 and 60 min later. The TSH causes the release of T_3 and T_4. The peak concentration of T_3, measured by radioimmunoassay is at 2 to 4 h (Lawton *et al.,* 1973) but the T_4 response is delayed. When T_4 is measured it is preferable to use a larger dose of TRH and after 40 mg orally, serum T_4 levels can be measured 6 or 24 h later. Measurement of T_3 or T_4 tests the whole pituitary-thyroid axis.

The normal response to 200 μg TRH intravenously when assessed by TSH measurement varies with the TSH method used, with sex, age and time of day. The effect of circadian rhythm is minimised by carrying out the test in the morning. Ormston (1972) quotes the following normal responses.

TSH (mU/l) after 200 μg TRH as mean and range

	Men	*Women*
Basal level	1.6 (<0.5—2.8)	1.4 (<0.5—2.7)
20 min	9.5 (3.5—15.6)	13.5 (6.5—20.5)
60 min	6.8 (2.0—11.5)	9.8 (4.0—15.6)

The significantly greater response in women is an oestrogen effect. The increment in TSH is less in the elderly but basal levels are higher and peak levels similar to younger people. Certain drugs can modify this normal response. ACTH, glucocorticoids, *l*-dopa and thyroid hormones all reduce the response whilst oestrogens, theophylline and antithyroid drugs all increase it.

In *hyperthyroidism,* the increased level of circulating thyroid hormone diminishes the response following TRH. With the submaximal dose of 200 μg i.v. no rise in TSH is seen in clinical hyperthyroidism while a normal response excludes the condition. However, other conditions may cause a diminished response. If toxic effects are apparent then the syndrome of T_3 toxicosis is a possibility. In patients apparently euthyroid the causes may be ophthalmic Graves' disease, multinodular goitre, autonomous thyroid adenoma, treated or subclinical thyrotoxicosis and hypothyroid patients receiving more than the necessary replacement dose of thyroxine. Patients who show an impaired TSH response are those who also show an impaired or absent suppression with T_3 (see below).

In *hypothyroidism* an increased response to TRH is apparent, and is sometimes delayed. Ormston (1972) quotes the following results for TSH

Thyroid Function Tests 25

as range (mean) in mU/l : basal 3 to 75 (24.5); at 20 min, 25 to 89 (60); at 60 min, 18 to 109 (56.8). The greatest rises occur in overt myxoedema but abnormal responses are seen in milder degrees of hypothyroidism associated with autoimmune thyroiditis, antithyroid drug administration, following partial thyroidectomy or radioiodine therapy, in endemic goitre and in thyroid enzyme defects. A normal response probably excludes hypothyroidism.

The test has also been used to assess *hypopituitarism*. Obvious hypothyroidism from this cause is associated with no response to TRH and a normal response excludes pituitary hypothyroidism. However, an absent response may not imply hypothyroidism but indicate a risk of its future development. This is often the case in treated acromegalics. In the rarer cases of hypothalamic disease with a normal pituitary and some hypothyroidism the response to TRH may be normal although delayed. In hyperpituitarism and in some cases of Cushing's syndrome, there is usually a diminished or absent response to TRH.

Stimulation and Suppression Tests. The availability of TSH allows stimulation of the thyroid gland to be studied directly and has been used to differentiate primary thyroid failure from failure secondary to hypopituitarism. TSH causes release of T_3 and T_4 from the thyroid which can be measured by a variety of methods as described earlier. It also increases the rate of uptake of radioactive iodide by the gland as assessed by the usual uptake methods. Williams *et al.* (1969a) measured T_4 by a competitive protein binding assay 24 h after giving 10 IU of TSH intramuscularly. The normal response was an increase in serum T_4 of at least 35 per cent above the basal level. The T_4 response was shown to correlate well with the uptake of radioiodine by the thyroid. In primary thyroid failure a reduced response is seen.

The administration of thyroid hormone results in suppression of TSH secretion from the anterior pituitary. This has been used to investigate cases in whom thyroid activity is autonomous and unresponsive to TSH. Initially studies of thyroid uptake of radioiodine before and after a course of thyroid extract or, later, T_3 were performed. The need to administer a radioisotope twice has been avoided by Williams *et al.* (1969b) who determined serum T_4 concentrations before and 9 days after commencing T_3 in a dose of 40 μg every eight hours for 7 days. The normal response is a fall to between 38 and 72 per cent of the initial value. Although this avoids radioisotopes it still involves giving T_3 to a patient who may already be thyrotoxic.

The introduction of TSH assays and the TRH test has reduced the need for these tests.

TESTS BASED ON THE ACTION OF THYROID HORMONES ON BODY TISSUES

The thyroid hormones influence the overall rate of metabolism of the body. The earliest tests used in thyroid disease were those which

26 *Practical Clinical Biochemistry*

demonstrated a change in metabolic rate. With the advent of the tests described in the preceding section these earlier tests have been much less used because the metabolic rate is also influenced by extra-thyroid factors and there are technical difficulties in achieving accurate results. Several workers, however, consider the determination of the basal metabolic rate (BMR) to be helpful still in certain cases.

In addition to a general influence on metabolic rate, thyroid hormones can affect the metabolism of particular groups of substances on particular tissues. The alteration in lipid metabolism has long been studied by measuring serum cholesterol and this is still a useful ancillary investigation. Abnormal thyroid activity is associated with a skeletal muscle abnormality resulting in the escape of enzymes from the muscle cell and their determination in serum is helpful. Other investigations which are occasionally used in thyroid disease include the glucose tolerance test (see Chapter 14, Vol. 1) and the excretion of creatine in urine (Chapter 17, Vol. 1).

I. Basal Metabolic Rate

Basal metabolism is the amount of energy required to maintain the body processes when a person is at complete physical and mental rest twelve to fourteen hours from the time when food was last taken. Such basal conditions afford a means of comparing metabolism in health and disease. They do not, however, correspond to the smallest energy needs of the body, since in sleep, energy requirements may sometimes fall below basal metabolism.

Energy requirements are now expressed in terms of the Joule (J). Because of the large amount of energy involved in basal metabolism it is more convenient to use kilojoules (kJ) or megajoules (MJ) = 10^6 J). Until the adoption of SI units, energy requirements were expressed in kilocalories, the large calorie (C) of physics, the energy required to raise the temperature of 1 kg of water from 15 to 16°C. One kilocalorie equals 4.186 kJ or for most purposes 4.2 kJ.

Factors Influencing Basal Metabolism

Basal metabolism in normal persons varies directly with size and with differences in the rate at which the body processes are taking place so that in drawing up normal standards both these factors have to be allowed for.

Most of the energy used under basal conditions is needed to maintain a constant body temperature which is above the surroundings. The energy is needed to balance the loss of heat by evaporation and radiation from the body surface. The basal energy production is thus much more closely related to body surface area than to body mass and comparisons between persons of different size is best made in terms of the rate of energy consumption per unit area, expressed in the unit $kJ\,m^{-2}h^{-1}$.

Thyroid Function Tests 27

In the second place BMR varies with the intensity at which the body processes are occurring. It is greater in men than in women by about 7 per cent, perhaps due to the thinner layer of subcutaneous fat in males. Then, again, the BMR is appreciably greater in children than adults; in young children by as much as 25 per cent. This, together with their greater relative surface area for their weight, makes the basal metabolism of children per unit weight considerably higher than that of adults. In older people the rate of metabolism falls when compared with that found in adults between 20 and 40 years old by as much as 20 per cent in the seventies.

The normal ranges for many years were those of Boothby and Sandiford (1929) and Boothby *et al.* (1936). However, more recently Robertson and Reid (1952) published revised figures, the result of 20 years work on normal persons in the London area. These are lower than those of Boothby and Sandiford for all ages except the youngest. This appears to be due to

TABLE 1,4
Normal Values for Basic Metabolic Rate
$(kJ\ m^{-2}h^{-1})$

Age (years)	MALES			FEMALES		
	Robertson and Reid	Fleisch	*Lewis *et al.* and †Shock	Robertson and Reid	Fleisch	*Lewis *et al.* and †Shock
3	252	215	*222	228	214	*214
4	242		217	226		208
5	236	206	212	222	203	203
6	227		207	217		197
7	218	198	197	210	190	191
8	210		192	203		185
9	202	189	187	194	179	180
10	195		182	185		174
11	189	180	178	177	176	168
12	183		†188	170		†172
13	179	177	185	164	169	167
14	175		182	158		159
15	172	175	179	154	159	149
16	169		172	151		143
17	166	171		148	152	
20	161	162		144	148	
25	155	157		143	147	
30	152	154		143	147	
40	149	152		136	146	
45	144	151		135	144	
50	142	150		134	142	
60	139	146		132	137	
70	136	141		129	133	
75	134	139			131	

N.B. Robertson and Reid also gave the limits for both sexes between which 95 per cent lie. These are roughly ±15 per cent of the mean values above.

28   *Practical Clinical Biochemistry*

the fact that whereas Robertson and Reid used the method outlined subsequently (p. 30) in which the measurement is repeated until consistent results are obtained, Boothby *et al.,* took "the first determination made for the individual unless at the time of the test and before its calculation it was noted as unsatisfactory for reasons of restlessness, observable nervous tension, or an elevated temperature." The element of training was thus deliberately excluded. Robertson pointed out that when successive determinations are to be made, this is not possible, but as nervous tension is not uncommon during the first test, especially in thyrotoxicosis, initial readings may be 10 to 20 per cent and more higher than those finally obtained. Robertson's technique is preferred. Another series of more recent figures are those of Fleisch (1951).

Normal ranges were also discussed by Dubois (1936), and by Peters and Van Slyke (1932, 1946). The BMR of children and adolescents has been specially studied by a number of workers (see, for example, Talbot, 1925, Lewis *et al.,* 1937, for children, and Shock, 1942, for a study of adolescents). There is general agreement that just after birth the BMR is low and that it rises during the first year or two of life to reach a peak, after which it slowly declines. The age at which the maximum occurs has been rather variously placed about two to three years, but from the work of Lewis *et al.,* it appears to occur before two years of age. Some workers have held that there is a rise at puberty.

The figures of Robertson and Reid and of Fleisch, together with those of Lewis *et al.* and of Shock for childhood and adolescence are given in Table 1,4.

Measurement of Basal Metabolic Rate

Both direct and indirect calorimetry have been used.

Direct calorimetry. The actual heat production is measured using a respiration chamber, of which only a few exist. Because of the elaborate apparatus required, this method is not used in routine work. Details are given in larger works on metabolism and nutrition.

Indirect calorimetry. The volume of oxygen consumed, or of the oxygen consumed and the carbon dioxide produced, are measured over an accurately timed period of a few minutes. From these the energy utilised can be calculated.

The volume of oxygen used by the body varies to some extent with the type of food metabolised. Thus, when carbohydrate is being used, the consumption of 1 litre of oxygen represents the production of 21.2 kJ (5.05 kcal). For fat and proteins the corresponding figures are 19.7 and 18.9 kJ (4.69 and 4.49 kcal) respectively. On an average mixed diet the consumption of 1 litre of oxygen by healthy persons represents the production of approximately 20.2 kJ (4.80 kcal). If we ignore the nature of the diet and use this figure to calculate the energy production, the error introduced will be between −5 and +6 per cent. Instead of converting

Thyroid Function Tests 29

consumption into kJ, tables can be drawn up giving the normal oxygen consumption for different heights and weights. The observed oxygen consumption in a particular case is compared with this normal and the result then reported as a percentage increase or decrease. This method is used in *closed circuit methods* of estimating BMR. The patient breathes in air or oxygen from a reservoir to which the expired air is returned through soda lime to absorb the carbon dioxide produced. The oxygen consumed is read directly as the decrease in volume of the gas in the reservoir.

For more accurate work it is necessary to take into account the type of nutrients metabolised. To do this, both the oxygen consumed and the carbon dioxide produced are measured, and the *respiratory quotient* calculated.

Respiratory quotient, RQ

$$= \frac{\text{Volume of carbon dioxide produced}}{\text{Volume of oxygen consumed}},$$

in a given period. This differs for the different nutrients. Thus, when carbohydrates are metabolised, the process may be represented

$$C_6H_{12}O_6 + 6O_2 \rightarrow 6CO_2 + 6H_2O$$

so that the RQ is exactly 1.00.

Fats contain a much greater proportion of hydrogen to oxygen than do carbohydrates, and so produce more water. Taking tripalmitin as example, we have

$$2C_{51}H_{98}O_6 + 145O_2 \rightarrow 102CO_2 + 98H_2O$$

giving a RQ of 0.7. This varies a little for different fats. For the mixture present in the human diet it is taken as 0.707.

The case of proteins is more complicated since they are not completely metabolised to carbon dioxide and water. Most of the nitrogen is excreted as urea in the urine. The RQ averages 0.80.

On an ordinary mixed diet the RQ is about 0.85. When the body is in the post-absorptive state it is about 0.82. It is clear that the RQ gives some indication of the type of food being consumed. When carbohydrate only is metabolised, the quotient is 1.00 and the energy equivalent of a litre of oxygen is 21.2 kJ. If only fat is being metabolised the RQ is 0.707 and the energy equivalent of a litre of oxygen is 19.7 kJ. It is thus possible to draw up a table giving the energy equivalents for the range of RQs from 0.70 to 1.00 for all mixtures of fat and carbohydrate. This respiratory quotient is termed the non-protein RQ. Such a table was given by Lusk (1924).

The non-protein RQ can be determined by measuring the oxygen consumption, the carbon dioxide production, and the urinary nitrogen excretion over a measured time. The excretion of 1 g of nitrogen

30 *Practical Clinical Biochemistry*

corresponds to the consumption of 5.94 litres of oxygen and the production of 4.76 litres of carbon dioxide thus giving the volume of oxygen and carbon dioxide associated with the protein metabolised. By subtracting these from the volumes found experimentally we can obtain the oxygen consumed and carbon dioxide produced by the metabolism of fat and carbohydrate. This gives us the non-protein RQ and from the table the energy equivalent of the oxygen consumed in their metabolism. The energy equivalent of the oxygen consumed in metabolising protein is 18.8 kJ (4.485 kcal). The total energy utilisation can then be calculated with as high a degree of accuracy as the collection of the expired air permits.

The amount of protein ordinarily metabolised is small compared with that of fat and carbohydrate. Only 10 to 12 per cent of energy is derived from protein when ordinary mixed diets are being taken. In most determinations the effect of protein is ignored. The error thus introduced is small. The RQ is calculated from the carbon dioxide expired and the oxygen consumed. The energy equivalent of a litre of oxygen is obtained using this RQ as though it were the non-protein RQ. The BMR can then be calculated and compared with the normal, and the percentage increase or decrease calculated.

This method of calculating the results can be used in the *open circuit methods.* In this the expired air is collected in a Douglas bag, and analysed for carbon dioxide and oxygen content in a gas analysis apparatus. The RQ can be calculated and the volume of oxygen used obtained from the known composition of ordinary air (inspired air) and the ascertained composition of the expired air.

The closed circuit method is so much simpler and quicker than the open circuit one that it is now almost exclusively used. Only this will be described.

Closed Circuit Method

The various forms of apparatus which are used for this method are all based on the original Benedict-Roth apparatus, shown diagrammatically in Fig. 1,4. The patient breathes a supply of oxygen contained in the reservoir A. As the patient breathes out and in the reservoir moves up and down. The circulation of oxygen is shown by the arrows. On its way to the mouthpiece the oxygen passes through a valve which shuts when the patient breathes out, so that the expired air is returned along the other tube and passes through soda lime to absorb the carbon dioxide before returning to the reservoir. The amount of oxygen in the reservoir thus falls steadily during the course of the experiment. The upper end of the reservoir is connected over a pulley with a weight W to which is attached a pen. This

Thyroid Function Tests

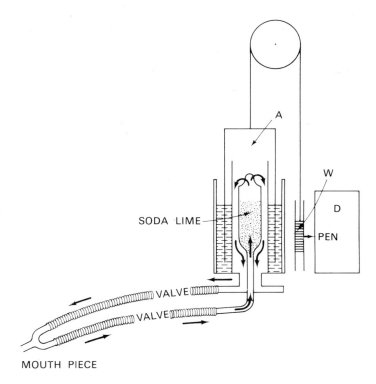

Fig. 1,4. Closed Circuit Apparatus for Basal Metabolism.

records the movements of the reservoir on a slowly rotating drum, D, on which a suitably calibrated paper is wrapped. Each movement of the pen up and down corresponds to a complete respiration, so that a line drawn along the crests or the troughs can be used to read the oxygen consumption. If such a line is to be drawn with sufficient accuracy, the size of the patient's respirations must be fairly uniform. In most cases it is possible to get the patient to breathe regularly enough. When this is not possible, an open circuit method has to be used.

The type of chart obtained is shown in Fig. 1,5. The volume of oxygen consumed per minute is easily calculated, and is then corrected to 0° C and 760 mm Hg pressure using the factor given in Table 1,6.

Variations in RQ are ignored and the consumption of a litre of oxygen corresponds to 20.2 kJ (4.82 kcal). From the patient's height and weight the surface area is found from Table 1,7 and hence the BMR can be calculated and compared with the normal values given. The result is usually expressed as a percentage increase or decrease of the normal for the age and sex.

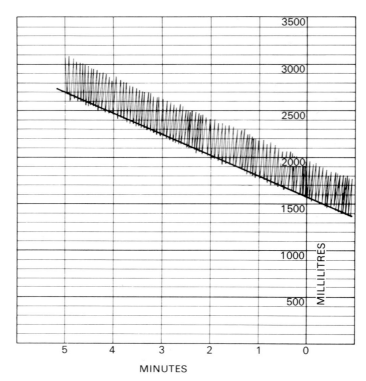

Fig. 1,5. Chart from Closed Circuit Apparatus.

TABLE 1,5

Water Vapour Pressure, mm Hg

°C	mm Hg	°C	mm Hg	°C	mm Hg
8	8.0	14	11.9	20	17.4
9	8.6	15	12.7	21	18.5
10	9.2	16	13.5	22	19.7
11	9.8	17	14.4	23	20.9
12	10.5	18	15.4	24	22.2
13	11.2	19	16.3	25	23.5

As an example the chart in Fig. 1,5 was from a female patient 32 years old, 55 kg weight, 162 cm tall. The surface area is thus 1.58 square metres (Table 1.7). From the chart it is seen that oxygen consumption was 2 700 to 1 590 ml = 1 110 ml, in 5 min, i.e. 222 ml/min. The barometric pressure was 754 mm Hg, temperature 16°C. The water vapour pressure was 13.5

Thyroid Function Tests 33

TABLE 1,6
Factors for Converting the Volume of Gas to $0°C$, $760\,mm\,Hg$

Pressure (mm Hg)	Temperature ($°C$)									
	8	10	12	14	16	18	20	22	24	26
720	0.920	0.914	0.908	0.901	0.895	0.889	0.883	0.877	0.871	0.865
725	0.927	0.920	0.914	0.907	0.901	0.895	0.889	0.883	0.877	0.871
730	0.933	0.927	0.920	0.914	0.907	0.901	0.895	0.889	0.883	0.877
735	0.940	0.933	0.926	0.920	0.914	0.907	0.901	0.895	0.889	0.883
740	0.946	0.939	0.933	0.926	0.920	0.914	0.907	0.901	0.895	0.889
745	0.952	0.946	0.939	0.933	0.926	0.920	0.913	0.907	0.901	0.895
750	0.959	0.952	0.945	0.939	0.932	0.926	0.919	0.913	0.907	0.901
755	0.965	0.958	0.952	0.945	0.939	0.932	0.926	0.919	0.913	0.907
760	0.972	0.965	0.958	0.951	0.944	0.938	0.931	0.925	0.919	0.913
765	0.978	0.971	0.964	0.958	0.951	0.944	0.938	0.931	0.925	0.919
770	0.984	0.977	0.970	0.964	0.957	0.951	0.944	0.938	0.931	0.925

Figures for intermediate values of temperature and pressure can easily be assessed.

Read the barometer, subtract from this the aqueous vapour pressure (Table 1,5), and use the pressure obtained to find the correction factor in the above table for the temperature at which the volume of gas was measured.

(Table 1,5) so the factor to convert to NTP was 0.92. Corrected volume = 222 × 0.92 = 204 ml. So

$$BMR(kJ\ m^{-2}\ h^{-1}) = \frac{204 \times 20.2 \times 60}{1.58 \times 1000} = 156.5$$

Average normal from Table 1,4 = 142

$$So\ BMR = \frac{14.5}{142} = +\ 10.2\ per\ cent.$$

Preparation of the Patient. Tests on Out-patients

Careful preparation of the patient is most important for reliable results. The patient must be in a state of complete rest, both physical and mental, and fasting for at least 12 h. It is convenient to do the test in the early morning. As regards physical rest, if there has not been any vigorous muscular activity, it is sufficient if the patient lies down for half an hour immediately before the test. With hospital in-patients this presents no difficulty. The test can either be done at the bedside or the patient taken in bed to a special room. With out-patients, the half-hour rest is less satisfactory since the effect of any strenuous exercise in raising the rate of metabolism may extend over several hours. There must be an element of doubt as regards the reliability of tests done on out-patients. Robertson

TABLE 1,7

Surface Area (in square metres) from Height and Weight

HEIGHT IN INCHES

HEIGHT IN CENTIMETRES	HEIGHT IN INCHES	WEIGHT IN KILOGRAMS 25	30	35	40	45	50	55	60	65	70	75	80	85	90	95	100	105
190	75						1.70	1.77	1.84	1.90	1.96	2.02	2.08	2.13	2.18	2.23	2.28	2.33
185	73					1.59	1.67	1.74	1.80	1.87	1.92	1.98	2.04	2.09	2.14	2.19	2.24	2.29
180	71				1.49	1.56	1.64	1.70	1.77	1.83	1.89	1.94	2.00	2.05	2.10	2.15	2.19	2.24
175	69			1.38	1.46	1.53	1.60	1.67	1.73	1.79	1.85	1.90	1.96	2.01	2.06	2.10	2.15	2.20
170	67		1.26	1.35	1.43	1.50	1.57	1.63	1.69	1.76	1.81	1.86	1.91	1.96	2.01	2.06	2.11	2.15
165	65	1.14	1.23	1.32	1.40	1.47	1.53	1.60	1.66	1.72	1.77	1.82	1.87	1.92	1.97	2.02	2.06	2.11
160	63	1.12	1.21	1.29	1.36	1.43	1.50	1.56	1.62	1.68	1.73	1.78	1.83	1.88	1.93	1.97	2.01	
155	61	1.09	1.18	1.26	1.33	1.40	1.47	1.53	1.58	1.64	1.69	1.74	1.79	1.84	1.88	1.93		
150	59	1.07	1.15	1.23	1.30	1.37	1.43	1.49	1.55	1.60	1.65	1.70	1.75	1.79	1.84			
145	57	1.04	1.12	1.20	1.27	1.34	1.40	1.45	1.51	1.57	1.61	1.66	1.71	1.75				
140	55	1.01	1.10	1.17	1.24	1.30	1.36	1.42	1.47	1.53	1.57	1.62	1.66					
135	53	0.99	1.07	1.14	1.21	1.27	1.32	1.38	1.43	1.49	1.53	1.58						
130	51	0.96	1.04	1.11	1.17	1.23	1.29	1.34	1.39	1.45	1.49							
125	49	0.93	1.01	1.08	1.14	1.20	1.25	1.31	1.36	1.41								
120	47	0.91	0.98	1.05	1.11	1.16	1.22	1.27	1.32									
115	45	0.88	0.95	1.02	1.07	1.13	1.18	1.23										
110	43	0.85	0.92	0.98	1.04	1.09	1.14											
105	41	0.82	0.89	0.95	1.01	1.06												
WEIGHT IN POUNDS		55	66	77	88	99	110	121	132	143	154	165	176	187	198	209	220	231

These figures are calculated from DuBois' formula: Surface area in square metres
= Height in $cm^{0.725}$ x Weight in $kg^{0.425}$ x 71.84 ÷ 10,000.
Values for heights and weights intermediate between those given can easily be assessed.

Thyroid Function Tests

(1944) made a careful study of BMR methods and concluded that reliable results can be obtained if determinations are made on successive days. He used a rest of half an hour lying on a couch and made duplicate measurements of 10 min duration each morning. His results on the second day agreed within 5 per cent in the great majority of cases and were rather lower than those obtained on the first morning. In the few cases in which there was not such agreement further estimations were carried out. These findings have been confirmed by other workers. The procedure suggested is as follows. After 30 min rest, lying down, on the first morning, make an estimation, and repeat after a further rest of 30 min. The second estimation is usually lower than the first. A third estimation is made, in the same way, on the second morning. If this agrees with the second test done on the first morning, the investigation can be stopped at this point. If it does not, a further estimation is done 30 min later. In the authors' experience it is rare for agreement not to be obtained by this time. Under such conditions sufficiently accurate estimations can be made on out-patients.

It is equally important that the patient should be in a state of mental rest. Disturbing influences should be excluded as far as possible and a few explanatory words to the patient on arrival should give the necessary reassurance. In any case, any apprehension should disappear after the first determination. The advantage of freedom from disturbance makes a special room desirable whenever possible. This should be normally heated.

The patient should not read or talk during the period of resting and should be quite comfortable so that movements arising from discomfort are not often made. The bladder should be emptied shortly before beginning the test so that any discomfort from a full bladder does not interfere.

INTERPRETATION

Table 1,4 gives the normal values. It is often convenient to report the results as the percentage change from the appropriate mean normal figure.

A high energy diet, particularly if it is rich in protein, raises BMR whilst a low energy diet, poor in protein as in malnutrition, often reduces it. Fever raises BMR by approximately 13 per cent for each $^{\circ}C$ rise. Increases in pregnancy and during lactation may reach + 30 per cent.

Becker (1971) points out that the BMR test is the only one measuring the effect of thyroid hormones on tissue metabolism generally and suggests that it still has a place in assessing thyroid activity when interfering substances make it difficult to interpret other tests. It may have a role in assessing response to therapy and be a useful index of the severity of thyroid abnormality, an attribute not always shared with such tests as the determination of PBI or iodine uptake studies. However, in the view of many workers the test is now obsolescent. Increases found in hyperthyroidism vary from normal to + 100 per cent or more. The disease is severe if BMR is increased more than + 50 per cent, very severe if it is over + 75 per cent. The test may be useful in cases of T_3 thyrotoxicosis with no increase in T_4 or PBI but with marked biological effects. The BMR is

36 *Practical Clinical Biochemistry*

reduced in hypothyroidism. In the severest cases values of -50 per cent are obtained, but the common range is from -15 to -35 per cent.

II. Serum Cholesterol and Creatine Kinase Determinations in Thyroid Disease

The serum cholesterol may be decreased in hyperthyroidism and is more consistently increased in myxoedema. In a recent series of patients in our hospital with T_4 values of less than 20 nmol/l (1.0 μg I/100 ml) the serum cholesterol was over 7.8 mmol/l (300 mg/100 ml) in 71 out of 102 cases. Fowler *et al.* (1970) reported that hypercholesterolaemia precedes all evidence of thyroid failure in patients with autoimmune thyroiditis. A fall of 1.55 mmol/l (60 mg/100 ml) in serum cholesterol after a period on L-thyroxine was considered by Hobbs *et al.* (1963) to be an objective test of thyroid insufficiency. A rapid fall in serum cholesterol after starting thyroxine treatment has been demonstrated in 3 of our cases: 9.19 to 6.22 mmol/l (355 to 240 mg/100 ml) in 3 weeks, 7.0 to 5.43 mmol/l (270 to 210 mg/100 ml) in 1 week, and 13.0 to 9.6 mmol/l (500 to 370 mg/100 ml) in 4 weeks.

The serum creatine kinase (CK) was reported increased in myxoedema by Craig and Ross (1963) and Griffiths (1963) and to be low in hyperthyroidism, a condition associated with muscle wasting. Doran and Wilkinson (1971) confirmed these somewhat anomalous findings. The serum CK found in hyperthyroidism is the isoenzyme characteristic of skeletal muscle. Doran and Wilkinson estimated the serum adenylate kinase (AK, myokinase) another muscle enzyme, which catalyses the interconversion of adenosine mono, di, and triphosphate:

$$2 \text{ ADP} \rightleftharpoons \text{ATP} + \text{AMP}$$

They found this increased in hyperthyroidism and decreased in myxoedema, the reverse of findings with CK. Skeletal muscle is the richest known source of AK and this is probably the source in thyrotoxicosis. It is suggested that the lack of any increase in CK is due to its selective inhibition by the abnormally high amounts of thyroid hormone. The increase in CK in myxoedema may be related to the associated hypothermia, a condition known to cause elevation of the serum enzyme.

There was a more marked increase in CK than of cholesterol in our series of patients of whom 72 out of 102 gave values greater than 10 units per ml, the upper limit of normal using the Hughes method (see Chapter 22, Vol. 1), the highest value being 190 units. The fall after starting treatment is again apparent, but more marked. In three cases the figures were 106 to 16, 56 to 10, and 39 to 31 units/ml, which suggests that CK determinations may be a better index of hypothyroidism. It must be remembered, however, that in all our patients there were extremely low concentrations of T_4.

Thyroid Function Tests

The Choice of Thyroid Function Tests and Their Interpretation in Thyroid Disorders

Investigational problems in thyroid disease fall into two groups, the assessment of thyroid size including irregularities of shape due to the presence of one or more tumours, and the assessment of thyroid activity. The clinician assesses the former and arrives at a clinical judgement of the activity. Laboratory investigations provide a more objective assessment of thyroid activity.

An increase in thyroid size is referred to as a goitre. A local tumour is a nodule but sometimes a multinodular goitre occurs. Increased activity or hyperthyroidism when producing clinically apparent effects is usually called thyrotoxicosis and is usually associated with a diffuse goitre (classical Graves' disease) but may occur in multinodular goitre or with an isolated nodule, due to an adenoma or carcinoma which is secreting T_3 and T_4 in an autonomous fashion. In most cases of thyrotoxicosis the increased thyroid activity is not due to an increased secretion of TSH but to the presence of a circulating immunoglobulin (IgG) known as long-acting thyroid stimulator (LATS). Milder degrees of hyperthyroidism may show little increase in gland size.

The combination of a goitre with the euthyroid or mildly hypothyroid state is often referred to as "non-toxic goitre" but is a mixed group. It includes endemic goitre arising from iodine deficiency, a genetic predisposition often seen as pubertal goitre, and the presence of natural goitrogens in the diet. Other cases of non-toxic goitre include dyshormonogenesis arising from congenital enzyme defects and the early stages of autoimmune thyroiditis. More localised enlargements arise with a non-toxic or "cold" adenoma or carcinoma.

Hypothyroidism is also seen with a gland of normal or reduced size. Such hypoactivity may be due to primary thyroid failure as in the later stages of autoimmune thyroiditis or after partial thyroidectomy or radioiodine therapy. Alternatively, it may be an expression of hypofunction of the pituitary or hypothalamus.

The laboratory investigation of thyroid disease is often straightforward but difficulties arise when the degree of abnormality is slight. Also many drugs interfere with some tests. These may affect thyroid or pituitary function altering hormone production directly but can also change the concentration of TBG or the binding of T_3 or T_4 to TBG. Other diseases may alter TBG concentration and increases are seen in pregnancy.

For most cases, particularly those with more marked clinical symptoms, the determination of serum T_4 or, less satisfactorily, PBI, provides clear evidence of the correctness of the diagnosis. Where facilities are available and doubt exists the neck uptake of radioiodine can be measured. This can be especially helpful in demonstrating either a toxic nodule or a "cold" nodule. The next most useful test is one of the T_3 uptake methods with calculation of the FTI. This extends the discriminating ability in the more doubtful areas at some extra cost. Where doubt still exists the other tests particularly those involving TSH or T_3 assays can be invaluable. Such tests are usually only available in specialised laboratories.

Problems arise in the use of T_4I and PBI methods from direct contamination with iodine-containing drugs. These are precipitated with the proteins and cause appreciable interference in PBI methods (see Acland, 1971, for a list of possible interfering materials). In our laboratory at least 1.5 per cent of specimens for PBI estimation showed gross contamination, with values between 4 and 40 μmol I_2/l (100 to 1 000 μg I/100 ml). Using similar criteria Cusick (1974) found 0.75 per cent gross contamination in 7 800 consecutive specimens. The number of less contaminated specimens giving results from within the normal range up to 8 μmol/l is uncertain but could be as high as 10 per cent. Cusick (1974) estimated the incidence of significant contamination at 16.7 per cent. The commonest interfering materials are radiographic contrast media but such readily available drugs as Enterovioform, used for the treatment of intestinal disorders, are a potentially greater problem. For some of these substances, several months or even years may elapse after administration before normal PBI values are obtained. Using the T_4I method, grossly contaminated specimens affect less than 0.1 per cent of results and show a characteristic behaviour (p. 14). This has usually been due to the use of Biloptin for cholecystography 24 to 48 h previously. The interference rate for CPB T_4 methods may be lower still but in all cases iodinated material can release a relatively massive amount of inorganic iodide, with an effect on thyroid function. It is imperative therefore that thyroid function tests be carried out before radiological investigations using iodine-containing material. Despite these deficiencies the PBI method is still widely used because it can be fully automated. But minor degrees of contamination cause appreciable uncertainty in interpretation and the method is better avoided and replaced by CPB T_4 or semi-automated T_4I methods. Commercial kit methods for both these incur similar costs, but if the manufacturer's columns are re-used, resin regenerated and reagents prepared the semi-automated T_4I method is much cheaper. Work simplication has been investigated for the CPB method (Seth, 1973) but the semi-automated T_4I method given here runs at 30 tests per hour (2 eluates per test) and that of Burnett *et al.* (1973) at 45 per hour. This compares very favourably with the fully automated PBI method, particularly when a screening run to eliminate contaminated specimens is taken into account. With the greater availability of radioimmunoassay methods for T_3 and T_4 these can compare favourably both in cost and time with these methods and will be increasingly used. (For discussion see Hoffenberg, 1975).

The effects of other forms of drug interference are complex but important. Table 1,8 shows the effect on T_4 determinations.

The T_3 resin uptake tests measure free TBG binding sites and if the TBG is reduced in amount, fewer sites are available. This could be interpreted as due to hyperthyroidism. When TBG is increased or drugs compete for TBG

Thyroid Function Tests

TABLE 1,8

Effect of Drugs on T_4 Determinations

---

(1) DRUGS CAUSING LOW T_4 VALUES

(a) *By inhibiting T_4 formation in the thyroid*
antidiabetic drugs—carbutamide, tolbutamide
antithyroid drugs—carbimazole (Neomercazole), methimazole, methyl (or propyl) thiouracil, perchlorate
anti TB drugs—isoniazid, PAS
anticonvulsants—aminoglutethimide
analgesics—oxyphenbutazone (Tanderil)
steroids-hydrocortisone, prednis(ol)one, DOCA
others—sulphonamides, lithium salts, phenindione (Dindevan), phenothiazines (large doses), and occasionally acetazolamide (Diamox)

(b) *By reducing the amount of TBG*
anabolic steroids—norethandrolone (Nilevar), oxymethalone (Adroyd, Anapolon)
androgens—testosterone and methyltestosterone
corticosteroids—cortisone and other glucocorticoids; ACTH

(c) *By displacing T_4 from binding sites on TBG*
analgesics—*aspirin*, phenylbutazone (Butazolidin)
anticonvulsants—diphenylhydantoin (Epanutin), mephenytoin

(d) *By PBI method interference*: mercury compounds including mercurial diuretics

(e) *Mechanism uncertain*: thiazide diuretics, reserpine (occasionally)

(2) DRUGS CAUSING HIGH T_4 VALUES

(a) *By increasing T_4 output from the thyroid*
iodides, lysergic acid derivatives

(b) *By increasing the amount of TBG*
oestrogens—natural and synthetic including diethylstilboestrol and ethinyl-oestradiol
progestogens—natural and synthetic including chlormadinone, norethynodrel
the contraceptive pill (also seen to some extent at ovulation and in luteal phase of cycle; more marked during pregnancy)

---

binding sites, the opposite occurs and hypothyroidism may be erroneously suspected. Competition with binding sites also increases the urinary excretion of T_3 and T_4.

In other conditions alteration of TBG concentration can occur. It is increased in pregnancy and also as a familial genetic fault. Decreased concentrations occur in starvation, as a genetic abnormality and in the nephrotic syndrome where the protein is lost in the urine. The latter circumstance increases the urinary T_3 and T_4 excretion.

40 Practical Clinical Biochemistry

Hyperthyroidism

The more marked degrees of thyrotoxicosis are reflected in increased levels of PBI, or T_4. Maximal values are approximately 1 000 nmol I_2/l (25 μg/100 ml) for PBI or 400 nmol/l (20 μg I/100 ml) for T_4. Results in excess of these are very suggestive of contamination. When the clinical diagnosis is classical Graves' disease, little more needs to be done. Radio-iodine uptake studies may be helpful in those cases with a toxic adenoma or functioning carcinoma. The high T_4 concentrations are associated typically with high saturation of TBG and a reduction in binding sites for T_3 in the T_4 uptake methods. The free thyroxine index is increased. T_3 suppression of iodine uptake or of circulating hormone does not occur. TSH levels are low and do not increase after TRH. When the clinical evidence of thyrotoxicosis is strong but the T_4 concentration and T_3 uptake are normal a likely diagnosis is T_3 thyrotoxicosis in which T_3 is produced preferentially (see review by Hollander and Shenkman, 1972). This is sometimes the early stage of the typical thyrotoxic state in which there is normally over-production of both T_3 and T_4. Thyroid uptake of radio-iodine may be normal but the TRH-TSH test is typical of thyrotoxicosis and the BMR is raised. Definitive diagnosis requires the determination of plasma T_3 level.

In subclinical thyrotoxicosis the main screening tests may give borderline results and confusion arises with anxiety states. At present the TRH-TSH test seems the best investigation on which to base a decision. If the main tests appear to indicate thyrotoxicosis when the patient is clinically euthyroid the possibility of drug interference should be considered.

Hypothyroidism

Where clinical symptoms of myxoedema are apparent the circulating hormone levels fall considerably. As iodine interference is more frequent with PBI methods, it is preferable to use T_4I or T_4 methods in which figures less than 20 nmol/l (1.0 μg I/100 ml) are often found. This decrease is associated with increased serum CK and cholesterol making the diagnosis almost certain. There is a low saturation of TBG and an increase in T_3 binding sites. The problem is then one of defining the cause of the hypothyroidism before commencing treatment.

Hypothyroidism occurring in the infant during the period when growth is normally rapid leads to *cretinism* with impaired skeletal and mental development. Sporadic cretinism is associated with thyroid aplasia but the incidence is increased in areas where endemic goitre is common. If the diagnosis is established by the tests already outlined immediate thyroxine treatment is needed to minimise the effects on the skeleton and brain. In the untreated case, serum alkaline phosphatase is low and rises on treatment even before bone growth is detectable. When the diagnosis is

Thyroid Function Tests 41

uncertain the rise in TSH under basal conditions and the increased response in the TRH-TSH test are helpful.

A group of genetic disorders involving an enzyme required for thyroid hormone synthesis Fig. 1,1 present as childhood goitre with varying degrees of hypothyroidism. For a detailed discussion see Stanbury (1972) but in brief the disorders are:

(a) Defect of the iodide carrier resulting in reduced concentration of iodine by the thyroid and also the salivary glands. This is a rare cause of hypothyroidism.

(b) Presumed peroxidase deficiency with failure to convert iodide to iodine. Although radio-iodine is quickly taken up by the thyroid it can rapidly be discharged by perchlorate. Hypothyroidism is present but is uncommon in the milder form with partial enzyme defect known as Pendred's syndrome in which goitre is linked with deaf-mutism as a recessive trait.

(c) Defect in coupling of iodotyrosines. Hypothyroidism is associated with rapid iodine uptake with prolonged retention in the thyroid and failure of perchlorate to discharge the iodine.

(d) Dehalogenase deficiency with increase in circulating and urinary MIT and DIT, rapid radio-iodine uptake by the thyroid and rapid discharge. If the deficiency is confined to the thyroid, hypo-thyroidism is unusual but occurs if the defect includes extra-thyroid dehalogenases.

(e) Defective release of T_3 and T_4. Circulating iodinated proteins include polypeptides containing MIT, DIT, T_3 and T_4. The patients are euthyroid or only mildly hypothyroid.

In adult hypothyroidism the differentiation is between primary thyroid failure and malfunction secondary to pituitary insufficiency. Primary thyroid failure sometimes develops after surgical or irradiation treatment of thyrotoxicosis and is also associated with auto-immune thyroiditis (Hashimoto's disease). There is a high incidence of thyroid antibodies in such cases. Secondary hypothyroidism is likely to be associated with insufficiency of adrenocortical and gonadal function. However, such findings are inconstant and a more definite decision is best made by determination of TSH. This is increased in primary thyroid failure and decreased in secondary hypothyroidism. In cases where the change is not marked, determination after TRH increases the discrimination. If the latter test is not available, the TSH stimulation test which is positive in secondary hypothyroidism can be used. Investigation of adrenal function may be misleading as adrenal function is not always reduced in the less severe forms of hypopituitarism. In primary thyroid failure the retardation of metabolic processes may delay steroid reduction leading to decreased excretion of 17-hydroxycorticosteroids and 17-oxosteroids. Although the plasma cortisol concentration is normal the rate of increase following ACTH is subnormal. Differentiation between primary and secondary hypo-

42 *Practical Clinical Biochemistry*

thyroidism is important as treatment with thyroxine alone in the latter may precipitate an adrenal crisis.

The milder degrees of hypothyroidism are less easily detected by the simpler thyroid function tests and may be difficult to diagnose clinically. The TRH-TSH test is currently the most satisfactory investigation. It is positive very early and can antedate the need for therapy.

"Non-toxic Goitre"

The various types of congenital goitre associated with enzyme deficiency are discussed earlier (p. 41). Auto-immune thyroiditis in its earlier stages is accompanied by thyroid enlargement. At this stage circulating thyroid hormone levels may well be normal but radio-iodine uptake is occasionally increased and thyroid antibodies are present in the majority of cases. An increase in T_3 binding sites on TBG is apparent early.

The commonest form of non-toxic goitre is endemic goitre. Causes include iodine deficiency, natural goitrogens, constitutional factors and, rarely, excessive iodine intake. The considerable increase in gland size is a consequence of the attempt to synthesise sufficient T_3 and T_4. The extra needs at puberty in the milder cases lead to enlargement at that age. In most cases the output of T_3 and T_4 is normal and the usual function tests are normal also. In a minority the TRH-TSH test reveals minor degrees of hypothyroidism. In most cases, however, the uptake of radio-iodine by the gland is increased. Thyroid antibodies are absent.

Thyroid Nodules

These comprise adenomas and carcinomas. The majority metabolise iodine less than normal tissue, and are revealed as "cold" areas on scanning the thyroid after uptake of radio-iodine. The few which produce increased amounts of T_3 and T_4 are discussed under thyrotoxicosis. In most cases other biochemical tests are not helpful in diagnosis of these tumours. One exception is that some medullary carcinomas of the thyroid occur in families in association with bilateral phaeochromocytomas.

References

Acland, J. D. (1958), *J. clin. Path.*, 11, 195.
Acland, J. D. (1971), *J. clin. Path.*, 24, 187.
Albert-Recht, F. and Frazer, S. C. (1961), *Clin. chim. Acta*, 6, 591.
Ashkar, F. S. and Bezjean, A. A. (1972), *J. Amer. med. Ass.*, 221, 1483.
Backer, E. T., Postmes, Th. J. and Wiener, J. D. (1967), *Clin. chim. Acta*, 15, 77.
Barker, S. B., Humphrey, M. J. and Soley, M. H. (1951), *J. clin. Invest.*, 30, 55.
Becker, D. V. (1971), see Werner, S. C. and Ingber, S. H., below, p. 269.
Boothby, W. M., Berkson, J. and Dunn, H. L. (1936). *Amer. J. Physiol.*, 116, 468.
Boothby, W. M. and Sandiford, I. (1929), *Amer. J. Physiol.*, 90, 290.
Braverman, L. E., Vagenakis, A. G., Foster, A. E. and Ingeber, S. H. (1971), *J. clin. Endocrinol.*, 32, 497.

Thyroid Function Tests

Burnett, D., Carpenter, B. T., Day, D. W., Hill, R. H. and Woods, T. F. (1973), *Clin. chim. Acta*, 46, 321.
Chan, V., Besser, G. M., Landon, J. and Ekins, R. P. (1972), *Lancet*, 2, 253.
Chan, V. and Landon, J. (1972), *Lancet*, 1, 4.
Chopra, I. J., Ho, R. S. and Lam, R. (1972), *J. Lab. clin. Med.*, 80, 729.
Clark, F., and Horn, D. B. (1965), *J. clin. Endocrinol. and Metab.*, 25, 39.
Craig, F. A. and Ross, G. (1963), *Metabolism*, 12, 57.
Cusick, C. F. (1974), *Ann. clin. Biochem.*, 11, 130.
Doniach, I. (1967), see McGowan, G. K. and Sandler, M. below, p. 309.
Doran, G. R. and Wilkinson, J. H. (1971), *Clin. chim. Acta*, 35, 115.
Dubois, E. F. (1936), "Basal Metabolism", 3rd Edition, Lea and Febiger, Philadelphia.
Evered, J. and Hall, R. (1972), *Brit. med. J.*, 1, 290.
Farrell, L. P. and Richmond, M. H. (1961), *Clin. chim. Acta*, 6, 620.
Fischl, J. (1956), *Clin. chim. Acta*, 1, 462.
Fleisch, A. (1951), *Helv. med. Acta*, 18, 23.
Foss, O. P. (1963), "Standard Methods in Clinical Chemistry", edited Seligson, D., Academic Press, 4, 125.
Foss, O. P., Hankes, L. V. and Van Slyke, D. D. (1960), *Clin. chim. Acta*, 5, 301.
Fowler, P. B. S., Swale, J. and Andrews, H. (1970), *Lancet*, 2, 288.
Galton, V. A. and Pitt-Rivers, R. (1959), *Biochem. J.*, 72, 310.
Gemmill, C. L. (1955), *Arch. Biochem. Biophys.*, 54, 359.
Griffiths, P. D. (1963), *Lancet*, 1, 894.
Hall, R. (1972), *Clin. Endocrinol.*, 1, 115.
Hamado, S., Kosako, T. and Torizuka, K. (1975), *Clin. chim. Acta*, 63, 129.
Hamolsky, M. W., Stein, M. and Freedberg, A. S. (1957), *J. clin. Endocrinol.*, 17, 33.
Hobbs, J. R., Bayliss, R. I. and Maclagan, N. F. (1963), *Lancet*, 1, 8.
Hoffenberg, R. (1975), *Ann. clin. Biochem.*, 12, 135.
Hollander, C. S. and Shenkman, L. (1972), *Brit. J. Hosp. Med.*, 8, 393.
Howorth, P. J. N., McKerron, C. G. and Marsden, P. (1975), *Ann. clin. Biochem.*, 12, 200.
Jørgensen, J. V. (1974), *Brit. med. J.*, 4, 533.
Kessler, G. and Pileggi, V. J. (1968), *Clin. Chem.*, 14, 811.
Kessler, G. and Pileggi, V. J. (1970), *Clin. Chem.*, 16, 382.
Lawton, N. F., Ellis, S. M. and Subi, S. (1973), *Clin. Endocrinol.*, 2, 57.
Lewis, R. G., Kinsman, G. M. and Iliff, A. (1937), *Amer. J. Dis. Child.*, 53, 348.
Lusk, G. (1924), *J. biol. Chem.*, 59, 41.
McGowan, G. K. (1975), *J. clin. Path.*, 28, 207.
McGowan, G. K. and Sandler, M. (1967), Symposium on the thyroid gland, Suppl., *J. clin. Path.*, 20, 309.
McIntyre, I. (1967), see McGowan, G. K. and Sandler, M., above, p. 399.
Miedema, K., Boelhouwer, J. and Otten, J. W. (1971), *Clin. chim. Acta*, 32, 367.
Mitchell, M. L. (1958), *J. clin. Endocrinol.*, 18, 1437.
Murphy, B. E. P., Patten, C. J. and Gold, A. (1966) *J. clin. Endocrinol. and Matab.*, 26, 247.
Oneal, L. W. and Simms, E. S. (1953), *Amer. J. clin. Path.*, 23, 493.
Oppenheimer, J. H. and Surks, M. I. (1971), see Werner, S. C. and Ingber, S. H. below, p. 52.
Ormston, B. J. (1972), *Front. Hormone Res.*, 1, 45.
Owen, J. A. (1970), *Clin. chim. Acta*, 29, 89.
Peters, J. P. and Van Slyke, D. D. (1932), "Quantitative Clinical Chemistry", vol. 1, Interpretations, (1946), 2nd edition, Baillière, Tindall and Cox, London.
Pileggi, V. J. and Kessler, G. (1968), *Clin. Chem.*, 14, 339.
Pitt-Rivers, R. (1967), see McGowan, G. K. and Sandler, M. above, p.318.
Reichlin, S. (1971), see Werner, S. C. and Ingber, S. H. below, p. 197.
Riley, M. and Gochman, N. (1964), *Clin. Chem.*, 10, 649.

44 Practical Clinical Biochemistry

Robbins, J. and Rall, J. E. (1967), in "Hormones in Blood", edited Gray, C. H. and Bacharach, A. ., 2nd edition, vol. 1, Academic Press.

Robertson, J. D. (1944), *Brit. med. J.*, 1, 617.

Robertson, J. D. and Reid, D. D. (1952), *Lancet*, 1, 940, 954.

Scholes, J. F. (1962), *J. Nucl. Med.*, 3, 41.

Scott, K. G. and Reilly, W. A. (1954), *Metabolism*, 3, 506.

Seligson, H. and Seligson, D. (1972), *Clin. chim. Acta*, 38, 199.

Seth, J. (1973), *Clin. chim. Acta*, 46, 431.

Shock, N. W. (1942), *Amer. J. Dis. Child.*, 64, 19.

Stanbury, J. B. (1972), in "The Metabolic Basis of Inherited Disease", edited Stanbury, J. B., Wyngaarden, J. B. and Frederickson, D. S., 3rd edition, McGraw-Hill, p. 223.

Sterling, K. (1971), in "Laboratory Diagnosis of Hormone Disease", edited Sundermann, F. W. and Sundermann, F. W. Jr., Adam Hilger, London, p. 252.

Talbot, F. B. (1925), *Physiol. Rev.*, 5, 477.

Tong, W. (1971), see Werner, S. C. and Ingber, S. H. below, p. 24.

Watson, D. and Lees, S. (1973), *Ann. clin. Biochem.*, 10, 14.

Watson, D., Lees, S. and Stafford, J. E. H. (1974), *Ann. clin. Biochem.*, 11, 1.

Wellby, M. L., O'Halloran, M. W. and Marshall, J. (1973), *Clin. chim. Acta*, 45, 255.

Welshman, S. W., Bell, J. F. and McKee, G. (1966), *J. clin. Path.*, 19, 510.

Werner, S. C. and Ingber, S. H., editors (1971), "The Thyroid", 3rd edition, Harper and Row.

Widdowson, G. M. and Northam, B. E. (1963), *Clin. chim. Acta*, 8, 636.

Widdowson, G. M. and Northam, B. E. (1964), *Clin. chim. Acta*, 9, 595.

Widstrom, G. and Bjorkman, M. (1958), *Acta med. Scand.*, 12, 1881.

Williams, E. S., Ekins, R. P. and Ellis, S. M. (1969), *Brit. med. J.*, 4, (a) 336; (b) 338.

Woeber, K. A., Soebel, R. J., Ingber, S. H. and Sterling, K. (1970), *J. clin. Invest.*, 49, 643.

Wolff, J. (1970), in "Biochemistry of Human Disease", edited Thompson, R. H. S. and Wootton, I. D. P., 3rd edition, Churchill, London, p. 379.

Yee, H. Y., Bowdell, J. and Jackson, B. (1971), *Clin. Chem.*, 17, 622.

Zieve, L., Vogel, W. C. and Schultz, A. L. (1956), *J. Lab. clin. Med.*, 47, 663.

Zak, B., Koen, A. M. and Boyle, A. J., (1953), *Amer. J. clin. Path.*, 23, 603.

Zak, B., Willard, H. H., Myers, G. B. and Boyle, A. J. (1952), *Analyt. Chem.*, 24, 1345.

CHAPTER 2

STEROID HORMONES
INTRODUCTION AND TECHNIQUES FOR C_{19} AND C_{21} STEROIDS

Chemistry of the Steroids

THE steroid hormones secreted by the adrenal cortex, ovary, testis, corpus luteum and placenta, are derivatives of the tetracyclic hydrocarbon cyclopentanoperhydrophenanthrene, $C_{17}H_{28}$, the carbon atoms of which are numbered as shown in formula I. Substitution of other groups for hydrogen occurs at various positions, most commonly on carbon atoms 3, 10, 11, 13, 16 and 17. Where further carbon atoms are introduced as at positions 10, 13 and 17, the latter as a side chain of two carbon atoms, these are numbered as in formula II and III. Common substituents are

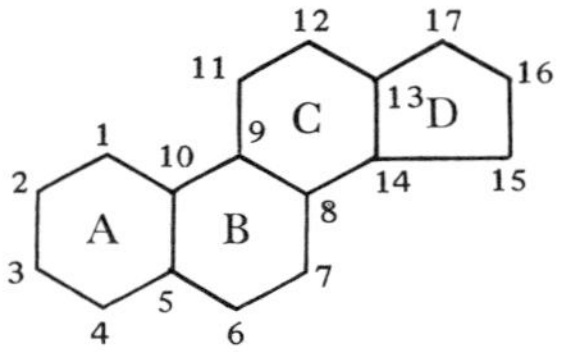

I 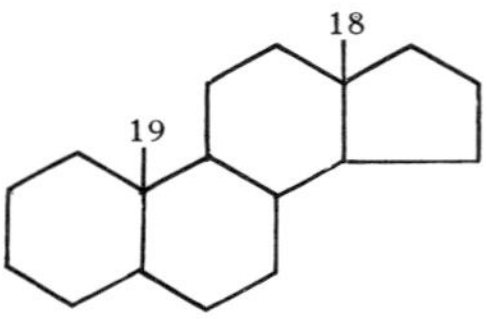   II   III

androstane   pregnane

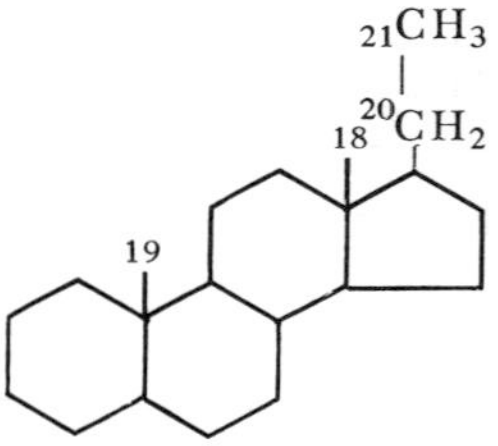

oxygenated groups either as hydroxyl or oxo commonly at positions 3, 11, 16, 17, 18, 20 and 21. The steroids can be classified into three groups according to the number of carbon atoms present.

C_{18} **Steroids**, the oestrogens. In these, ring A in formula I is aromatic and there is a methyl group on C-13. The parent hydrocarbon is *oestrane* (IV). The common human oestrogens are oestrone (V), oestradiol-17β (VI), and oestriol (VII), formed mainly in the ovary in females of reproductive age, but also by the fetoplacental unit (see p. 113). The hydroxyl on C-3 is phenolic and so is weakly acidic, a property used in their separation from neutral steroids.

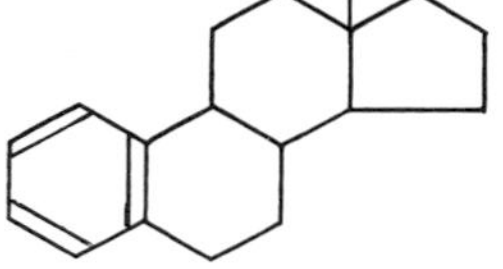

IV   V

oestrane   oestrone

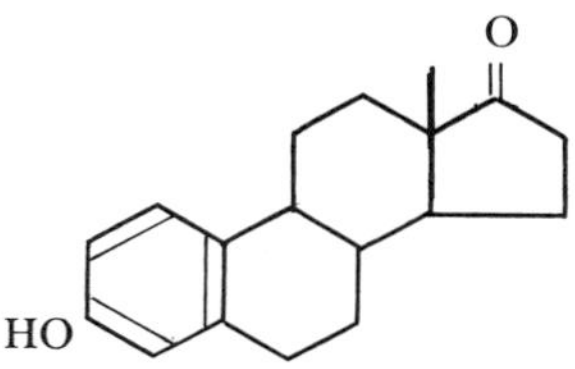

46 — Practical Clinical Biochemistry

VI
oestradiol-17β

VII
oestriol

C_{19} **Steroids,** the androgens, have methyl groups on C-10 and C-13 of formula I, the hydrocarbon nucleus being *androstane* (II). Some are androgenic, the most potent of these being testosterone (XXI, Fig. 2,1) secreted by the testis. It is a C_{19} steroid with a hydroxyl on C-17, most of the others having a 17-oxo group (formerly termed 17-keto) which is used for their detection and estimation. These 17-oxosteroids, hereafter abbreviated to 17-OS, include androsterone (XL) and aetiocholanolone (XLI), metabolites of testosterone (Fig. 2,2), and 17-OS secreted by the adrenal cortex, for example, dehydroepiandrosterone (XVIII, Fig. 2,1) and 11-β-hydroxyandrostenedione (XXII, p. 47). There is also a group, mostly 11-oxygenated, which includes metabolites of C_{21} steroids, such as 11-β-hydroxyaetiocholanolone (XLIII, Fig. 2,2) from cortisol (XVI, Fig. 2,1).

C_{21} **Steroids,** have the basic structure of formula III, the parent hydrocarbon being pregnane. Active hormones include progestogens such as progesterone (IX, Fig. 2,1) produced by the corpus luteum and by the placenta in pregnancy, and products of the adrenal cortex such as aldosterone (XII, Fig. 2,1) and cortisol (XVI). The main differences occur in the 2-carbon side chain at C-17, and the possibility of hydroxyl substitution at C-11, 17 and 21. The side chain may be a simple ketone as in progesterone, an α-ketol as in aldosterone, or a hydroxyl on C-17 may form a substituted dihydroxyacetone. Note that cortisol is derived from progesterone by introducing hydroxyl groups at C-11, 17 and 21.

The active hormones and precursors undergo metabolism (see p. 52) mainly without loss of carbon atoms to give a group of C_{21} steroids from the adrenal cortex referred to as corticosteroids, of which the subgroup 17-hydroxycorticosteroids (17-OHCS) includes important metabolites of cortisol and its precursors.

It will be seen that in addition to the three double bonds in ring A of the C_{18} steroids important double bonds may be present between C-4 and 5 and between C-5 and 6 in some C_{19} and C_{21} steroids.

For a useful introduction to the chemistry of steroids see Klyne (1957).

Steroid nomenclature

Systematic steroid nomenclature giving precise information on their structure uses a set of conventions. As such standardised names are

Steroid Hormones   47

cumbersome, commonly occurring steroids are often referred to by trivial names. In naming steroids we first take the name of the basic hydrocarbon, oestrane, androstane or pregnane. The nature, position, and if relevant, the configuration of all substituents on this nucleus are then indicated by prefixes or suffixes together with the position of any double or triple bonds. Substituents are most commonly: —OH, prefix hydroxy- or suffix —ol; =O, prefix oxo-, or suffix -one. Their position is indicated by numbering as in formulae I, II and III. A further problem is the "configuration" of monovalent substituents as the basic hydrocarbons possess a number of actual or potential asymmetric carbon atoms on which stereoisomerism can arise.

The main rules governing nomenclature are:

1. As the basic ring structure is approximately flat it can be considered as lying in the plane of the page with the hydrogen atoms projecting above and below it. Two isomers can result at carbon atoms to which two hydrogen atoms are attached according to whether the substituted group (a) projects below the plane of the paper, the α configuration with the bond shown ---- (as in VII) or (b) projects above the plane of the paper, the β configuration with the bond shown ——— (as in VI and VII). Carbon atoms in steroid hormones on which substituents occur in different configurations are mainly positions 3, 5, 16, 17 and 20.

In the naturally occurring steroids, carbon atoms at C-10 and C-13 and the two-carbon side chain at C-17 are all in the β-configuration as is the H atom at C-8. Hydrogen atoms at C-9 and C-14 are always α. Thus at the junctions of rings B/C and C/D (see formula I) the two groups on the C atoms common to both rings project on opposite sides; the rings are joined in the *trans* configuration. The junction of the rings A/B is variable as the configuration of the H atom at C-5 can be α or β corresponding to the *trans* or *cis* linkage of these two rings. Thus the pregnane nucleus can be either 5α-pregnane (formerly *allo*-pregnane) or 5β-pregnane. Similarly androstane can be either 5α-androstane or 5β-androstane (formerly aetiocholane). As oestrane does not possess a 5-H atom this problem does not arise.

Isomerism at C-3 and C-5 is particularly important in connection with steroid metabolites. Most physiologically active steroids have the Δ^4-3 ketone group in ring A (XXIII). This undergoes reduction to tetrahydro derivatives (XXIV-XXVII) in the liver.

XXII

11 β-hydroxyandrostenedione

XXIII

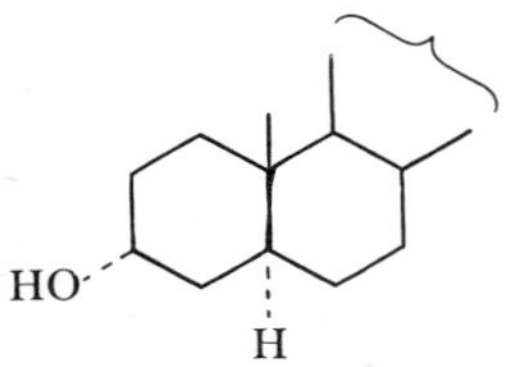

48   *Practical Clinical Biochemistry*

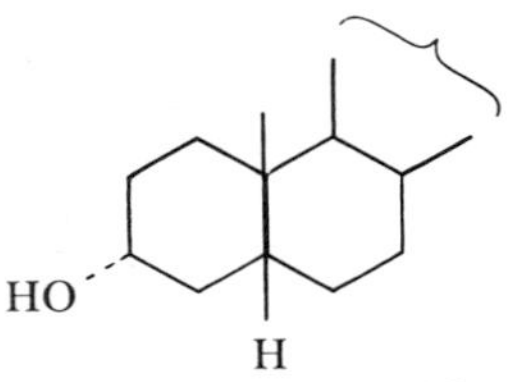

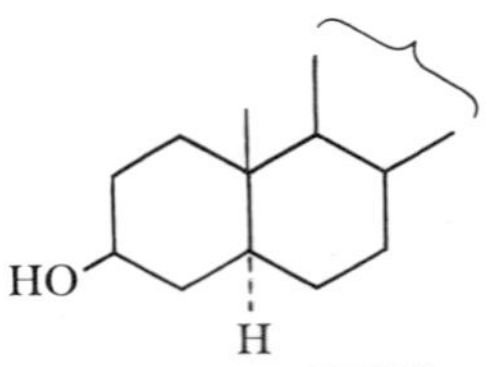

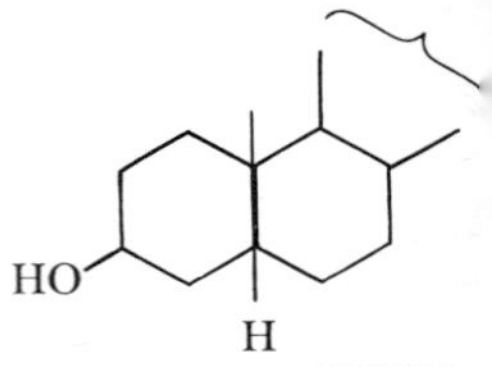

XXIV	XXV	XXVI	XXVII
3α,5α	3α, 5β	3β,5α	3β,5β

Of the four possible isomers the 3α, 5β (XXV) is preferentially formed in the metabolism of progestogens and adrenocortical steroids. The 5α isomer occurs less frequently as in *allo*pregnanediol (XXXI) (see opposite).

2. When a double bond is present the position can be indicated in a trivial name by using Δ as, for example Δ^5-pregnenolone (VIII) which shows the double bond is between carbons 5 and 6. In the full form the suffix of the basic hydrocarbon is changed from -ane to -ene and the position of the double bond shown by putting the lower number of the two C atoms in front of the suffix. Thus Δ^5-pregnenolone in full is 3β-hydroxypregn-5-en-20-one. If there is no prefix to the hydrocarbon name, the number is used in front of the whole name, e.g. progesterone (IX) is 4-pregnene-3,20-dione, If the double bond links two C atoms not numbered consecutively the number of the second must be specified. Thus for a double bond between C-9 and C-11 this could be indicated as $\Delta^{9(11)}$ or $-9(11)$en-.

3. When substituted groups are present the basic hydrocarbon structure retains the *e* if the suffix begins with a vowel but otherwise omits it. Thus

pregnanolone (XXVIII) 3α-hydroxy-5β-pregn*an*-20-*o*ne
pregnanediol (XXIX) 5β-pregn*ane*-3α, 20α-*d*iol

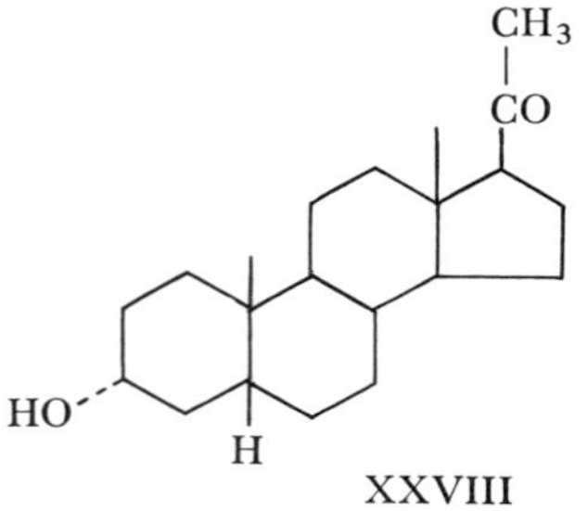

XXVIII
pregnanolone

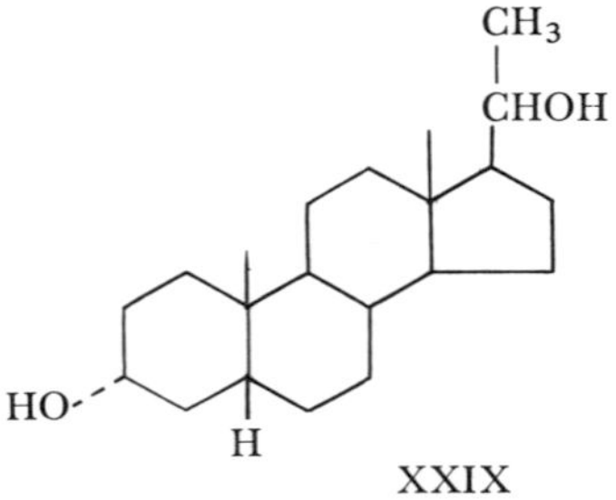

XXIX
pregnanediol

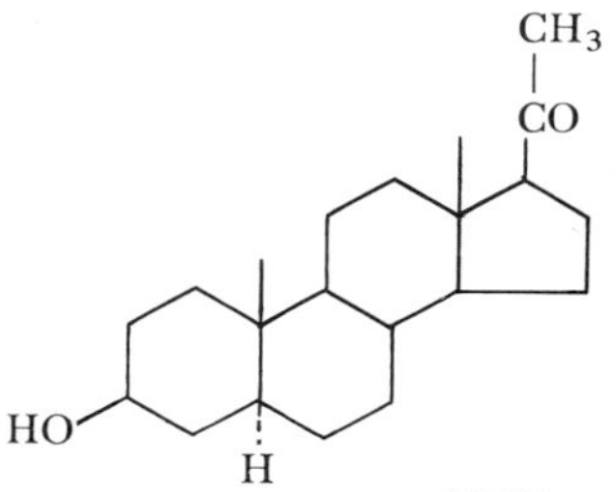

Steroid Hormones 49

XXX
allopregnanolone

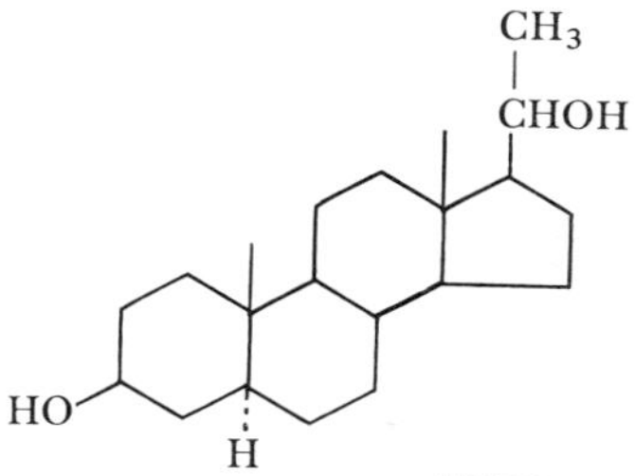

XXXI
allopregnanediol

4. When the substituents are all of the same type, i.e. hydroxyl or oxo, the group structure takes precedence as in pregnanediol above, but when more than one type of substituent is present hydroxyl precedes the group name and the oxo is indicated by a suffix as in pregnanolone. Systematic and trivial names of hormones and precursors are given in Table 2,1. Their structures are shown in Fig. 2,1.

TABLE 2,1
Steroid Nomenclature. Adrenocortical Hormones and Precursors

C_{18} *Steroids*

V	Oestrone	3-hydroxyoestra-1,3,5(10)-trien-17-one
VI	Oestradiol-17β	oestra-1,3,5(10)-triene-3,17β-diol
VII	Oestriol	oestra-1,3,5(10)-triene-3,16α,17β-triol

C_{19} *Steroids*

XVIII	Dehydroepiandrosterone (DHA)	3β-hydroxyandrost-5-en-17-one
XIX	Δ^5-Androstenediol	5-androstene-3β,17α-diol
XX	Δ^4-Androstenedione	4-androstene-3,17-dione
XXI	Testosterone	17α-hydroxyandrost-4-en-3-one
XXII	11β-Hydroxyandrostene-dione	11β-hydroxyandrost-4-ene-3.17-dione

C_{21} *Steroids*

VIII	Δ^5-Pregnenolone	3β-hydroxypregn-5-en-20-one
IX	Progesterone	4-pregnene-3,20-dione
X	Deoxycorticosterone	21-hydroxypregn-4-ene-3,20-dione
XI	Corticosterone	11β,21-dihydroxypregn-4-ene-3,20-dione
XII	Aldosterone	11β,21-dihydroxy-pregn-4-ene-3,18,20-trione
XIII	17-Hydroxypregnenolone	3β,17α-dihydroxypregn-5-en-20-one
XIV	17-Hydroxyprogesterone	17α-hydroxypregn-4-ene-3,20-dione
XV	11-Deoxycortisol Compound S	17α,21-dihydroxypregn-4-ene-3,20-dione
XVI	Cortisol, Compound F, Hydrocortisone	11β,17α,21-trihydroxypregn-4-ene-3,20-dione
XVII	Cortisone, Compound E	17α,21-dihydroxypregn-4-ene-3,11,20-trione

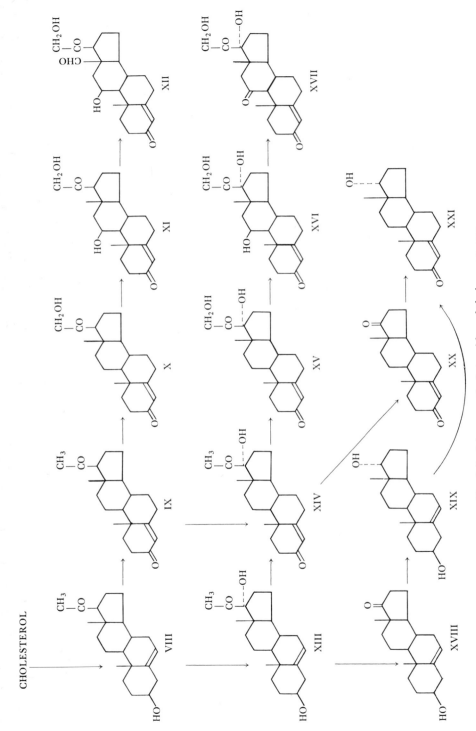

Fig. 2.1. Adrenocortical steroids and their precursors.
Systematic and trivial names corresponding to the numbered formulae appear in Table 2.1.

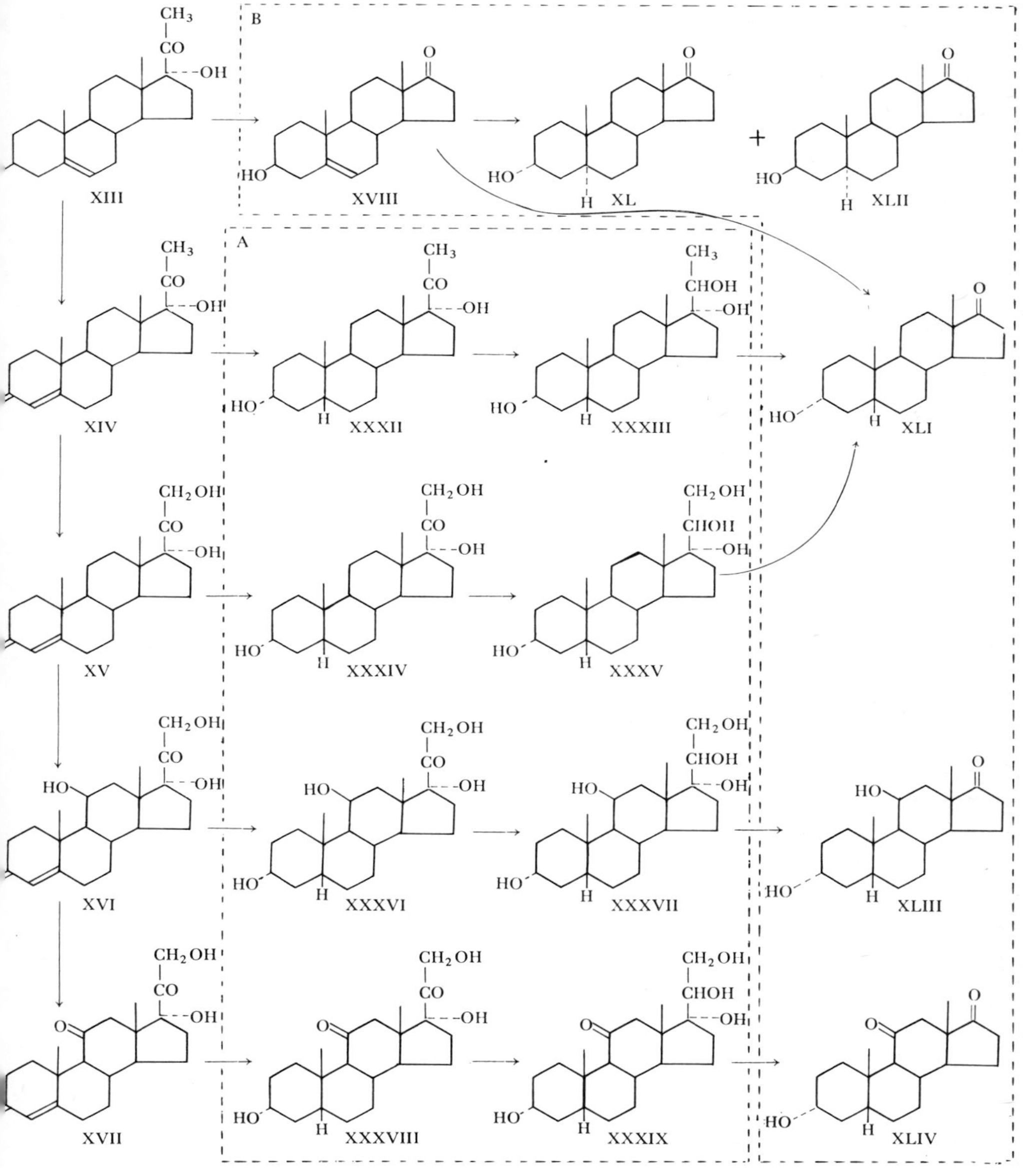

Steroid Hormones

Fig. 2,2. Adrenocortical Hormones and their Metabolites.
Trivial and systematic names corresponding to the numbered formulae appear in Tables
36.1 and 36.2. The metabolites enclosed in area A are major components of the urinary
17-oxogenic steroids in normal or pathological states. The substances in area B are
17-oxosteroids.

Practical Clinical Biochemistry

52

Metabolism of Steroids

Inactivation of secreted hormones is achieved by chemical change in the steroid nucleus and by conjugation with glucuronic or sulphuric acid. These changes occur mainly in the liver. The products are then excreted in the urine.

Most active hormones possess the Δ^4-3-ketone group or less commonly the Δ^5-3-hydroxy structure as in DHA and some foetal steroids, though the oestrogens possess neither. A common change is reduction of these groupings to the 3-hydroxy-steroid without a double bond in rings A or B as in Fig. 2,2. In addition, interconversion of 11-hydroxyl and 11-oxo groups is common and reduction of the oxo group at C-20 can occur in some corticosteroids. Common metabolites are therefore tetrahydro and hexahydro derivatives as conjugates. The introduction of additional hydroxyl groups, especially at C-6 is less common but well recognised. Finally, corticosteroids may undergo loss of the side chain at C-17 with production of 17-OS. Several of these changes are common to androgens, progesterone and corticosteroids. Oestrogens are largely conjugated before excretion but further hydroxylation is known.

Further reference is made to the synthesis and metabolism of adrenocorticosteroids and their precursors and metabolites in Chapter 3. The systematic and trivial names of common metabolites are given in Table 2,2.

TABLE 2,2

Steroid Nomenclature. Metabolites of Adrenocortical Hormones

C_{19} *Steroids*

XL	Androsterone	3α-hydroxy-5α-androstan-17-one
XLI	Aetiocholanolone	3α-hydroxy-5β-androstan-17-one
XLII	Epiandrosterone	3β-hydroxy-5α-androstan-17-one
XLIII	11β-Hydroxyaetiocholanol-one	3α,11β-dihydroxy-5β-androstan-17-one
XLIV	11-Oxoaetiocholanolone	3α-hydroxy-5β-androstane-11,17-dione

C_{21} *Steroids*

XXVIII	Pregnanolone	3α-hydroxy-5β-pregnan-20-one
XXIX	Pregnanediol	5β-pregnane-3α,20α-diol
XXX	Allopregnanolone	3β-hydroxy-5α-pregnan-20-one
XXXI	Allopregnanediol	5α-pregnane-3β,20αdiol
XXXII	17-Hydroxypregnanolone	3α,17α-dihydroxy-5β-pregnan-20-one
XXXIII	Pregnanetriol	5β-pregnane-3α,17α,20α-triol
XXXIV	Tetrahydro S	3α,17α,21-trihydroxy-5β-pregnan-20-one
XXXV	Hexahydro S	5β-pregnane-3α,17α,20α,21-tetrol
XXXVI	Tetrahydro F	3α,11β,17α,21-tetrahydroxy-5β-pregnan-20-one
XXXVII	α-Cortol	5β-pregnane-3α,11β,17α,20α,21-pentol
XXXVIII	Tetrahydro E	3α,17α,21-trihydroxy-5β-pregnane-11,20-dione
XXXIX	α-Cortolone	3α,17α,20α,21-tetrahydroxy-5β-pregnan-11-one

Steroid Hormones 53

General Techniques Used in Steroid Determinations

Two main approaches have been used, the analysis of plasma or serum and of urine.

Plasma. In this the steroids determined are almost always the secreted hormones even though a major part, being protein bound, may be biologically inactive. A relatively simple fluorimetric method for plasma cortisol is described later (p. 73). Other hormones may be present in lower concentrations so that current methods mostly use radioimmunoassay or competitive protein binding. Whatever the method the analysis gives information only about the concentration at the time of sampling. Plasma hormone concentrations may vary physiologically as with circadian rhythms or in response to external stimuli so the time and circumstances of collection are important in interpreting results.

Urine. Urinary steroids are mostly metabolites of the primary hormones and are excreted mainly as conjugates. As there may be several metabolites of a particular hormone one approach has been to employ a suitable group reaction given by all or most members of such a group and relatively specific for it. Alternatively, metabolites may be separated by appropriate extraction or chromatography before being individually determined, a general type of group reaction may be applied to the purified fraction, or further specificity may be achieved by a selective reaction for an individual steroid. Examples of such techniques are given later for different steroids. In general, the analysis of urinary steroids usually implies the collection of a 24 h sample of urine. The result then gives the average excretion over this period of time. The fluctuation in circulating steroid levels is avoided but at the expense of a less direct assessment of the hormone.

Hydrolysis of Steroid Metabolites

The 3-hydroxyl group produced by reduction of the Δ^4-3-ketone is conjugated with glucuronic or sulphuric acid in the liver before excretion. Unlike the free hormones which, being insoluble in water circulate attached to plasma proteins, these are water soluble and have a high renal clearance. As a result almost all the urinary steroids are present in conjugated form. Less than 0.1 per cent may be excreted in the free form so the determination of urinary conjugates gives the best indication of the total secretion of the steroid. In order to obtain the steroids in a suitable organic solvent the conjugates have first to be hydrolysed to liberate the free steroids. However, the various steroids differ widely in their stability to hydrolytic procedures. While some molecules such as 17-OS without a Δ^5 bond, one of the first groups to be determined, are relatively stable to hydrolysis with hot acid, this completely destroys others. With hot acid, steroids may also undergo chlorination or dehydration without affecting the 17-oxo group. This may not matter when 17-OS are being determined (see p. 58) but cannot be used if individual steroids are determined.

P.C.B.(II)—3

54 *Practical Clinical Biochemistry*

1. **Hot acid hydrolysis of sulphates and glucuronides.** This, the earliest, crudest and most destructive method of hydrolysis, can only be used if the group required for subsequent reaction is unaffected. The acid used is usually hydrochloric acid in a final concentration of at least 10 per cent by volume of the concentrated acid and heating is either by refluxing or by immersion in boiling water in lightly stoppered tubes. Total neutral 17-OS, oestrogens and pregnanediol conjugates can be hydrolysed under these conditions but metabolites of 17-OHCS are destroyed.

The 17-oxo group is undamaged in steroids such as DHA or 11-oxygenated 17-OS which are present as conjugates in urine or are derived from 17-OHCS conjugates following treatment with borohydride-metaperiodate. However, although the 17-oxo group reacts in the Zimmerman reaction the rest of the molecule may be so modified that it behaves differently in separative procedures and may give different colour equivalents. Thus about 40 per cent of DHA sulphate under these conditions yields DHA, the rest being dehydrated or chlorinated to give substances with different polarities, which therefore behave differently when chromatographed. At pH values nearer neutrality up to 70 per cent may be converted to the 6β-hydroxy-3,5-cyclo derivative. The proportion of artefacts found varies according to the pH and presence of chloride, so that when this metabolite is being determined the hydrolytic procedure must be carefully chosen.

The amount of 11-hydroxy and 11-oxosteroids normally present as 17-OS conjugates in urine is not great and may be not significant quantitatively in the determination of total 17-OS. Where 11-oxygenated 17-OS have been formed during the determination of 17-OHCS however this is not so. Under normal conditions about 90 per cent of the 17-OHCS in urine arise from the 11-oxygenated steroids cortisol and cortisone and their metabolites. During their determination the side chain is removed with bismuthate or metaperiodate to give the corresponding 17-OS. Strong acid hydrolysis of these steroids dehydrates the 11-hydroxy compound to give the unsaturated $\Delta^{9(11)}$ compound (see XLV, p. 56). This behaves more like aetiocholanolone both chromatographically and in the Zimmermann reaction. Misleading results may then be obtained depending on the proportion of 11-judroxy material present originally. Of much greater consequence, however, is the fact that the 11-oxygenation· index for the diagnosis of congenital adrenal hyperplasia (see pp. 72, 92) and reliable separation of 11-oxygenated and 11-deoxy material cannot be obtained by chromatography.

2. **Mild hydrolysis conditions for sulphates.** In the method of Lieberman and Dobriner (1948) urine is acidified to pH 1, placed in a continuous extractor with ether and the hydrolysis continued for 3 days. The ether then contains all the liberated steroids. Although this requires more complicated apparatus than the following method the extract is not contaminated with so much pigment.

Steroid Hormones 55

A more commonly used procedure is that of Burnstein and Lieberman (1958) in which urine is brought to molar concentration with sulphuric acid and extracted three times with ethyl acetate. The combined ethyl acetate extract contains all the sulphates as well as an appreciable concentration of acid. The sulphates are hydrolysed on standing at $37°$ C, overnight.

Another procedure is that of Fotherby (1959) who observed that sulphates of Δ^5-3β-hydroxysteroids can be hydrolysed by heating at approximately neutral pH whereas the sulphates of other steroids are not affected.

3. **Enzymic hydrolysis of glucuronides.** This has been used for the hydrolysis of glucuronides of steroids such as 17-OHCS which are destroyed by hot acid hydrolysis (p. 54). The enzyme β-glucuronidase which effectively hydrolyses steroid glucuronides can be obtained commercially as a beef liver preparation (Ketodase, Warner Chilcot) or in more potent form as an extract from the visceral hump of the limpet. The latter preparation also contains a sulphatase which can be inhibited by the addition of phosphate if separation between steroid sulphates and glucuronides is required. The presence of sulphatase is an advantage, however, if total steroids are to be determined. The enzyme can be added directly to the urine or the conjugates concentrated by first extracting them into ether-ethanol (Edwards *et al.*, 1953). A concentration of 1 500 units per ml urine has been recommended for unextracted urine whereas it was shown by Bell and Varley (1960) that as little as 335 units per ml buffer is sufficient for hydrolysis of pregnanetriol conjugates.

A more potent glucuronidase, developed from a specially selected strain of *Esch. coli*, has an activity 10 times as great as that produced from *Helix pomatia* and urine conjugates can be hydrolysed in 1 to 2 h at $37°$ C without extraction. This product is obtainable from API Laboratory Products Ltd., Philpot House, Rayleigh, Essex, England.

4. **Other methods.** The commonest method for hydrolysis of corticosteroid glucuronide metabolites is to use metaperiodate which simultaneously oxidises the glucuronides and removes the side chain at C-17 in the procedure for 17 oxogenic steroids (p. 66). The glucuronide residue is replaced by a formyl group which is readily hydrolysed under mild alkaline conditions without affecting the steroid molecule.

Group Reactions for C_{19} Steroids. The Use of the Zimmermann Reaction

One of the most widely known reactions in steroid chemistry is the Zimmermann reaction for 17-OS (Zimmermann, 1935). Methods for their determination in urine are mostly modifications of Callow's original

56   *Practical Clinical Biochemistry*

method (Callow *et al.*, 1938). The 17-oxo group is not itself involved in the reaction which takes place at the adjacent 16 methylene group:

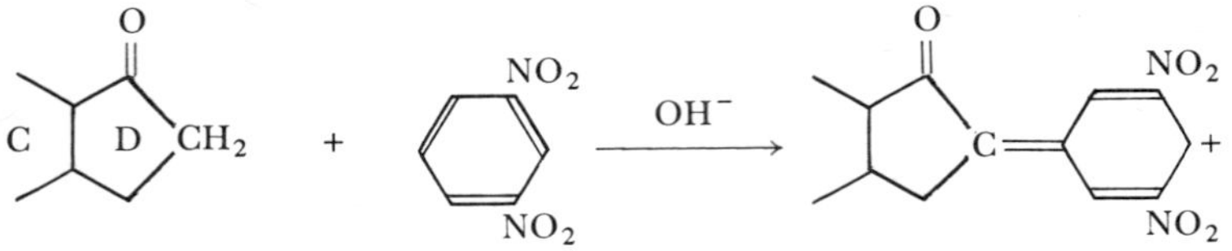

The reagents required for this reaction are absolute ethanol, *m*-dinitro benzene and strong alkali.

Colour Equivalents of 17-oxosteroids

All 17-OS give purple colours with the Zimmermann reagents but their intensity is influenced by other groups present in the molecule and the type of alkali used. If the extinction is corrected by one of the methods described later, the final extinction depends on the correction procedure. Androsterone (XL), aetiocholanolone (XLI) and dehydroepiandrosterone (XVIII) give approximately equal molar extinction whichever procedure is used. Another oxo group at C-3 and especially at C-11 has an enhancing effect particularly when ethanolic potassium hydroxide is used but a hydroxyl group at C-11 reduces the molar extinction. Such compounds when treated with hot acid undergo dehydration. Thus 11β-hydroxy-aetiocholanolone (XLIII) gives 9(11)-dehydroaetiocholanolone (3α-hydroxyandrost-9(11)-en-17-one, XLV) with a colour equivalent

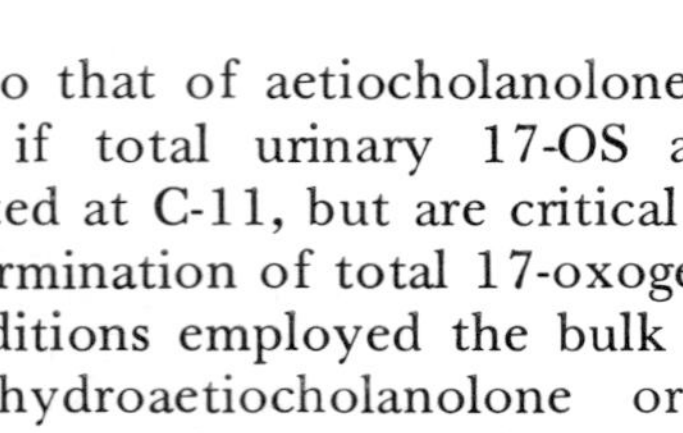

9(11)-dehydroaetiocholanolone

XLV

similar to that of aetiocholanolone. These considerations are of academic interest if total urinary 17-OS are being estimated as most are not substituted at C-11, but are critical if the Zimmermann reaction is used in the determination of total 17-oxogenic steroids (see p. 66). Depending on the conditions employed the bulk of the steroid estimated will be either 9(11)-dehydroaetiocholanolone or 11-β-hydroxyaetiocholanolone. The approximate colour equivalents of the steroids involved are: aetiocholanolone (XLI) 100; 11β-hydroxyaetiocholanolone (XLIII) 75; 11-oxo-aetiocholanolone (XLIV) 130; 9(11)-dehydroaetiocholanolone (XLV) 100.

Steroid Hormones

Correction Procedures to Eliminate Interfering Chromogens

When the Zimmermann reaction is applied to acid-hydrolysed urine extracts, appreciable colour can arise from non-steroid substances causing over estimation unless some correction procedure is used.

1. **Preliminary purification of crude extract.** This, the most effective way to correct for non-steroid chromogens, is unsuitable for use in routine investigations. Girard Reagent T, trimethylacetohydrazine, condenses with ketones in glacial acetic acid solution to give water-soluble derivatives which may be separated from non-steroid contaminants by partition between ether and water (Girard and Sandulesco, 1936). The ketonic steroids can then be recovered by hydrolysis with aqueous acid and extraction into an organic solvent.

2. **Mathematical correction procedures.** These assume that the interfering materials behave identically in all urines. This is not always valid but in practice agreement is obtained using two procedures.

(a) *The Talbot correction* (Talbot *et al.*, 1942) used the equation suggested by Fraser *et al.* (1941) although the equation usually quoted derives from constants obtained by Engstrom and Mason (1943). Two extinction readings are made at approximately 520 and 430 nm using green and violet filters. The purple Zimmermann product absorbs strongly in the green but has low extinction at the shorter wavelength. Interfering substances show greater extinction in the violet than in the green. Then:

$$\text{Corrected extinction at } 520 \text{ nm} = \frac{K_s(G - K_i V)}{K_s - K_i}$$

$$\text{where} \qquad K_s = \frac{E_{520} \text{ for the standard}}{E_{430} \text{ for the standard}},$$

and K_i is the same ratio for the interfering chromogens. G and V are the observed readings at 520 and 430 nm. Engstrom and Mason found 2.4 and 0.6 for K_s and K_i respectively and if these figures are used:

$$\text{Corrected extinction at } 520 \text{ nm} = \frac{\text{observed } E_{520} - 0.6 \text{ observed } E_{430}}{0.73}$$

K_s can easily be determined, K_i can be obtained from urines which contain almost no 17-OS, as in Addison's disease (Talbot *et al.*) or by using the non-ketonic fraction obtained from the Girard reaction (Engstrom and Mason). As K_s and K_i may vary with different filters, Talbot *et al.* recommended users to obtain the values for their own instrument. If K_s is near 2.4 the use of this type of formula will probably be satisfactory especially if the formula is also applied to the standard. Although the observed reading at 520 nm will be close to the corrected reading the calculation is simplified as the factor 0.73 can be ignored.

(b) *The Allen correction* (Allen, 1950) has a more general application than that of Talbot. Readings are made at the wavelength corresponding to

58 *Practical Clinical Biochemistry*

the peak extinction and equidistant on each side of it, in this instance 520, 440 and 600 nm. It cannot be used with filter instruments as the resolution is not sufficiently great. The assumption is made that the interfering chromogen has a linear absorption spectrum over the wavelength range. Then:

$$\text{Corrected reading at } 520 \text{ nm} = E_{520} - \tfrac{1}{2}(E_{440} + E_{600})$$

Corrected readings are usually made for both test and standard and the ratio is calculated from $2E_{520} - (E_{440} + E_{600})$ for each.

3. **Solvent partition procedures.** These most recently introduced methods depend on the partition of the Zimmermann chromogen between aqueous ethanol and ether or dichloromethane. The interfering chromogens remain in the aqueous phase and the Zimmermann chromogens pass into the organic layer. These are the most satisfactory procedures in that reading at only one wavelength is required but occasionally substances are encountered which still cause interference.

Determination of Urinary Neutral 17-Oxosteroids

Much work has been done on this determination. The subject was reviewed by Callow (1950), and by Mason and Engstrom (1950). In 1951 a Medical Research Council Committee on Clinical Endocrinology published a method which it was hoped would make the results of different laboratories more strictly comparable. This was replaced in 1963 by a modified technique in which dichloroethane was used to extract the steroids (Drekter *et al.*, 1952; Norymberski *et al.*, 1953; Gray *et al.*, 1969) instead of carbon tetrachloride used in earlier methods. This is used in the technique given below in which tetramethylammonium hydroxide is used as alkali in the colour development.

Reagents. 1. Chloroform.

2. Concentrated hydrochloric acid.

3. 1,2-Dichloroethane (May and Baker). Impurities can increase the blank in the final colour reaction and may impair the precision of the determination. To purify, redistil from a flask containing $\frac{1}{20}$th its volume of concentrated sulphuric acid, carrying out the procedure under a fume hood as the vapour is toxic.

4. Sodium hydroxide 2.5 mol/l.

5. Absolute ethanol (aldehyde-free). The quality of the ethanol is important in obtaining low reagent blanks. British Drug Houses Analar or Burroughs R.R. ethanol are satisfactory without further purification and should be used throughout the determination. Attempts to purify cruder ethanol have given uncertain results.

6. *m*-Dinitrobenzene in ethanol 20 g/l. Use British Drug Houses material specially purified for 17-OS determination or, less satisfactorily, recrystallise the usual grade before use. The solution is best freshly prepared but can be kept 1 to 2 weeks in a brown glass-stoppered bottle in the dark.

Steroid Hormones 59

Methods for purifying ethanol and *m*-dinitrobenzene (Callow *et al.*, 1938) do not seem to be needed with the above products; it is rare for trouble to arise from this. If it does, obtain a fresh supply.

7. Tetramethylammonium hydroxide, Hopkins and Williams. This is supplied as a 250 g/l aqueous solution.

8. Standard solution of dehydroepiandrosterone, 0.90 mmol/l. Dissolve 25.9 mg DHA in 100 ml ethanol.

9. Aqueous ethanol. Mix 3 volumes ethanol with 7 volumes water.

10. Ether.

Technique. Collect a 24 h specimen of urine. This should be kept cold. It is not necessary to add a preservative if the determination can be done soon after completing the collection. Alternatively add sufficient chloroform to saturate the specimen (M.R.C. Committee, 1963) shaking each time more urine is added.

Dilute the 24 h specimen to 2 litres and to 10 ml of this add 2 ml hydrochloric acid in a 50 ml glass-stoppered centrifuge tube and place in a boiling water bath for 10 min. Cool, add 10 ml dichloroethane and shake mechanically for 15 min. Centrifuge. Remove the upper aqueous layer by suction and wash successively with 2.5 ml water and 2.5 ml sodium hydroxide. Filter the dichloroethane extract through a fluted filter paper then transfer 6 ml to a suitable glass-stoppered tube. Evaporate in a boiling water bath in a fume cupboard. Add a few chips of glass if bumping occurs. Dry in a desiccator. Add 0.2 ml ethanol, mix to dissolve, then add 0.2 ml *m*-dinitrobenzene reagent and 0.2 ml tetramethylammonium hydroxide. If a batch is being done it is convenient to add 0.4 ml of a mixture of equal volumes of these last two freshly prepared before use. At the same time treat 0.2 ml standard (0.18 μmol) and 0.2 ml ethanol (for the blank) in the same way. Keep these in the dark at $25°C$ for 1 h. Then to each add 2 ml aqueous ethanol followed by 5 ml ether, stopper, shake for 15 sec, allow the ether layer to separate and then decant it into a cuvette. Read the test and standard against the reagent blank at 515 nm or using a green filter.

Calculation. Urinary 17-oxosteroids (μmol/24 h)

$$= \frac{\text{Reading of unknown}}{\text{Reading of standard}} \times 0.18 \times \frac{2\,000}{10} \times \frac{10}{6}$$

$$= \frac{\text{Reading of unknown}}{\text{Reading of standard}} \times 60$$

To convert to mg/24 h multiply μmol/24 h by 0.29.

For a standard curve set up the following:

17-Oxosteroids (μmol/24 h)	0	12	24	36	48	60
Standard solution (ml)	0	0.04	0.08	0.12	0.16	0.20
Ethanol (ml)	0.2	0.16	0.12	0.08	0.04	0
			Treat as described above			

60 *Practical Clinical Biochemistry*

For higher values it may be possible to extend the curve a little further using a standard double the strength, otherwise repeat using a smaller volume of the dichloroethane extract.

Notes 1. *Acid interference.* As the Zimmermann reaction is alkali dependent, especial care must be taken to avoid acid contamination. Traces of acid round the neck of the reaction tube or in the cuvette will cause a rapid decrease in colour in the organic extract as the alkali is mainly left behind in the aqueous phase. It is only observed if solvent partition is used. Both reaction tubes and cuvettes should be kept for this determination only.

2. *The alkali used.* Originally ethanolic potassium hydroxide was used and difficulty was experienced preparing a satisfactory reagent but this is essential if colour correction formulae are to be applied. Non-linear curves are obtained with aqueous reagents (Edwards, 1961). A satisfactory potassium hydroxide solution can be prepared by the method of Wilson and Carter (1947). Hamburger (1952) used this as follows. Bring 50 ml absolute ethanol to the boil, add 40 mg ascorbic acid and 10 g finely powdered potassium hydroxide, stir to dissolve for no more than a minute, cool, filter through a sintered glass filter, standardise, adjust to 2.5 mol/l and store in a refrigerator in small bottles. If satisfactory when prepared this will keep for 2 to 4 weeks. Use 0.2 ml instead of the tetramethyl-ammonium hydroxide.

Because of this difficulty, James and de Jong (1961) and Corker *et al.* (1962) investigated the quaternary ammonium bases tetramethyl ammonium hydroxide and benzyl trimethyl ammonium hydroxide. Commercially available products give more intense colours and nearly colourless blanks if the reaction products are extracted into an organic solvent as described above. As benzyl trimethyl ammonium hydroxide gives more variable blanks tetramethyl ammonium hydroxide is preferred.

Tetramethyl ammonium hydroxide   Benzyl trimethyl ammonium hydroxide

3. Dehydroepiandrosterone is the most satisfactory standard (Mason and Engstrom, 1950). Run a standard with each batch.

4. Hormone metabolites other than 17-OS may also give some colour with the Zimmermann reagent. Thus the small increases reported in pregnancy are probably due to 20-oxosteroids resulting from the increased production of progesterone.

5. *Drug interference.* Various drugs reduce 17-OS excretion by influencing their metabolism. These include the phenothiazines, phenytoin, morphine and the contraceptive pill. Probenecid is especially likely to produce figures as low as half the usual value (Friend, 1968). Other drugs

Steroid Hormones 61

have been reported to interfere directly in the Zimmermann reaction. Not all these drugs will interfere with all variants of this reaction but the effects should be borne in mind when unexpected results are obtained. Preferably the drug should be discontinued and the test repeated but direct tests of its interference by the drug or its metabolites in a normal subject can be tried. Oestrogens and reserpine have been reported to give falsely low results. High results are seen with antibiotics: cloxacillin, erythromycin, nalidixic acid, oleandomycin and penicillin. Also involved are quinidine and spironolactone. Varying results followed treatment with barbiturates, chlordiazepoxide, meprobamate and the phenothiazines.

INTERPRETATION

The 17-OS determined by this method are metabolites formed from hormones of the testis and adrenal cortex. Some of the androsterone and aetiocholanolone arises from the testis, a wider variety of 17-OS from the adrenal cortex.

In males the amount excreted is thus a measure of the combined testicular and adrenocortical secretion of androgens, in the female of those from the adrenal cortex only. On average about twice as much is derived from the adrenal cortex as from the testis. Since both the adrenal cortex and testis are under the hormonal control of the anterior pituitary, changes in urinary 17-OS excretion are found in diseases involving the anterior pituitary, adrenal cortex or testis.

Androgen secretion increases at puberty and is associated with the development of male secondary characters and active spermatogenesis. Androgens also affect somatic growth causing protein anabolism reflected in increased muscle and skeletal growth and, later, closure of the epiphyses.

Adult normal 17-OS values can be summarised as follows:

Males   31 to 83 μmol/24 h (average 52 μmol/24 h)
       or 9 to 24 mg/24 h (average 15 mg/24 h)
Females   18 to 59 μmol/24 h (average 35 μmol/24 h)
       or 5 to 17 mg/24 h (average 10 mg/24 h)

These figures are for young adults aged about 25 years, at which time 17-OS excretion is at a maximum. A slow fall follows thereafter with advancing years. Thus Hamburger (1948) found at 50 years an average daily output of 35 μmol (10 mg) with a range of 18 to 63 μmol (5 to 18 mg) for men and of 21 μmol (6 mg) with a range of 10 to 31 μmol (3 to 9 mg) in women. See also Levell *et al.* (1957) and the M.R.C. Committee on Clinical Endocrinology (1963).

Before puberty the excretion is the same in both sexes. It is very low in the first year of life rising slowly during childhood roughly as follows:

From	0 to 1 year	. . .	less than 3.5 μmol	(less than 1 mg)
	1 to 5 years	. . .	1.4 to 6.3 μmol	(0.3 to 1.8 mg)
	5 to 7 years	. . .	2.8 to 9.5 μmol	(0.8 to 2.6 mg)
	7 to 10 years	. . .	4.5 to 12.0 μmol	(1.3 to 3.5 mg)
	10 to 12 years	. . .	6.3 to 17.5 μmol	(1.8 to 5.0 mg)

Decreased excretion of 17-OS is found when there is hypo-activity of the adrenal cortex (see p. 102) pituitary or testis.

Hypogonadism may either be due to disease of the gonad or be secondary to a reduction in the secretion of the gonadotrophic hormone of the pituitary due to hypopituitarism. It is only in these latter cases that really low figures for 17-OS excretion are found. In primary hypogonadism in males adrenal cortical steroids are little affected so that there is only a reduction in testicular hormones. Since only about a third of the urinary 17-OS are derived from these, findings are in the lower part of the normal range or are slightly reduced. In females primary ovarian failure has no effect on 17-OS excretion but again this is low or absent if the hypogonadism is due to hypopituitarism.

In hypogonadism due to primary ovarian or testicular failure there is increased secretion of gonadotrophins by the pituitary, whereas in secondary hypogonadism due to hypopituitarism, gonadotrophins are low or absent.

Increased excretion of 17-OS is most characteristic of increased activity of the adrenal cortex (see p. 90) but increase may be found in some tumours of the testis. Thus greatly increased excretion has been found associated with interstitial cell tumours, but in other testicular tumours normal or reduced amounts are excreted.

Effect of drugs. Following administration of testosterone propionate about 50 per cent of it appears in the urine as 17-OS. Methyl testosterone, however, is not converted to 17-OS.

More Selective Colour Reactions for C_{19} Steroids

Greater specificity in the determination of 17-OS has been sought using several other reagents. Pincus (1943) used antimony trichloride in acetic acid which on heating yields a blue colour with saturated 17-OS but not with dehydroepiandrosterone. Some C_{19} steroids with a 17-hydroxyl group contribute a certain amount of colour and although good agreement with the Zimmermann reaction can be obtained when ketonic fractions are used, the reagent is unpleasant and the complex nature of the absorption curve makes application of correction formulae difficult. Munson *et al.* (1948) introduced the Pettenkoffer reagents, furfural and sulphuric acid, in an effort to achieve a differential estimation of dehydroepiandrosterone. This gives a blue colour on heating. Patterson (1947) used sulphuric acid alone for the detection of large amounts of dehydroepiandrosterone excreted by some patients with adrenal tumours. The Pettenkoffer reagents were also used by Fotherby (1959) who combined them with the chromatographic separation on alumina for the estimation of DHA in urine. This method can be made more sensitive with the use of the Oertel reagent (6 volumes concentrated sulphuric acid, 1 volume ethanol, 2 volumes water; Oertel and Eik-Nes, 1959) with which a yellow colour develops immediately. The readings are made at 365, 405 and 445 nm and an Allen correction applied.

Steroid Hormones

Testosterone and Androstenedione

The only methods which give a true indication of androgen production are those for plasma testosterone and androstenedione. The 17-OS derived from these and excreted in the urine are far outweighed by adrenal DHA and its derivatives. Methods for the estimation of plasma testosterone and androstenedione are not widely available for routine use. These include double isotope dilution (Gandy and Peterson, 1968), electron capture GLC using halogenated derivatives (Kirschner and Coffman, 1968), competitive protein binding (Andre and James, 1972) and radioimmunoassay (Dufau *et al.,* 1972) (see p. 135).

Group Reactions for C_{21} Steroids

As we have seen (p. 46) C_{21} steroids fall into two groups, the "progestogens" including progesterone and substances derived from it, and "corticosteroids" arising from the adrenal cortex. Side chains in the former have either a 20-ketone as in progesterone (IX) and the pregnanolones (XXVIII and XXX) or a 20-hydroxyl as in the pregnanediols (XXIX and XXXI). The simple ketone side chain is relatively inert though it gives some colour with the Zimmermann reaction, and both resist hot acid hydrolysis.

However, we are concerned here with the C_{21} steroids formed during metabolism of the adrenocortical hormones and their precursors. It is necessary to consider how the reagents used for group estimation of corticosteroids affect the six possible side chains which can occur. These (Fig. 2,3) are:

(a) 21-deoxyketols (XLVII) derived from 17-hydroxyprogesterone (XIV).

(b) 17,20-glycols (XLVIII) including pregnanetriol (XXXIII) and its 11-oxo derivative.

(c) dihydroxyacetones (XLIX) examples of which are cortisol (XVI), cortisone (XVII), compound S (XV) and their tetrahydro derivatives (XXXVI, XXXVIII and XXXIV).

(d) glycerols (L) such as cortol (XXXVII), cortolone (XXXIX) and hexahydrocompound S (XXXV).

(e) 20,21-ketols (LI), corticosterone (XI) and aldosterone (XII).

(f) 20,21-glycols (LII).

An early method, now obsolete, for "reducing steroids" used the reduction of an alkaline copper reagent or phosphomolybdic acid by α-ketols. Another reaction, the basis of a popular method in the United States for determining "17-hydroxycorticosteroids", used the characteristic yellow colour given by the dihydroxyacetones with phenylhydrazine in sulphuric acid—the Porter-Silber reaction. However, it is the behaviour towards oxidising and reducing agents which has been most used.

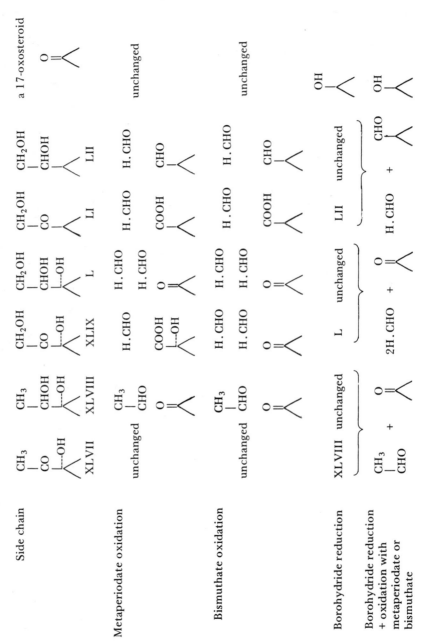

Fig. 2,3. Reactions of side chains of C_{21} steroids and of 17-oxosteroids with various oxidising and reducing agents.

Steroid Hormones

(a) Reaction with Oxidising Agents

Metaperiodate was the first oxidising agent used (Talbot and Eitingon, 1944). The products are shown in Fig. 2,3. All side chains except 21-deoxyketols which are unchanged and 17,20-glycols, which form acetaldehyde, give formaldehyde which can be distilled over and reacted with chromotropic acid ("formaldehydogenic steroids"). The acetaldehyde can be estimated in the same way if glycine is added to hold the formaldehyde (Cox, 1952). This method does not differentiate between 17-hydroxy and 17-deoxysteroids, and the 21-deoxyketols important in congenital adrenal hyperplasia (see p. 91) are excluded. Of the major products only the 17,20-glycols and the glycerols but not the important dihydroxyacetones yield the easily estimated 17-OS.

An important advance was made by Norymberski (1952) who introduced bismuthate as oxidising agent. The dihydroxyacetones are now included, those excluded being the 17-deoxysteroids (LI and LII) and the 21-deoxyketols (XLVII). The native 17-OS are unaffected so the total steroids estimated by the Zimmermann reaction include the native 17-OS present in the urine. If these are determined separately the increment represents those produced during the oxidation, now termed 17-oxogenic steroids (originally 17-ketogenic steroids) and hereafter designated 17-OGS. Thus

17-oxogenic steroids = total 17-oxosteroids − native 17-oxosteroids.

The precision of the determination of 17-OGS is clearly somewhat less than that of a single 17-OS determination as it involves two determinations.

(b) Reduction with Borohydride

In order to include the 21-deoxyketols Appleby *et al.* (1955) introduced borohydride as a general reducing agent for oxo groups. For 17-OHCS this has the advantage of reducing 21-deoxyketols to 17,20-glycols thus making it possible to include them in the group determination of total 17-OGS. This term is used to differentiate them from the 17-OHCS as used in the United States for the steroids determined by the Porter-Silber reaction (referred to on p. 63). As borohydride also converts the native 17-OS to the corresponding 17-hydroxy compounds which do not react in the Zimmermann reaction it made possible the determination of total 17-OGS using a reduction-oxidation sequence before applying the Zimmermann reaction.

(c) Reduction and Oxidation Sequence

1. **Borohydride-bismuthate.** This determines total 17-OGS using a simple 17-OS determination of the steroids remaining after borohydride reduction followed by bismuthate oxidation. At the same time there may be oxidation of the glucuronide residue to a formyl group. The need to use

66   *Practical Clinical Biochemistry*

acid hydrolysis of the oxidation products is still controversial. Unless it can be shown for a given batch of bismuthate that similar results are obtained with and without acid hydrolysis, reliable removal of glucuronide cannot be assumed. It is probably safer to accept that after bismuthate oxidation, acid hydrolysis is still necessary with consequent probable modification of the steroid molecule (see p. 54).

2. **Borohydride-metaperiodate.** The major objection to the use of metaperiodate was its inability to convert the dihydroxyacetones (XLIX) to 17-OS. Borohydride, however, converts the dihydroxyacetones to the glycerol derivatives (L, Fig. 2,3) so that oxidation can then proceed. The use of metaperiodate by Few (1961) has decided advantages over bismuthate. It is cheaper and can be used in aqueous solution and not as a solid requiring constant agitation during the reaction. Also it reliably removes the glucuronide residue under the reaction conditions. Further acid hydrolysis is not required so that subsequent modification of the molecule is avoided. This is important when the products are separated either by solvent partition or chromatography for the determination of the oxygenation index, or by GLC for steroid excretion patterns (see later). As the end product is now almost entirely 11β-hydroxyaetiocholanolone the nature of the alkali used in the Zimmermann reaction is of greater significance. Factors may have to be introduced to allow for the much lower chromogenicity of this compound (see p. 56) than that of the 11-deoxy, oxo or dehydro derivatives.

Thus with the borohydride-bismuthate-hot acid hydrolysis sequence the resulting steroids are 9(11)-dehydroaetiocholanolone (XLV, p. 56) and perhaps a little 11-oxoaetiocholanolone (XLIV, Fig. 2,2) with colour equivalents of at least 100 (see pp. 54 and 56). With the borohydride-metaperiodate sequence without acid hydrolysis the product is almost entirely 11 β-hydroxyaetiocholanolone (XLIII) with a colour equivalent of about 75. As 17-OGS are usually reported as dehydroepiandrosterone equivalents it is essential with these newer procedures to incorporate a correction in the calculation to compensate for this reduced chromogenicity. Provided this is done very good agreement can be demonstrated between the older method using bismuthate and acid hydrolysis, with ethanolic potassium hydroxide for colour development and the newer method using borohydride-metaperiodate and tetramethyl ammonium hydroxide.

Determination of Urinary Total 17-Oxogenic Steroids Using Borohydride and Metaperiodate (Few, 1961).

Ketone groups in steroids are reduced using borohydride. Oxidation with metaperiodate converts 17-hydroxy C_{21} steroids to 17-OS, and 3-glucuronides to 3-formyl derivatives. These are hydrolysed by cold alkali, the free 17-OS extracted into dichloroethane and traces of oxidising agent removed with dithionite before carrying out the Zimmermann reaction.

Steroid Hormones 67

Reagents. 1. Potassium borohydride, 100 g/l in 100 mmol/l sodium hydroxide, prepared freshly before use.

2. Acetic acid, 250 ml glacial acid diluted to 1 litre with water.

3. Sodium metaperiodate, 100 g/l solution in water. Prepare freshly.

4. Sodium hydroxide, 2.5 and 1 mol/l.

5. 1,2-Dichloroethane (as p. 58).

6. Sodium dithionite, approximately 25 g/l in 1.25 mol/l sodium hydroxide.

Standard solution of dehydroepiandrosterone and reagents for the Zimmermann reaction as for 17-OS (reagents 5 to 10, pp. 58 and 59).

Technique. Dilute a 24 h urine specimen to 2 litres, measure 5 ml into a 50 ml glass-stoppered tube and adjust to pH 7.0 with acetic acid or sodium hydroxide. Add 0.5 ml potassium borohydride solution and allow to stand, preferably overnight, but at least 2 h at room temperature. Then add, drop by drop, 0.25 ml acetic acid and, after standing 15 min, add 2 ml sodium metaperiodate and 0.5 ml 1 mol/l sodium hydroxide. Check the pH, adjusting if necessary to between 6.5 and 7.0 using narrow range indicator paper. Incubate at 37°C for an hour. Then add 0.5 ml 2.5 mol/l sodium hydroxide and leave at 37°C for another 15 min. Cool to room temperature, add 10 ml dichloroethane, stopper and shake mechanically for 15 min. Centrifuge, remove the urine layer by suction, and filter the extract through No. 1 Whatman filter paper into a 30 ml glass-stoppered tube. Add 2.5 ml alkaline dithionite, stopper and shake for a minute. Again remove the aqueous layer by suction and filter the extract into a test tube. Measure 6 ml filtrate into a 15 ml stoppered tube, evaporate to dryness in a boiling water bath in a fume cupboard and proceed with the colour development as for 17-OS (p. 59).

Calculation. Urinary total 17-oxogenic steroids (μmol/24 h)

$$= \frac{\text{Reading of unknown}}{\text{Reading of standard}} \times 0.18 \times \frac{2\,000}{5} \times \frac{10}{6} \times 1.33$$

$$= \frac{\text{Reading of unknown}}{\text{Reading of standard}} \times 160$$

To convert to mg/24 h multiply μmol/24 h by 0.29.

Determination of Urinary 11-Deoxy-17-Oxogenic Steroids Using Hexane Extraction (Whigham, 1968)

Reagents. As above for total 17-OGS but substituting hexane for dichloroethane.

Technique. Take 10 ml of urine and double all the reagent volumes in the above procedure for 17-OGS. Instead of using 10 ml dichloroethane add 20 ml hexane to extract the deoxysteroids and, after washing, evaporate 15 ml of this to dryness for the Zimmermann reaction.

68   *Practical Clinical Biochemistry*

Calculation. Urinary 11-deoxy-17-oxogenic steroids (μmol/24 h)

$$= \frac{\text{Reading of unknown}}{\text{Reading of standard}} \times 0.18 \times \frac{2\ 000}{10} \times \frac{20}{15}$$

$$= \frac{\text{Reading of unknown}}{\text{Reading of standard}} \times 48$$

As aetiocholanolone and DHA have approximately the same colour equivalent the factor of 1.33 in the calculation of total 17-OGS is not used. To convert to mg/24 h multiply μmol/l by 0.29.

Notes on Methods for Total 17-Oxogenic Steroids and 11-Deoxy-17-Oxogenic Steroids

1. When large amounts of 11-deoxy-17-OGS are being produced, as in congenital adrenal hyperplasia, total 17-OGS are over-estimated in the standard procedure because of the use of the factor 1.33 to correct for the colour characteristics of 11β-hydroxyaetiocholanolone.

Correction for the 11-deoxy fraction can be made as follows:

$$\text{Corrected total 17-OGS} = \text{total 17-OGS} - \tfrac{1}{3} \times (\text{11-deoxy-17-OGS})$$

When total 17-OGS and 11-deoxy-17-OGS were estimated by us in 80 consecutive urine specimens, the mean total 17-OGS excretion was 33 μmol/24 h (range 7.3 to 65) or 9.6 mg/24 h (range 2.1 to 18.7). The mean 11-deoxy-17-OGS was 3.5 μmol/24 h (range 0.3 to 12.5) or 1.01 mg/24 h (range 0.1 to 3.6) and the mean corrected 17-OGS figure was 32 μmol/24 h (range 6.6 to 65) or 9.3 mg/24 h (range 1.9 to 18.7). Under normal conditions therefore, the different chromogenicity causes no significant difference. In contrast, when investigating cases of congenital adrenal hyperplasia or after metopirone administration to patients with Cushing's syndrome overestimation of 34 to 52 μmol/24 h or 10 to 15 mg/24 h occurs.

2. *Effect of glucose on 17-oxogenic and 11-deoxy-17-oxogenic steroid methods.* Glucose in amounts over 5 g/l significantly decreases the result by using up the metaperiodate. It is important to test all urine specimens for glucose. Errors due to its presence can be avoided either by increasing the amount of metaperiodate twofold for each 20 g/l glucose above 5 g/1 or by removing the glucose. Prepare a suspension of yeast (1 in 3) in water after washing three times to remove any sugar. Take 1 ml of this suspension, centrifuge, drain thoroughly, add 8 to 10 ml urine and incubate at 37° C until the Clinistix test is negative. Finally centrifuge and carry out determinations as described previously on the supernatant fluid.

Another technique is to extract the conjugated steroids by the method of Edwards *et al.,* as in the method for pregnanetriol (p. 78). After evaporating the extract add 5 ml water and proceed as described above.

Steroid Hormones 69

3. *Incubation temperature.* Whigham (1968) and Trafford and Makin (1972) used elevated incubation temperatures thereby reducing the overall time of the methods.

	Above method	Whigham	Trafford & Makin
Borohydride reduction	At least 2 h at room temperature	45 min at 56°C	15 min at 50°C
Destruction of excess borohydride with acetic acid	15 min at 37°C	5 min at 56°C	15 min at 50°C
Metaperiodate oxidation	60 min at 37°C	10 min at 56°C	20 min at 50°C

This elevation of temperature increases the speed of operation without detracting from the reliability of the results. In 43 consecutive paired estimations by the above method and Whigham's carried out in our laboratory there was no significant difference between the mean values or standard deviation. The standard error of the difference was 0.38 μmol (0.11 mg)/24 h for urinary 17-OGS ranging from 13 to 66 μmol (3.7 to 19 mg)/24 h.

4. *Formyl derivatives.* In Trafford and Makin's method, alkali is not added to hydrolyse the formates as they separate the formyl derivatives on GLC. When estimations are done after metopirone administration, metopirone derivatives are extracted from alkaline reaction mixtures and interfere with both colorimetric and GLC determinations. It is then advisable to reacidify before extracting the steroids. Satisfactory results can be obtained by adding 1 ml concentrated hydrochloric acid just before the dichloroethane. The interference is worse when ethanolic potassium hydroxide is used as the base but is not entirely eliminated when tetramethylammonium hydroxide and partition procedures are used.

5. *Dichloroethane purity.* Purity of this reagent is critical for good precision. It is not sufficient to check that dichloroethane gives no colour with concentrated sulphuric acid as is shown by our results in Table 2,3. A single urine with high concentrations of 17-OS and 17-OGS was used with

TABLE 2,3

Effect of Dichloroethane Purity on 17-Oxogenic Steroid Results

Dichloroethane Batch	Urinary steroids (mg/24 h) as mean (S.D.)		
	17-OS	17-OS + 17-OGS	17-OGS (by difference)
A	65 (1.0)	182 (2.5)	117 (2.7)
		195 (2.0)	130 (2.3)
B	62 (3.3)	194 (9.8)	132 (10.4)
		196 (14.1)	134 (14.5)
C	64 (0.8)	177 (3.0)	113 (3.1)

A—previous batch of dichloroethane, purified with concentrated sulphuric acid.
B—new batch of dichloroethane as received.
C—batch B after purification with concentrated sulphuric acid.

Practical Clinical Biochemistry

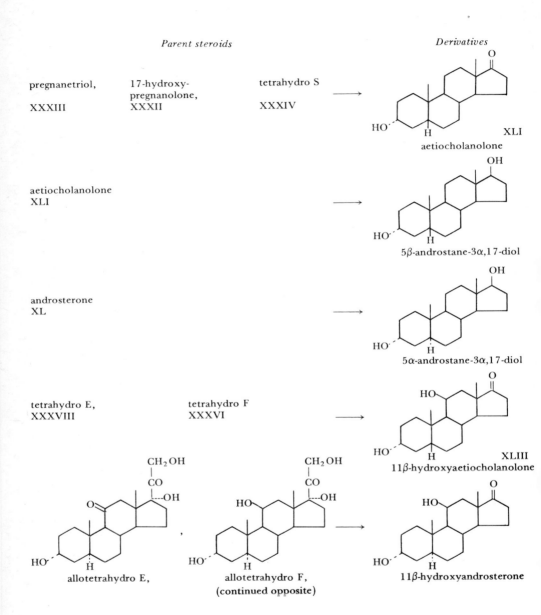

three batches of dichloroethane. Quadruplicate colour development was done using amounts of extract giving extinctions close to that of the standard so as to reduce errors of measurement. The 17-OGS method involved bismuthate oxidation, ethanolic potassium hydroxide in the Zimmermann reaction with a Talbot correction and separate 17-OS determination.

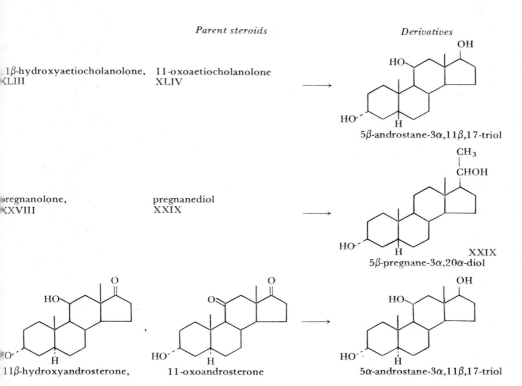

Fig. 2,4. Products derived from urinary steroids by reduction with borohydride followed by metaperiodate oxidation. The products are arranged in order of polarity, the least polar being at the top. For detailed names and formulae see earlier figures and Table 2,2.

The poor precision of batch B in both determinations is apparent as is the improvement after treatment with sulphuric acid. The effect on the final result for 17-OGS involves the errors of both determinations. Impure dichloroethane causes an unacceptable deterioration in precision. The overall precision will be worse than the figure quoted. The experimental conditions were such as to isolate the role of dichloroethane purity.

6. *Drug interference.* Various drugs may modify cortisol metabolism and indirectly alter the excretion of 17-OGS. Thus long-term therapy with barbiturates, phenytoin or phenylbutazone increases the excretion of 6-hydroxycortisol thereby reducing the 17-OGS figure as the former metabolite is not included in the extraction method. Phenothiazines, morphine, and pentazocine (Fortral), also reduce 17-OGS excretion, but aspirin in large doses increases their output. The effects of oestrogens and the contraceptive pill are variable.

72 *Practical Clinical Biochemistry*

Other drugs interfere directly in the method. Some of these have already been mentioned as interfering with the Zimmermann reaction (p. 60). In addition, acetazolamide, digoxin, glutethimide and quinidine may give high results. Interference in the metaperiodate oxidation has been reported for meglumine salts used as radiographic contrast media (Nelson *et al.*, 1968), an effect also seen in the determination of normetadrenaline (p. 207).

Normal range. The approximate range for total 17-OGS is 21 to 69 μmol/24 h (6 to 20 mg/24 h). Values for adult males are on average a little higher than for adult females, 28 to 70 μmol/24 h (8 to 20 mg/24 h) compared to 21 to 63 μmol/24 h (6 to 18 mg/24 h). Values are lower in childhood and are the same for both sexes.

Oxygenation Index and Steroid Profiles

Other features of the steroid molecule other than the 17-oxo group may be of diagnostic interest or be used to achieve separation. Thus in the rapid and early diagnosis of congenital adrenal hyperplasia (p. 91) it is desirable to separate 17-OS bearing an oxygen function at C-11 from the 11-deoxy-17-OS. The development of GLC methods for steroids permits the measurement of substances which do not possess the 17-oxo group whether naturally occurring or formed during chemical modification. As would be expected the retention time is influenced by the polarity. A complete list of C_{19} steroids derived from urine steroid metabolites using the borohydride-metaperiodate sequence is given in Fig. 2,4 in order of increasing polarity and retention time using an SE 30 column (Trafford and Makin, 1972).

When urinary metabolites have been treated with borohydride followed by metaperiodate the 17-OS present are derived from two groups: 11-deoxy compounds particularly aetiocholanolone from 17-hydroxypregnanolone, pregnanetriol and tetrahydro compound S; 11-hydroxy compounds from the metabolites of normal adrenal metabolism namely tetrahydro E and F and allotetrahydro E and F. These two groups were originally separated on silica gel columns before applying the Zimmermann reaction. The ratio of 11-deoxy to 11-hydroxy derivatives was termed the 11-oxygenation index by Morris (1959). Solvent extraction was employed by Few (1968) and Whigham (1968), the latter using chloroform to extract the total 17-OS and hexane the 11-deoxy fraction. Several workers have used GLC for the determination of the oxygenation index and for steroid profile studies (Quazi *et al.*, 1971; Makin and Trafford, 1971; Cook, 1972; Craig and Chamberlain, 1972; and Trafford and Makin, 1972).

Determination of Individual C_{21} Steroids

In addition to the above group reactions for 17-OS more specific methods for individual steroids are available. Two such particularly useful methods are the fluorimetric technique of Mattingly for steroids with an

Steroid Hormones 73

11-hydroxyl group, which has been used to give a measure of the plasma cortisol since this in most cases forms by far the largest component of these, and a method for pregnanetriol using a more elaborate chromatographic separation before applying a relatively non-specific colour reaction.

Determination of Plasma 11-Hydroxycorticosteroids. Fluorimetric Method (Mattingly, 1962)

Unconjugated protein-bound cortisol and corticosterone are extracted into dichloromethane. The extract is back extracted with a sulphuric acid–ethanol reagent and the resulting fluorescence read. A cortisol standard is treated similarly. Though corticosterone gives about four times as much fluorescence as cortisol it is present in much smaller concentration so the results are expressed as plasma cortisol. The optimum activation wave-length for this is about 470 nm which requires a zinc lamp. However, if a mercury lamp is used satisfactory results can be obtained using the 436 nm line. If necessary the quantities given below can be modified to suit the instrument available.

Although individual "cortisol" results may be of somewhat doubtful value the method gives valuable information in studies of diurnal rhythm and when following the response to some stimulus. In such cases background interference is reasonably constant so that increments are significant.

Reagents. 1. Dichloromethane, British Drug Houses. Purify further as follows. Allow to stand several days over concentrated sulphuric acid, shaking occasionally. Wash with one-tenth its volume of 1 mol/l sodium hydroxide, then twice with distilled water (about 200 ml/l). Dry for 24 h over anhydrous sodium sulphate. Distil, collecting the fraction between 39 and 40°C. Keep in the dark. However, the FDPC grade (BDH) solvent is satisfactory without further purification.

2. Concentrated sulphuric acid, Analar.

3. Ethanol, British Drug Houses Analar or Burroughs R.R.

4. Fluorescence reagent. Add 7 volumes concentrated sulphuric acid slowly to 3 volumes ethanol while cooling under running water or in iced water. The reagent obtained should be colourless. If it is yellowish purify the ethanol (Peterson *et al.*, 1955) or obtain a fresh batch. The reagent keeps up to a month at room temperature, or may be mixed freshly.

5. Cortisol standards, in purified ethanol. Dissolve 10.86 mg cortisol in 10 ml ethanol. Dilute 1 ml of this to 100 ml with ethanol. These solutions are stable at 4°C for several months. Prepare the working standard by diluting 1 ml of the latter to 10 ml with water as required. This contains 3.0 μmol/l.

Technique. Collect 10 ml of blood in a heparinised tube. Separate the plasma as soon as possible and store at 0 to 4°C but not frozen, since this may produce a precipitate causing low results. Plasma may be kept up to

74   *Practical Clinical Biochemistry*

72 h. If it cannot be separated at once keep the blood in the refrigerator up to 12 h.

Pipette 2 ml of heparinised plasma into a 250 ml stoppered conical flask or glass-stoppered tube, add 15 ml dichloromethane and shake gently for 5 to 10 min or invert some 30 times, so that no emulsion forms. Centrifuge and remove the supernatant plasma by suction. Treat 2 ml water and 1 ml working standard plus 1 ml water in the same way. These extracts will keep at least 24 h at 0 to 4°C.

Fluorimetry. Careful timing is necessary to keep non-specific plasma fluorescence as low and uniform as possible. Not more than six tests plus standard and blank should be run in one batch. At one minute intervals beginning with the blank add 10 ml of the extract to 5 ml of the fluorescence reagent in a suitable glass-stoppered tube and shake vigorously for 20 sec. Carefully suck off the supernatant layer. The interface between the two phases may be difficult to see but it usually appears blue in colour and is best seen with the interface at eye level. Then carefully transfer the acid extracts to separate cuvettes for reading.

Read the fluorescence at 530 nm exactly 15 min after mixing with the fluorescence reagent placing the cuvettes in the instrument in good time to allow any adjustments to be made. Zero the instrument with the blank in position using the backing off control. One minute later, with the standard in position, set the instrument at a convenient reading using the sensitivity controls. Then read the tests at minute intervals.

Calculation. Plasma cortisol (nmol/l)

$$= \frac{\text{Reading of unknown}}{\text{Reading of standard}} \times 3.0 \times \frac{1000}{2} \quad \text{i.e.} \times 1500$$

To convert to μg/l multiply nmol/l by 0.36.

Determination of Urinary 11-Hydroxycorticosteroids (Mattingly *et al.,* 1964)

The above technique has been applied to urine by Mattingly *et al.* again with a degree of specificity which is surprising, though it appears that interfering substances may occasionally be present.

Reagent. Sodium hydroxide, 1 mol/l.

Other reagents are as above.

Technique. Collect a 24 h specimen of urine kept cool. If the test cannot be done soon after completing the collection keep a portion frozen. Centrifuge if the urine is turbid. Extract a 2 ml sample with 15 ml dichloromethane in a glass-stoppered tube. Remove the upper aqueous layer by suction then shake well for about 20 sec with 2 ml sodium hydroxide. Stand for the layers to separate (about 10 min) or centrifuge and remove the soda layer by suction. Add 10 ml of the extract to the fluorescence reagent. Shake vigorously for 20 sec. Remove the upper layer, transfer the acid layer to a cuvette and read the fluorescence as above.

Steroid Hormones 75

Calculation. Urinary cortisol (nmol/24 h)

$$= \frac{\text{Reading of unknown}}{\text{Reading of standard}} \times 3.0 \times \frac{\text{Volume of 24-h urine (ml)}}{2}$$

Notes for both plasma and urinary 11-hydroxycorticosteroids. 1. The glassware must be scrupulously clean. It is best to keep a set of tubes only for these determinations. Wash these initially with detergent or nitric acid, then with tap water and with distilled water; subsequently after use a thorough rinsing with tap water followed by distilled water is sufficient.

2. Automatic pipettes are recommended for measuring the dichloromethane and fluorescence reagents. Otherwise plug the pipette with cotton wool to prevent contamination if rubber bulbs are used with ordinary pipettes so as to avoid high results.

3. Separation of the two phases before fluorimetry can be simplified and the method made more suitable for batch analyses if modified extraction tubes are used. These consist of a suitably sized stoppered tube to the base of which a standard diameter fluorescence cell is fused. After the extraction, the heavier acid reagent fills the cell allowing measurements to be made without removing the upper phase. The cover of the cell compartment in the fluorimeter requires modification. This type of tube was first described for the Kober reaction (p. 124) by Brown *et al.* (1968) and can be made to individual specification by J. J. McCulloch & Son, 313 Shettleston Road, Glasgow, E.1, Scotland.

4. *Choice of solvent.* Dichloromethane may not be the most suitable solvent for extraction of cortisol. Usui and Kawamoto (1970) found it extracted most of the cortisol but a variable amount of 20-dihydrocortisol from urine and preferred dichloroethane for extracting cortisol and ethyl acetate for total fluorogens. Sammons *et al.* (1969) investigated the use of chloroform and found it to give greater stability and to be cheaper.

5. *Solvent purity.* Waddecar (1968) found the sensitivity for the standard decreased as the dichloromethane aged and Lever (1971) showed this was due to the formation of formaldehyde from dichloromethane in the presence of moisture and daylight. Formaldehyde at a concentration of less than 2 μg/l causes quenching and hence standards with low readings. As protein in plasma reacts with the formaldehyde this removes the interference and gives normal fluorescence, resulting in over-estimation. Lever showed that washing three volumes of the reagent with one volume of saturated sodium bisulphite, rinsing with water, drying over anhydrous sodium sulphate and distilling, removed the impurities and gave a reagent as good as that obtained by the method recommended by Mattingly and given above. Store the distillate (39 to 40° C) over anhydrous sodium sulphate. In other cases interfering materials can cause an increase in the blank reading. These can be removed by distillation.

6. *Effect of drugs and other interfering substances.* Interference giving high results due to interfering fluorogens can be caused by administration of spironolactone, fucidic acid, or mepacrine and is difficult to eliminate. Similar problems arise in haemolysed specimens.

Occasionally plasma extracts are pigmented in which case an additional alkaline wash can be incorporated after removing the supernatant plasma. To each tube, including the standard and blank, add 2 ml 100 mmol/l sodium hydroxide, shake for a few seconds and centrifuge. Non-specific yellow pigments usually pass into the alkaline layer. Remove this and carry out the rest of the determination as described.

Impurities in the heparin can also cause trouble. Benzyl alcohol is present in some commercial heparins and interferes. Traces of phenol or o-cresol in other heparins react with impurities in dichloromethane (Verjee, 1971) giving spuriously high results. When serum is used such interference is eliminated. The emission spectrum of the interfering product is identical with that from cortisol. The purity of dichloromethane is thus critical particularly when specimens are received from different sources possibly using different batches of heparin.

Falsely high results in the determination of plasma cortisol have been reported due to the non-specific fluorescence of cholesterol (Graef and Staudinger, 1970) and following heavy smoking (Kershbaum *et al.,* 1968).

Gross contamination is rare and obvious. The original method is simple and sufficiently specific for the purposes for which it is intended provided adequate attention is paid to details.

7. *Choice of wavelength.* The best excitation wavelength for the cortisol fluorogen is 470 nm with optimal emission setting between 520 and 530 nm depending on the instrument used. There is no major emission line in the mercury arc at this wavelength but in our experience adequate sensitivity is obtained using the mercury 436 nm line in the Locarte fluorimeter with a Balzer 438 nm interference filter for the excitation and the interference wedge set at 530 nm for the emission. Mattingly stressed and we agree that extraneous fluorescence from interfering chromogens is kept to a minimum providing timing is accurate and readings are made at about 15 min after mixing. Interfering substances have caused little trouble and the precision of the method has remained satisfactory over a long period. Usui *et al.* (1970) read at 468/520 nm after 30 min. They suggest that if excitation at 436 nm is used, fluorescence readings (F) should be made at 470 and 520 nm to obtain a corrected reading using $k = 0.3$ in the following equation:

$$F \text{ (corrected)} = F \text{ (436/520)} - k \times F \text{ (436/470)}$$

They also find that F (468/520) increases with time and recommend correction of the 30 min reading to allow for this. If the excitation wavelength is 436 nm this is achieved by using $k = 0.55$ in the equation above.

On the other hand Koch *et al.* (1973) find correction factors unsatisfactory and believe wavelengths below 450 nm should not be used to avoid non-specific interference. They recommend a filter arrangement using

Steroid Hormones 77

475 nm which would include some contribution from the mercury line at 490 nm with low but adequate sensitivity.

Using a Baird Atomic spectrophotofluorimeter with a xenon lamp and diffraction gratings for both excitation and emission wavelengths we found the final results for duplicates read at the same time against the same standard were virtually identical for the 436/520 nm and 470/520 nm combinations. These results were almost the same as those obtained on the same specimens with the Locarte fluorimeter using the 436/530 combination.

Normal ranges. *Plasma 11-hydroxycorticosteroids* by the above technique range from 220 to 750 nmol/l, mean 470 (80 to 270 μg/l, mean 170). Often referred to as *"cortisol"* this contains a small proportion of corticosterone. There is a considerable diurnal variation (see p. 83) and there can be appreciable variation from day to day in the same patient. The plasma cortisol appears to fall only slightly with age, unlike the 17-OS and 17-OGS. It is suggested this is due to a slower degradation in older people.

Plasma cortisol is largely bound to plasma proteins, in particular to cortisol-binding globulin or transcortin. Certain drugs can alter the concentration of this protein and thus alter the total plasma cortisol without changing the amount of free cortisol. The situation is analogous to that with thyroid hormones and TBG (see Chapter 1). The concentration of transcortin is increased by oestrogens, the contraceptive pill, and in pregnancy. It is decreased on administration of androgens.

Other drugs may interfere with normal controlling mechanisms for cortisol secretion (p. 82). Plasma cortisol concentration is reduced by dexamethasone which inhibits the hypothalamus and by *l*-dopa (p. 194) which reduces ACTH output. Increases in plasma cortisol occur for 24 h or so after taking cortisone, after ingestion of ethanol, and during anaesthesia, especially using ether. Lithium salts also have the same effect. Some central nervous system stimulants modify the diurnal rhythm; dexamphetamine increases evening levels and methylamphetamine morning.

Finally stress can temporarily increase plasma cortisol. Admission to hospital often results in increases for the first day or so. After surgical operation the same may be seen and repeated venepunctures are a potent stimulus in some patients.

The normal range for *urinary cortisol* was given by Mattingly *et al.* (1964) as 215 to 1 030 nmol/24 h (78 to 372 μg/24 h) with a mean for males of 630 nmol/24 h (229 μg/24 h) and for females of 490 nmol/24 h (178 μg/24 h). These workers also compared the daily "cortisol" by this method with the cortisol secretion rate and found a better correlation between these than between the latter and the 17-OGS output. A daily excretion of 610 nmol (220 μg) or less gave a 95 per cent probability that the cortisol secretion rate was normal or low, one above 1 400 nmol (500 μg) a 66 per cent probability that the cortisol excretion rate was increased.

78 *Practical Clinical Biochemistry*

Determination of Urinary Pregnanetriol (Bell and Varley, 1960)

This is a modification of the method of Stern (1957). Conjugates are extracted by the method of Edwards, Kellie and Wade (1953; see also Kellie and Wade, 1957) and hydrolysed by glucuronidase. The free pregnanetriol is extracted into benzene and applied to an alumina column with the same activity as that for determining pregnanediol. After elution and evaporation the product is assayed colorimetrically using the colour given with sulphuric acid.

Reagents. 1. Ammonium sulphate, A.R.

2. Ethanol. British Drug Houses Analar is satisfactory. Otherwise, to remove aldehydes reflux for several hours with sodium hydroxide (5 g/100 ml) and zinc dust (5 g/100 ml), distil and redistil.

3. Ether. British Drug Houses Analar is satisfactory. Otherwise, to remove peroxides shake with saturated ferrous sulphate solution, then wash with water. The ether can be used wet for extraction.

4. Extraction mixture, ether–ethanol 3 : 1 by volume.

5. Ammonium acetate, pH 5, approximately 100 mmol/l. Dissolve 7.7 g ammonium acetate in water, make to a litre and adjust to pH 5 with glacial acetic acid.

6. Ketodase, Warner Chilcot beef liver glucuronidase containing 5 000 Fishman units per ml.

7. Benzene. British Drug Houses Analar distilled and saturated with water.

8. Alumina, see pregnanediol method (p. 132).

9. Sodium hydroxide–saline solution. Dissolve 250 g sodium chloride in 1 litre, 1 mol/l sodium hydroxide.

10. Elution mixtures, ethanol in benzene, 8, 30, and 100 ml/l.

11. Concentrated sulphuric acid, British Drug Houses Analar.

12. Standard pregnanediol, 5β-pregnane-$3\alpha,20\alpha$-diol, 600 μmol/l ethanol. Dissolve 19.2 mg in 100 ml ethanol. This reagent is only needed if pregnanediol is determined simultaneously.

13. Standard pregnanetriol, 5β-pregnane-3α, 17α, 20α-triol, 600 μmol/l ethanol. Dissolve 20.2 mg in 100 ml ethanol.

Technique. Measure one-hundredth of the volume of a 24 h specimen of urine, collected without preservative, into a suitable separating funnel. With total volumes of over a litre dilute to 20 ml; of under a litre to 10 ml. Add 5 g solid ammonium sulphate per 10 ml diluted urine and shake until completely dissolved. Extract three times with half its volume of ether–ethanol, pool the extracts, allow to drain to remove as much water as possible and evaporate to dryness under reduced pressure on a boiling water bath.

Dissolve the dry residue and wash from the evaporating flask into a suitable tube with 10 ml ammonium acetate buffer. Quickfit and Quartz tubes, 150 × 18 mm with B19 stoppers are suitable. Add 1 ml of Ketodase

Steroid Hormones 79

and incubate for 4 h at $37°$ C. Cool, then extract three times by shaking with 10 ml benzene; if an emulsion forms break by centrifuging. Transfer the benzene layers to a separating funnel and wash the pooled extracts twice with 10 ml sodium hydroxide–saline solution, twice with water, and then drain.

Prepare the column as described for pregnanediol on p. 133. Apply the benzene extract to the column and allow to run until the liquid layer just disappears into the sand. Wash with 20 ml of ethanol in benzene, 30 ml/l then elute the pregnanetriol with 15 ml of ethanol in benzene, 100 ml/l. Evaporate the eluate to dryness on a boiling water bath with a slight negative pressure. A water pump can be used in conjunction with a small air leak.

Dry the residue in a desiccator for an hour and add 3 ml concentrated sulphuric acid. At the same time treat 60 nmol pregnanetriol, contained in 0.1 ml standard solution, in the same way. Mix thoroughly and place the tubes in a water bath at $25°$ C for at least an hour. For high values of pregnanetriol it is necessary to take a suitable aliquot of the eluate. Dissolve in 5 ml ethanol and pipette the required amount and evaporate to dryness again, and add the sulphuric acid. After colour development read at 400, 435 and 470 nm.

Calculation. An Allen correction is applied (see p. 57). So:

$$\text{Corrected reading} = 2E_{435} - (E_{400} + E_{470})$$

Then, Urinary pregnanetriol (μmol/24 h)

$$= \frac{\text{Corrected reading of unknown}}{\text{Corrected reading of standard}} \times 6.$$

If an aliquot has been taken make the necessary adjustment.

To convert to mg/24 h multiply μmol/24 h by 0.336.

Notes. 1. If pregnanediol is to be determined on the same extract, first wash the column with 25 ml ethanol in benzene, 8 ml/l. Discard this eluate. Then follow with 12 ml ethanol in benzene, 30 ml/l. This contains the pregnanediol.

2. By treating the aliquot of urine diluted as above with borohydride (freshly prepared potassium borohydride solution containing 100 mg in 1 ml water per 20 ml diluted urine) any 17-hydroxypregnanolone is reduced to pregnanetriol so that the subsequent estimation gives the total of these two compounds. Allow to stand overnight and then proceed as described above.

Normal range. Normal adults excrete up to 6 μmol/24 h (2 mg/24 h) of pregnanetriol. Similar amounts are found in Cushing's syndrome but increases up to 300 μmol/24 h (100 mg/24 h) are seen in adults and children with congenital adrenal hyperplasia (see p. 91). In the newborn, during the first few weeks of life when it is necessary to establish the diagnosis in cases of salt losing congenital adrenal hyperplasia (CAH) (see

80   *Practical Clinical Biochemistry*

p. 91), the concentration is less than 0.3 μmol/l (0.1 mg/l) in random urine specimens obtained from normal infants. Little additional 17-hydroxypregnanolone is found in normal persons but in CAH, treatment with borohydride may double the pregnanetriol determined as above.

REFERENCES

Allen, W. H. (1950), *J. clin. Endocrinol.*, **10**, 71.

Andre, C. M. and James, V. H. T. (1972), *Clin. chim. Acta*, **40**, 325.

Appleby, J. I., Gibson, G., Norymberski, J. K. and Stubbs, R. D. (1955), *Biochem. J.*, **60**, 453.

Bell, M. and Varley, H. (1960), *Clin. chim. Acta*, **5**, 396.

Brown, J. B., Macnaughton, C., Smith, M. A. and Smyth, B. (1968), *J. Endocrinol.*, **40**, 175.

Burnstein, S. and Lieberman, S. (1958), *J. Amer. chem. Soc.*, **80**, 5253.

Callow, N. H., Callow, R. K. and Emmens, C. W. (1938), *Biochem. J.*, **32**, 1312.

Callow, R. K. (1950), *Androgen and Adrenocortical Hormone Group Steroids, Hormone Assay*, edited C. W. Emmens, Academic Press, p. 363.

Cook, D. (1972). *Clin. chim. Acta*, **40**, 43.

Cope, C. L. (1972), *Adrenal Steroids and Disease*, Pitman Medical Publishing Co., London.

Corker, C. S., Norymberski, J. K. and Thow, R. (1962), *Biochem. J.*, **83**, 583.

Cox, R. I. (1952), *Biochem. J.*, **52**, 339.

Craig, A. and Chamberlain, J. (1972), *Ann. clin. Biochem.*, **9**, 67.

Drekter, I. J., Heisler, A., Scism, G. R., Stern, S., Pearson, S. and MacGavack, T. H. (1952), *J. clin. Endocrinol.*, **12**, 55.

Dufau, M. L., Catt, K. J., Tsuvuhava, T. and Ryan, D. (1972), *Clin. chim. Acta*, **37**, 109.

Edwards, R. W. H. (1961), in "The Adrenal Cortex", editors G. K. McGowan, and M. Sandler. Pitman Medical Publishing Co., London, p. 56.

Edwards, R. W. H., Kellie, A. E. and Wade, A. P. (1953), *Mem. Soc. Endocrinol.*, **2**, 53.

Engstrom, W. W. and Mason, H. L. (1943), *Endocrinology*, **33**, 229.

Few, J. D. (1961), *J. Endocrinol.*, **22**, 31.

Few, J. D. (1968), *J. Endocrinol.*, **41**, 213.

Fotherby, K. (1959), *Biochem. J.*, **73**, 339.

Fraser, R. W., Forbes, A. P., Albright, F., Sulkowitch, H. and Reifenstein, E. C., Jr. (1941), *J. clin. Endocrinol.*, **1**, 234.

Friend, D. G. (1968), *Practitioner*, **200**, 153.

Gandy, H. M. and Peterson, R. E. (1968), *J. clin. Endocrinol.*, **28**, 949.

Girard, A. and Sandulesco, G. (1936), *Helv. chim. Acta*, **19**, 1095.

Graef, V. and Staudinger, H. (1970), *Z. Chem. klin. Biochem.*, **8**, 368.

Gray, C. H., Baron, D. N., Brooks, R. V. and James, V. H. T. (1969), *Lancet*, **1**, 124.

Hamburger, C. (1948), *Acta Endocrinol.*, **1**, 19.

Hamburger, C. (1952), *Acta Endocrinol.*, **99**, 129.

James, V. H. T. and de Jong, M. (1961), *J. clin. Path.*, **14**, 125.

Kellie, A. E. and Wade, A. P. (1957), *Biochem. J.*, **66**, 196.

Kendal, J. W., Elams, M. L. and Stott, A. K. (1968), *J. clin. Endocrinol. Metab.*, **28**, 1373.

Kersbaum, A., Pappajohn, D. J. and Bellett, S. (1968), *J. Amer. med. Ass.*, **203**, 275.

Kirshner, M. A. and Coffman, G. D. (1968), *J. clin. Endocrinol.*, **28**, 1347.

Klyne, W. (1957), "The Chemistry of the Steroids", Methuen, London; Wylie & Sons, New York.

Koch, T. R., Edwards, L. and Chilcot, M. E. (1973), *Clin. Chem.*, **19**, 258.

Levell, M. J., Mitchell, F. L. Payne, C. G. and Jordan, A. (1957), *J. clin. Path.*, **10**, 72.

Steroid Hormones 81

Lever, M. (1971), *Clin. chim. Acta,* 31, 291.
Lieberman, S. and Dobriner, K. (1948), *Recent Progr. Hormone Res.,* 3, 371.
Mason, H. L. and Engstrom, W. W. (1950), *Physiol. Rev.,* 30, 321.
Makin, H. J. L. and Trafford, D. J. H. (1971), *Clin. chim. Acta,* 32, 299.
Mattingly, D. (1962), *J. clin. Path.,* 15, 374.
Mattingly, D., Dennis, P. M., Pearson, J. and Cope, C. L. (1964), *Lancet,* 2, 1046.
Medical Research Council Committee on Clinical Endocrinology (1951), *Lancet,* 2, 585.
Medical Research Council Committee on Clinical Endocrinology (1963), *Lancet,* 1, 1415.
Morris, R. (1959), *Acta Endocrinol.,* 32, 596.
Munson, P. L., Jones, M. E., McCall, P. J. and Gallagher, T. F. (1948), *J. biol. Chem.,* 176, 73.
Nelson, J. C., Krueger, G. G., Wilcox, B. B. and Thompson, W. P., (1968) *J. clin. Endocrinol. and Metab.,* 28, 1515.
Norymberski, J. K. (1952), *Nature,* 170, 1074.
Norymberski, J. K., Stubbs, R. D. and West, H. F. (1953), *Lancet,* 1, 1276.
Oertel, G. W. and Eik-Nes, K. (1959), *Anal. Chem.,* 31, 98.
Patterson, J. (1947), *Lancet,* 2, 580.
Peterson, R. E., Wyngaarden, T. B., Guerra, S. L., Brodie, B-B. and Bunim, J. J. (1955), *J. clin. Invest.,* 34, 1779.
Pincus, G. (1943), *Endocrinology,* 32, 176.
Quazi, Q. H., Hill, G. J. and Thompson, M. W. (1971), *Clin. chim. Acta,* 31, 435.
Sammons, H. G., Almond, S. J. and Botterill, V. M. (1969), *Ann. clin. Biochem.,* 6, 169.
Stern, M. I. (1957), *J. Endocrinol.,* 16, 180.
Talbot, N. B., Berman, R. A. and Maclachlan, E. A. (1942), *J. biol. Chem.,* 143, 211.
Talbot, M. E. and Eitingon, I. V. (1944), *J. biol. Chem.,* 154, 605.
Trafford, D. J. H. and Makin, H. L. J. (1972), *Clin. chim. Acta,* 40, 421.
Usui, T. and Kawamoto, H. (1970a), *Clin. chim. Acta,* 30, 595.
Usui, T. and Kawamoto, H. and Shirmao, S. (1970b), *Clin. chim. Acta,* 30, 663.
Verjee, Z. H. M. (1971), *Clin. chim. Acta,* 33, 268.
Waddecar, J. (1968), *Proc. Ass. clin. Biochem.,* 5, 133.
Whigham, W. R. (1968), *Clin. Chem.,* 14, 675.
Wilson, H. and Carter, P. (1947), *Endocrinology,* 41, 417.
Zimmermann, W. (1935), *Z. physiol. Chem.,* 233, 257.

CHAPTER 3

STEROID HORMONES.
THE HYPOTHALAMIC-PITUITARY-ADRENAL AXIS

THE adrenal cortex synthesises various steroid hormones and releases these into the adrenal vein. The major groups are the C_{19} steroids, adrenal androgens and the C_{21} steroids, the adrenocorticoids. The C_{18} oestrogens produced by the adrenal play only a minor role in the normal state. The adrenocorticoids play a major role in controlling carbohydrate and electrolyte metabolism. The relative activity of different naturally occurring steroids for these two functions varies widely. Those primarily influencing carbohydrate metabolism are called *glucocorticoids*; those having a major role in electrolyte metabolism *mineralocorticoids*. Cortisol is the most important of the former in man, and aldosterone of the latter. Synthetic steroids also show both activities in varying degree. Thus dexamethasone (XLVI) and prednisolone (XLVII) are potent glucocorticoids used in adrenal function tests, 9α-fluorocortisol (fludrocortisol, XLVIII) is a potent mineralocorticoid.

dexamethasone prednisolone fludrocortisol

In disease the production of androgens, glucocorticoids or mineralocorticoids may be abnormal. Both hypersecretion and hyposecretion are known and result from a variety of diseases affecting complex controlling mechanisms which influence adrenal steroid production.

Control of Glucocorticoid Secretion

The highest co-ordinating centre is the *hypothalamus* which secretes corticotrophin releasing hormone (CRH), a short chain polypeptide, into the hypophyseal portal system. CRH stimulates the *anterior pituitary* to produce adrenocorticotrophic hormone (ACTH), a peptide hormone containing 39 amino acid residues. Physiological activity begins to occur with a peptide containing 16 amino acids from the N-terminal end and does not increase further after 20. Different species have variations in the amino acids between positions 25 and 32, but the remaining chain is common to

Adrenocortical Function Tests

all species. There is therefore the possibility of immunological reactivity when using ACTH gels of animal origin. The synthetic N-terminal peptide of 24 amino acids, tetracosactrin (Synacthen, Ciba Laboratories Ltd., Horsham, Sussex, England) is the more potent and immunologically safer substance. ACTH released into the circulation stimulates the *adrenal cortex* to secrete glucocorticoids, largely cortisol. Cortisol exerts its biological effect on the body tissues and has an important feed-back inhibition on CRH secretion by the hypothalamus so that there is a finely balanced control of ACTH and hence of cortisol production. Other influences, especially stress, can directly stimulate the hypothalamus to release CRH, overriding the normal feed-back. In addition there is a well-marked circadian rhythm of ACTH and cortisol due to varying sensitivity of the feed-back and secreting systems.

Control of Mineralocorticoid Secretion

Aldosterone secretion is only controlled to a minor degree through the hypothalamic-anterior pituitary-adrenal (HPA) axis. ACTH can stimulate aldosterone production but the major role is believed to be taken by the renin-angiotensin system. Renin is stored in the granular cells of the juxtaglomerular apparatus in the kidney. This is close to the afferent arteriole of the renal glomerulus and is sensitive to the degree of stretching of the arteriolar wall. If the blood volume should contract, this stretch diminishes and renin is released into the circulation. Renin is an enzyme which converts the plasma protein, angiotensinogen, into the decapeptide, angiotensin I, and thence into angiotensin II, an octopeptide. Angiotensin II has a constrictive effect on most arterioles thereby reducing the vascular bed and increasing the blood pressure. It also directly stimulates the adrenal cortex to secrete aldosterone which plays a major role in the renal retention of sodium and water. This retention expands the extracellular fluid space and, usually, the plasma volume. The overall process modifies the circulation and eventually replenishes the blood volume. Once this is achieved, a normal cardiovascular system and normal kidney no longer combine to release renin, i.e. there is a negative feed-back system. Abnormal function of the renin-angiotensin-aldosterone system can result in electrolyte abnormalities (see Chapter 23, Vol. 1).

Control of Adrenal Androgen Production

Adrenal androgen production is controlled by the CRH-ACTH system in the same way as that of glucocorticoids. The C-17 side chain of Δ^5-pregnenolone is removed (Fig. 2,2) to form dehydroepiandrosterone (DHA) and its sulphate which are secreted daily into the adrenal vein at an estimated rate of 70 to 105 μmol (20 to 30 mg), similar to that of cortisol but many times greater than that of aldosterone (approximately 0.6 μmol or 200 μg). These adrenal androgens have weak androgenic potency, about

84   *Practical Clinical Biochemistry*

5 per cent that of testosterone compared with about 20 per cent for androstenedione and about 1 per cent for 11β-hydroxyandrostenedione. Although free testosterone can be produced directly by adrenal tissue as well as by peripheral conversion of adrenal androstenedione, the testis produces daily 24 μmol (7 mg) of testosterone and 3.5 μmol (1 mg) of androstenedione + DHA. The major components of urinary 17-oxosteroids (17-OS) are derived from adrenal 17-OS of weak androgenic potency and not from the testis. The importance of this androgenic effect in the normal human is uncertain but overproduction of adrenal androgens can lead to virilism (see p. 94). The contribution of adrenal androgens to overall anabolic activity is not clear but these effects include growth stimulation, positive nitrogen balance and counteraction of the catabolic effect of cortisol on proteins. Reduction of muscle mass in Addison's disease and increased muscular development and skeletal growth in the adrenogenital syndrome are well recognised manifestations of abnormal androgen activity.

Adrenocorticosteroid Metabolism: Synthesis and Catabolism

Fig. 2,1 shows the interrelationships of the C_{19} and C_{21} steroids. A study of the precursors of cortisol and their metabolites (Fig. 2,2) clarifies the patterns of excretion seen in the various diseases associated with abnormal production of this hormone. Pregnenolone (VIII) derived from cholesterol is hydroxylated by a 17α-hydroxylase giving 17-hydroxypregnenolone (XIII). This is degraded to the C_{19} steroid, DHA (XVIII), which is secreted and partly excreted as such but is also metabolised to aetiocholanolone (XLI) and androsterone (XL). 17-Hydroxypregnenolone is converted to 17-hydroxyprogesterone (XIV) which is catabolised to its tetrahydro derivative, 17-hydroxypregnanolone (XX III) (see p. 51), and finally to pregnanetriol (XXXIII). 17-Hydroxyprogesterone can also undergo 21-hydroxylation to give Compound S (XV) and finally 11-hydroxylation to produce cortisol (XVI). Both these hormones undergo subsequent catabolism similar to 17-hydroxyprogesterone. The resultant 3-hydroxy-5β steroids are conjugated with glucuronic acid in the liver producing water-soluble derivatives which are excreted in the urine. They all possess one or other of the side chains discussed in Chapter 2, p. 64, and are thus capable of being converted to the corresponding 17-OS using the borohydride-metaperiodate sequence. The end products of this reaction (Fig. 2,4) demonstrate the difference between the 11-deoxy derivatives of the precursors and the 11-hydroxy metabolites of cortisol.

TESTS USED IN DISEASES AFFECTING THE HYPOTHALAMIC-PITUITARY-ADRENOCORTICAL AXIS

Knowledge of the control of glucocorticoid secretion and details of cortisol synthesis and degradation has led to the development of several

Adrenocortical Function Tests

tests which assess the functioning of different parts of the HPA system. The majority involve measurement either of circulating cortisol or of its metabolites as urinary total 17-oxogenic steroids (17-OGS). The measurements are either made without special modification of the patient's state or after a deliberate attempt to influence the HPA system.

The hypothalamus can be stimulated either by stress (insulin stimulation test) or by reduction of the circulating plasma cortisol (metopirone test); it can be suppressed by administration of a potent glucocorticoid (dexamethasone suppression test). The normal hypothalamus will respond by altering the output of CRH and hence of ACTH and cortisol. The ability of the adrenal cortex to respond to ACTH can be directly assessed by administering the natural hormone or Synacthen (stimulation tests). In all such tests, a disease process damaging a particular part of the system is reflected as failure to respond to the appropriate stimulus. A tumour affecting one of the three main glands is often overactive and unresponsive to the normal controlling mechanism. The tests are therefore important in assessing both hypo- and hyper-activity of the total system and in defining which particular part is affected.

Insulin Stimulation Test

The stress of hypoglycaemia stimulates the hypothalamus to release CRH which causes a marked increase in plasma ACTH. Provided the adrenal cortex is functional an increase in plasma cortisol results. It can be induced most easily and controllably by the administration of insulin. In normal individuals a blood glucose level below 2.2 mmol/l (40 mg per 100 ml) elicits a marked response. The actual mode of stimulation of the hypothalamus is uncertain but the plasma cortisol response is elicited only in the presence of an intact HPA axis and the insulin stimulation test is used to assess its integrity. In addition hypoglycaemia is a potent stimulus for growth hormone secretion and one of the earliest indications of hypothalamic or pituitary hypofunction is an absent or impaired response of growth hormone to insulin-induced hypoglycaemia.

Procedure. Give the patient nothing to eat or drink on the morning of the test which starts between 0900 and 1000 h. As the test is not without risk, supervise the patient closely and have a sterile solution of 50 per cent glucose and a 20 ml syringe available for immediate intravenous injection should the need arise. James and Landon (1971) consider the risks justified in view of the valuable information obtained from the test and point out that much larger doses of insulin were regularly given to patients receiving insulin coma therapy in psychiatric treatment. As with any adrenal investigation where repeated sampling of blood is required it is best to insert an intravenous cannula at least 30 min before the start of the test.

The dose of insulin, sufficient to reduce the blood glucose to below 2.2 mmol/l (40 mg/100 ml) without causing serious side effects, varies and is best related to the tentative diagnosis and the weight of the subject. For normal individuals a dose of 0.15 units/kg suffices but is reduced to

P.C.B.(II)—4

86 *Practical Clinical Biochemistry*

0.1 unit/kg for patients expected to have increased insulin sensitivity as in HPA hypo-function and in severe malnutrition such as anorexia nervosa. The dose is increased to 0.2 to 0.3 units/kg for obese patients and those with decreased insulin sensitivity as in Cushing's syndrome or acromegaly.

After sufficient time has elapsed after the insertion of the cannula for a return to resting conditions a base-line sample is collected. If desirable a second sample is taken after 30 min. Transfer samples for blood glucose to small fluoride-containing tubes and plasma cortisol samples to lithium heparin tubes. For ACTH and growth hormone determinations centrifuge the latter as soon as possible, remove 1 ml aliquots and store frozen. Inject the insulin intravenously as a single dose drawing blood into the syringe and re-injecting at least twice to administer the full dose. Take further blood samples at 30, 40, 60 and 90 min. At the end of the test 20 ml of 50 per cent glucose can be administered intravenously or a high carbohydrate meal given.

The blood glucose falls first. For a normal subject given 0.15 units/kg this should be less than 2.2 mmol/l (40 mg/100 ml) in the 30 min sample and still be below 2.8 mmol/l (50 mg/100 ml) at 45 min with a return to normal at about 120 min. The increase in plasma cortisol follows the fall in glucose and reaches a peak at about 90 min. The response is similar to that obtained for the same subject using the short Synacthen stimulation test (p. 88). The maximum value should exceed 560 nmol/l (200 μg/l) and the increment over the basal level should exceed 195 nmol/l (70 μg/l).

Metopirone (Metyrapone) Test

This substance, SU4885, 2-methyl-l,2-bis-(3'-pyridyl)-propan-l-one, inhibits 11-hydroxylation in the adrenal cortex and so reduces its production of cortisol. If the HPA axis is intact the normal feed-back mechanism increases ACTH output stimulating the adrenal cortex.

Inhibition of 11-hydroxylation is incomplete and after the initial fall in cortisol the increased production of ACTH increases cortisol production to near normal or even to slightly elevated values. 11-Deoxysteroid formation, particularly of Compound S, is usually appreciably increased but sometimes it balances the previous production of cortisol giving little increase in total steroid output. The result depends on the method used to assess this response. As plasma "cortisol" by the Mattingly technique (see p. 73) depends on the presence of the 11-hydroxyl group, the normal response is a decrease. Plasma "cortisol" measured by the Porter-Silber reaction depends on the presence of the dihydroxyacetone group, still present in

Adrenocortical Function Tests

Compound S so an increase is expected. Urinary 17-OS output is increased by the ACTH. Total 17-OGS determined by the borohydride-metaperiodate sequence also increase as Compound S is measured by this method. For the same reason Porter-Silber chromogens increase. When the diminution of cortisol production is balanced by increased Compound S output the total steroid output is an insensitive index of response so it is better to separate the 11-deoxy and 11-hydroxy fractions and estimate directly the products derived from Compound S.

Procedure. The usual amount of metopirone is 4.5 g given orally with milk or food as six doses of 750 mg 4-hourly over 24 h. The patient should be warned that he may experience slight nausea and dizziness after each dose. This is lessened if the drug is taken with milk. Give children a smaller amount (6 ×15 mg/kg) with a minimum of 250 mg 4-hourly. Collect four 24 h specimens of urine. The first two are control days, the metopirone being given on the third day. Determine the total 17-OGS in each specimen.

Metopirone has several features which have reduced its use recently. Nausea, malabsorption or vomiting may result in inadequate plasma levels. The drug is metabolised rapidly with a half life of 30 min so the dose must be given regularly without omissions. Drugs such as phenytoin increase the clearance of metopirone. All these factors may lead to apparent failure of response. The variable response shown in Table 3,7 may represent inadequate control over timing of the dose. In patients with an adrenal adenoma or carcinoma the test can produce extremely severe symptoms when the profound decrease in cortisol production is not balanced by an early increased release of ACTH due to long term suppression of the pituitary. For the investigation of hypopituitary states there are more suitable tests, such as insulin stimulation, which can be used to assess the whole HPA system and not only the feed-back control.

Normal response. Using the Porter-Silber reaction Liddle *et al.* (1959) found a mean increase in plasma 17-hydroxy-corticosteroids from 280 to 640 nmol/l (100 to 230 µg/l) 20 h after beginning to give metopirone. With urinary total 17-OGS the maximal increase may occur on the day after metopirone is given. Gold *et al.* (1960) found a mean daily excretion of 118 µmol (range 76 to 162) or 34 mg (range 22 to 47) in males for the 24 h after metopirone, an average increase of 62 µmol/24 h (18 mg/24 h). For females, the mean excretion of 80 µmol/24 h with range 66 to 90 µmol/24 h (23 mg/24 h, range 19 to 26) represented an average increase of about 38 µmol/24 h (11 mg/24 h). Whigham (1968) found mean values of 29, 86, and 170 µmol/24 h (8.3, 25, and 49 mg/24 h) for total 17-OGS on the control day, the day of metopirone dosage and the next day; increases over the control day of 3 and 6 times respectively. Corresponding excretions for 11-deoxy-17-OGS were 4.0, 57 and 124 µmol/24 h (1.14, 16.5 and 36 mg/24 h), increases of 14.5 and 31 fold. On both days, therefore, the relative increase of the 11-deoxy fraction was five times as great as that of the total 17-OGS.

ACTH Stimulation Tests

For many years these used highly purified animal ACTH preparations, mostly porcine. Administration of the gel was either intramuscularly, 30 units three times per day for example, or intravenously by infusion of 25 units in 500 ml saline administered over an accurately timed period of 2 or 4 h. The response was assessed either from the daily output of 17-OGS or by plasma corticosteroid estimation. ACTH gel itself had the disadvantages of uncertain standardisation and rate of release. Occasionally severe side-effects occurred, probably due to different immunological properties of ACTH from different sources. The pure synthetic product, Synacthen, avoids these disadvantages and is short acting. For more prolonged stimulation it is adsorbed onto zinc phosphate as Synacthen Depot. Three forms of Synacthen stimulation test are used for the investigation of adrenocortical function.

(a) **Short Synacthen or Synacthen Screening Test.** In this, the original form of the test (Wood *et al.*, 1965), the response is assessed by determining plasma cortisol (Mattingly technique). The patient need not fast and the test can be carried out as an out-patient procedure. With the patient at rest take 5 to 10 ml of blood into a heparinised bottle. Give 250 μg Synacthen, dissolved in about 1 ml sterile water or isotonic saline, intramuscularly into the deltoid and collect a second blood sample 30 min later and preferably a further sample at 1 h, to avoid relying on a single determination to assess the response.

Normal persons have resting levels between 220 and 720 nmol/l (mean 415) or 80 and 260 μg/l (mean 150) for bloods taken at about 0900 h with a lower limit down to about 140 nmol/l (50 μg/l) later in the day. Thirty minutes after the injection an increase of not less than 195 nmol/l (70 μg/l) with a concentration of at least 500 nmol/l (180 μg/l) regardless of initial concentration should be obtained.

This simple procedure should only be used for screening purposes. An impaired response requires investigation by more prolonged ACTH stimulation. The procedure is also of value in the serial assessment of any depression of adrenocortical function in patients who are, or have been, receiving corticosteroid therapy.

(b) **Five-hour Synacthen Test.** Landon *et al.* (1964) used a continuous infusion of 100 μg Synacthen over 5 h and determined the plasma cortisol before and at hourly intervals during the infusion. Infusion can be avoided by using Synacthen Depot. In either case the subject need not fast. Begin the test at about 1000 h and after taking the basal blood sample, inject 1 mg Synacthen Depot intramuscularly. Take further samples after 30 min and then hourly for 5 h. As serial specimens are needed it is advisable to insert an indwelling cannula. In either test, the amount of Synacthen, greatly in excess of that required for maximal response, ensures an accurate assessment of the reserve capacity of the adrenal cortex. The test gives a more thorough stimulus than the 30 min test and avoids relying on a single

Adrenocortical Function Tests

30 min sample. The plasma "cortisol" should rise to between 1 020 and 1 820 nmol/l (370 and 660 μg/l) after Synacthen Depot and to between 1 000 and 1 660 nmol/l (360 and 600 μg/l) after Synacthen infusion.

(c) **Three-day Synacthen Test.** This test for which the patient is admitted to hospital replaces the prolonged administration of ACTH gel. The test can be monitored either by daily output of total 17-OGS or in combination with the short Synacthen test and plasma cortisol determinations.

1. Collect two 24 h specimens as control urines for total 17-OGS and on days 3, 4, and 5 inject 1 mg of Synacthen Depot collecting 24 h specimens continuously over this period. James and Landon (1971) quote the following results for 25 normal subjects.

	Control	Day 3	Day 4	Day 5
μmol/24 h	47 ± 11.5	153 ± 30	204 ± 35	224 ± 39
mg/24 h	13.5 ± 3.3	44.4 ± 8.6	59.1 ± 10.1	65.0 ± 11.2

The advantage over the shorter tests is in the differentiation between primary and secondary adrenocortical insufficiency (p. 103).

2. Carry out a short Synacthen test on day 1 and then inject 1 mg of Depot Synacthen on days 1, 2 and 3. On day 4 repeat the short Synacthen test. Patients with primary adrenocortical insufficiency show no response to either short test. Those with secondary adrenal atrophy will show some improvement on the second test but Depot Synacthen may need to be administered for some time before an adequate response is obtained.

Dexamethasone Suppression Test

Since the output of ACTH is normally controlled by the production of cortisol by the adrenal, administration of exogenous glucocorticoid suppresses ACTH secretion. Cortisol itself can be used but an oral dose of about 100 mg/day is required to suppress the normal production. This dose gives approximately 40 mg/day of metabolites estimated as total 17-OGS. The synthetic steroid prednisolone (XLVII) has a potency about four times and dexamethasone (9α-fluoro-16α-methylprednisolone, XLVI), approximately 50 times that of cortisol. Thus 2 mg/day of dexamethasone can suppress the normal pituitary but the effect of its metabolites on the total 17-OGS excretion is minimised and as dexamethasone possesses a methyl substituent at C-16, the methylene group normally present in this position is not available to take part in the Zimmermann reaction.

Two forms of dexamethasone suppression test are used. A short test involves administration of a single dose just before midnight followed by a plasma cortisol estimation at 0900 h the following morning. The prolonged test involves giving the steroid over several days followed by the determination of 17-OGS.

90   *Practical Clinical Biochemistry*

Procedure 1. Give a single oral dose of 1 or 2 mg between 2200 and 2400 h. Pavlatos *et al.* (1965) used 1 mg and collected a specimen of blood at 0800 h. For normal individuals the usual range of plasma cortisol (Porter-Silber method), 280 to 670 nmol/l (101 to 243 μg/l), was reduced to 125 nmol/l (45 μg/l) after dexamethasone. Similar values were obtained for obese patients and those suffering from disease other than Cushing's syndrome. James and Landon (1971) used a 2 mg dose of dexamethasone under similar conditions and regarded plasma cortisol figures of less than 180 nmol/l (65 μg/l) at 0900 h as a normal response, representing a fall of at least 70 per cent from the basal level.

Neither method differentiates between the different causes of Cushing's syndrome but they are useful screening tests in differentiating simple obesity from them.

Procedure 2. For this investigation the patient is admitted to hospital. Successive 24 h collections of urine are required. Collect two basal 24 h specimens for total 17-OGS estimation, then give 0.5 mg of dexamethasone 6 hourly (2 mg/day) for 2 to 3 days, followed by doses of 2 mg 6 hourly (8 mg/day) for a further period of 2 to 3 days if Cushing's syndrome is strongly suspected.

In normal subjects urinary total 17-OGS fall to less than 172 μmol/day (5 mg/day) irrespective of control levels when the lower dose is used whereas over 90 per cent of patients with Cushing's syndrome whatever the aetiology fail to respond at this level. The higher dose is used to differentiate Cushing's syndrome due to hyperplasia from the other causes (see later p. 95).

THE STUDY OF ADRENOCORTICAL DYSFUNCTION

The determination of plasma cortisol and urinary 17-OS and 17-OGS alone or in combination with stimulation and suppression tests forms the basis of the investigation of adrenal dysfunction. Complications arise in cases where the steroids are not the usual ones. Plasma cortisol determinations may include other circulating steroids and urinary total 17-OGS do not only include cortisol metabolites. In normal persons the two upper pathways from XIV and XV in Fig. 2,2 are minor contributors and 17-OGS largely reflect cortisol metabolite excretion. But with a negative feed-back system, any reduction in cortisol production increases ACTH output and if the reduction is due to an enzyme block in the cortisol synthetic pathway, precursors produced before the block must increase. These will be catabolised and excreted. Often the excretions of 17-OS and total 17-OGS are then much greater than in diseases where the symptoms are due to overproduction of cortisol.

Adrenocortical Hyperfunction

This includes congenital adrenal hyperplasia (CAH) and other causes of virilism, Cushing's syndrome, hyperaldosteronism and certain extra-adrenal

Adrenocortical Function Tests 91

disorders. CAH is usually due either to 21-hydroxylase deficiency resulting in increased production along the pathway from XIV (Fig. 2,2) or to 11-hydroxylase deficiency with increased activity along the pathway from XV. Cases of adrenocortical carcinoma occur with one or other of these enzyme deficiencies. Both CAH and adrenal carcinoma may produce virilising effects but some milder cases of virilism have still other changes in adrenal function. In Cushing's syndrome there is overproduction of cortisol from adrenocortical hyperplasia, adenoma or carcinoma. It may also be seen in a severe form as the "ectopic ACTH syndrome" associated with extra-adrenal tumours (p. 102). CAH, virilism and Cushing's syndrome can be investigated by the procedures described earlier.

The metabolites of aldosterone are not included in the urinary 17-OGS so that different techniques have to be used in studying patients with hyperaldosteronism. Plasma aldosterone concentration is very low and best measured by immunological methods. The controlling mechanism is different (p. 83) but radio-immunoassay methods are available for angiotensin and renin. Hypersecretion can result either from an adrenal tumour, usually an adenoma, or from increased stimulation of a normal cortex by the renin-angiotensin mechanism. The former condition occurs in primary aldosteronism (Conn's syndrome) and is characterised by moderate increases in plasma and urinary aldosterone concentrations with feed-back suppression of plasma renin and angiotensin levels. The presence of hypokalaemia and metabolic alkalosis helps in the diagnosis. Increased secretion due to increased plasma renin and angiotensin concentrations is seen in secondary aldosteronism in which the output of aldosterone may be greater than in Conn's syndrome. Secondary aldosteronism may arise in the nephrotic syndrome, cirrhosis of the liver, congestive cardiac failure and severe hypertension. In some cases a hypokalaemic alkalosis is again present.

Congenital Adrenal Hyperplasia

21-Hydroxylase deficiency. This type of CAH occurs in two forms. Both produce virilism but in the more serious form there is also salt loss. This can cause death within 3 to 4 weeks after birth if not diagnosed and effectively treated, whereas virilisation does not endanger life and is of varying severity. Its effects differ in the two sexes. Both may show increased somatic growth seen as increased muscularity and stature in the first decade with early closure of the epiphyses. In the female, the external genitalia may be grossly abnormal at birth causing uncertainty regarding the sex, but in less severe cases the main effect may be primary amenorrhoea. In the male, precocious genital development is seen in some, the "infant Hercules" type, but lesser changes often pass unnoticed.

The salt losing type of CAH presents as such a baby who suddenly develops vomiting and dehydration during the second week of life leading to circulatory collapse. Serum potassium is markedly increased sometimes to 7 to 9 mmol/l. At this stage 17-OS, 17-OGS and pregnanetriol determinations or even the oxygenation index may not be helpful. The production of abnormal steroids is not itself serious but they produce sodium depletion which as with any other cause of sodium loss requires immediate replacement; administration of a salt-retaining steroid such as deoxycorticosterone acetate or fludrocortisol is required. At this stage cortisol or other pituitary suppressive steroid should be withheld. Once the child's electrolyte balance has been corrected and maintained, collection of urine for steroid estimation can be delayed for 12 to 14 days by which time there will be excretion of unequivocally large amounts of 17-hydroxy-progesterone metabolites. If suppressive steroids are given before adequate time has elapsed, biochemical confirmation of salt-losing CAH can be very difficult. Table 3,1 gives the excretion of steroids obtained under different circumstances. Untreated patients with salt-losing CAH excrete large amounts of 20-oxosteroids probably derived from pregnenolone (VIII) which do not give the true purple colour of a normal 17-OS in the Zimmermann reaction but a more brick red colour. A rise in pregnanetriol excretion may be equivocal up to about 8 days but reaches 15 to 18 μmol/l (5 to 6 mg/l) urine at 14 days rising several fold more by 3 weeks when salt has been given without suppressive steroids. Obviously the 17-OGS will be high; we have seen excretion of 45 μmol/24 h (13 mg/24 h) at 21 days of life. The oxygenation index, normally about 0.15, rises rapidly from about 0.5 to more than 2 during this period. It is claimed that this determination is quicker and more reliable than pregnanetriol measurements as it can be done on random specimens of urine. It may be superior in diagnosing virilising CAH at an early age or in CAH due to 11-hydroxylase deficiency,where pregnanetriol is not increased, but is not for rapidly confirming a diagnosis of salt-losing CAH. At three weeks old the difference in pregnanetriol excretion between less than 0.3 μmol/l (0.1 mg/l) for a normal child or the child with abnormal genitalia from other causes and 60 to 90 μmol/l (20 to 30 mg/l) in the salt-repleted but unsuppressed salt-losing CAH is obvious. A 2 h incubation with glucuronidase is adequate and the result, negative or positive, can be known within 4 h of receiving the specimen.

The child with salt-losing CAH is always at risk from a sudden crisis due to severe sodium deficiency in association with a relatively mild infection or inadvertent reduction of salt intake. It is easy to underestimate the usual amount of salt these children take and rapid deterioration may occur if the child is taken away from his family environment. It is also necessary to increase the steroid intake temporarily above the usual maintenance dose. The need can be monitored by following the pattern of steroid excretion. See also Hill (1961).

Virilising congenital adrenal hyperplasia. Though not potentially fatal, early diagnosis is desirable so that treatment can be started to ensure proper bone growth and development.

In the *female* if anatomical deformity is present at birth the oxygenation index may be more reliable for diagnosis than the rather low excretion of

Adrenocortical Function Tests

pregnanetriol. Preliminary borohydride reduction includes 17-hydroxy-pregnanolone in the pregnanetriol estimation and helps to make the estimation more reliable at this time. The female presenting with primary amenorrhoea due to CAH usually shows the highest levels of urinary 17-OGS and 17-OS, sometimes over $350 \mu mol/24$ h $(100$ mg/24 h) (Table 3,1). GLC shows the 17-OS to be DHA and its metabolites with derivatives of 17-hydroxy-pregnenolone. 17-OGS are overestimated in the standard procedure since the product, aetiocholanolone, has a greater colour equivalent than the 11-hydroxy derivative (p. 56). Pregnanetriol excretion

TABLE 3,1

Urinary Steroid Excretion in 21 Patients with Congenital Adrenal Hyperplasia

Case No.	Age	17-OS†		17-OGS†		Pregnanetriol A				Pregnanetriol B			
	days	(a)	(b)	(a)	(b)	(a)	(b)	(c)	(d)	(a)	(b)	(c)	(d)
I Untreated salt-losing patients													
1	8	26	7.5	28	8.0	3.9	1.3	18	6.0	11	3.6	49	16.5
	16	24	7.0	45	13.0	9.8	3.3	66	22.0	27	9.0	178	60
2	17	23	6.7	39	11.2	6.9	2.3	13	4.2				
3	2							3	1.0				
	8					1.3	0.44	24	8.0	2.4	0.8	45	15
	18					4.8	1.6	13	4.2	5.7	1.9	15	5.0
II Virilised patients													
i Infants													
4	6 months							36	12				
5	7 months							21	7.2				
ii Precocious puberty (males)													
6		54	15.5	138	40	43	14.5						
7		35	10.3	91	26.5	27	9.2						
8		42	12.2	107	31	50	16.8						
9		36	10.5	117	34	44	14.6			53	17.9		
10		130	38	169	49								

		17-OS†		17-OGS†		Pregnanetriol			
		(a)	(b)	(a)	(b)	(a)	(b)	(a)	(b)
iii Primary amenorrhoea (females)									
11 Cases	mean	185	53.7	263	76.7	100	33.3	128,285, 345	43,96, 115
	range	89-380	26-110	124-585	36-170	36-163	12.2-55	(3 cases)	

(a) $\mu mol/24$ h (b) mg/24 h (c) $\mu mol/l$ (d) mg/l
A = pregnanetriol determination without borohydride reduction.
B = preliminary borohydride reduction, results include 17-hydroxypregnanolone. In the 3 amenorrhoea cases the mean percentage increase was 86.
†17-OS = 17-oxosteroids; †17-OGS = 17-oxogenic steroids.

94 *Practical Clinical Biochemistry*

may be over 150 μmol/24 h (50 mg/24 h) and if 17-hydroxypregnanolone is included may exceed 300 μmol/24 h (100 mg/24 h).

The *male* patient is rather more difficult to identify at birth but may present at early school age with precocious growth, a bone age greatly in excess of actual age and radiological evidence of early epiphyseal closure but the clinical pattern varies. A boy of 5 years old has been seen with a bone age of 14 but another 16-year-old patient, with two sisters with CAH, was almost 6 feet tall yet excreted 250 μmol/24 h (72 mg/24 h) of 17-OS, 360 μmol/24 h (105 mg/24 h) of 17-OGS and 120 μmol/24 h (40 mg/24 h) of pregnanetriol.

The suppression test is positive and shows that the abnormal steroid output is due to CAH and not an adrenal adenoma or carcinoma. It is convenient to use prednisone rather than dexamethasone for this as it will usually be used in treatment later. Once an adequate dose for suppression has been found this can be continued. Then progress is assessed and the dose of prednisone adjusted by measuring steroid excretion regularly.

Plasma 11-hydroxycorticosteroids may be normal and show a diurnal rhythm; they also show a response to ACTH administration. It should be clearly understood that the steroid being measured is not all cortisol.

11-Hydroxylase deficiency. In this rare form of CAH, large amounts of metabolites of Compound S are excreted. The corresponding 17-deoxysteroid, deoxycorticosterone is also excreted in excess and causes the hypertension seen in this condition but virilisation is not prominent. The most suitable means for differentiation is the oxygenation index which is raised even when urinary pregnanetriol is normal or near normal. Again, suppression should occur with prednisone. Confusion may occur with cases of adrenal carcinoma producing Compound S. Suppression tests are negative in carcinoma but positive in CAH. One patient with a carcinoma excreted daily 17-OS, 520 μmol (150 mg); total 17-OGS, over 1 050 μmol (300 mg), including large amounts of tetrahydro S. However, pregnanetriol excretion was only 45 μmol (15 mg) and there was no clinical evidence of excessive cortisol production. Total 17-OGS excretion was over 2 400 μmol/24 h (700 mg/24 h) terminally.

Adrenal Virilism Not Due to Congenital Adrenal Hyperplasia

Virilism due to congenital enzyme deficiencies has been discussed. Acquired virilism is seen in some cases of adrenal carcinoma. Patients with Cushing's syndrome usually have only mild symptoms of virilism. The virilising effects are usually due to an increased plasma testosterone concentration arising from ACTH responsive tissue. The amount is only small so that urinary excretion of total 17-OS in many cases is normal or only slightly increased. The best method for demonstrating excess androgen production is to determine plasma testosterone and androstenedione. Urinary testosterone is less suitable because other metabolic transformations may produce an increase. If the overproduction is adrenal in origin

Adrenocortical Function Tests

the products will be mainly DHA and its sulphate so at near normal 17-OS excretion the proportion of DHA increases greatly. DHA determinations (Fotherby, 1959) require care with the method of hydrolysis as it is not excreted as glucuronide. Androgens also arise from the polycystic ovary in the Stein-Leventhal syndrome.

Simple virilism usually affects females in early reproductive life producing excessive hirsutism. Although 17-OS excretion may be normal, these patients have a higher average output than non-hirsute controls. Bush and Mahesh (1959), suggest that the cortisol/androgen ratio is genetically determined and that hirsutism occurs when this is low. This is confirmed using the ratio of total 17-OGS to 17-OS output. The normal ratio of 0.8 to 1.2 falls to 0.2 to 0.5 in simple virilism. A low ratio with hirsutism and amenorrhoea strongly suggests the diagnosis even when the 17-OS excretion is normal or near normal. Treatment with suppressive steroids such as prednisone (7.5 mg/day) often restores regular ovulatory menstrual cycles when hirsutism is accompanied by ovarian disturbances. The effect on the hirsutism is not so satisfactory.

Cushing's Syndrome

Excessive production of cortisol results in the clinical picture of Cushing's syndrome. Most cases are due to adrenocortical hyperplasia arising from overproduction of ACTH by a non-neoplastic anterior pituitary. Less common causes are adrenal adenoma or carcinoma, anterior pituitary basophil adenoma or the "ectopic ACTH syndrome". In the fully developed form, Cushing's syndrome includes hypertension, salt retention, increased appetite with truncal obesity, florid face and decreased carbohydrate tolerance with hyperglycaemia, glycosuria and increased gluconeogenesis from protein. Increased protein catabolism is shown by peripheral wasting, thinning of the skin and subcutaneous connective tissues with livid striae developing over areas where a lot of fat has been deposited, and by osteoporosis. The increased output of cortisol is not usually accompanied by increased androgenic activity and only mildly virilising effects such as slight increase in facial hair occur although secondary amenorrhoea is common. Mental changes are important in some cases. More severe forms of the disorder are seen with adrenal carcinoma or the "ectopic ACTH syndrome" when the greatly increased cortisol secretion may show sufficient mineralocorticoid activity to produce hypokalaemic alkalosis. Adrenal carcinomas also vary in their adrenal androgen production. Some cases show marked virilisation.

Investigation of Suspected Cushing's Syndrome

Tests to confirm the diagnosis first study the adrenal production of cortisol. Evidence that this is increased may be obtained by determining the plasma cortisol diurnal rhythm and urinary 17-OGS and 17-OS. If these

96 *Practical Clinical Biochemistry*

suggest a diagnosis of Cushing's syndrome a dexamethasone suppression test is done. A metopirone stimulation test should only be used when really essential to make the diagnosis since it may have severe side-effects especially in cases of adrenal tumour and of the ectopic ACTH syndrome.

Collection of specimens. Collect 24 h specimens of urine continuously throughout the whole period of the tests. Keep aliquots of each day's specimen in the refrigerator so that if needed they can be examined later. After at least one day to allow the stress arising from admission to hospital to subside, collect specimens of blood for plasma cortisol at 2400 h and 0900 h on successive days. Determine the urinary 17-OGS and 17-OS on the urine specimens.

Plasma cortisol. The normal diurnal rhythm shows minimal values around midnight rising to a maximum at about 0900 h then falling gradually during the day. An early feature of Cushing's syndrome is an increase in cortisol production during the later part of the day. The difference between the samples at 0900 h and 2400 h can be markedly reduced or absent even when the 0900 h figure is still normal. In severe cases both are increased above normal. Table 3,2 compares the results in

TABLE 3,2

Plasma Cortisol Concentrations in Patients with Cushing's Syndrome due to Adrenal Hyperplasia and in Normal Individuals

	No.	Mean (and range) plasma cortisol	
		0 900 h	2 400 h
Cushing's syndrome	32	640 nmol/l (360-1 340) [or 215 µg/l (95-325)]	610 nmol/l (420-1 250) [or 205 µg/l (140-420)]
Normals	40	580 nmol/l (280-970) [or 195 µg/l (95-325)]	195 nmol/l (45-475) [or 65 µg/l (15-160)]

Cushing's syndrome due to hyperplasia with a group of normal persons. Morning results are similar but at 2400 h only one normal had a plasma cortisol over 420 nmol/l (150 µg/l) while all but three of the patients with Cushing's syndrome had plasma values above this. Values between 1 250 and 1 950 nmol/l (450 and 700 µg/l) have been obtained in patients with adrenal hyperplasia during severe exacerbations of the syndrome. In 6 patients with adrenal tumours morning values were 650 to 1 330 nmol/l (235 to 480 µg/l) while 6 patients with the ectopic ACTH syndrome had results of 1 050 to 2 600 nmol/l (380 to 950 µg/l). In all tumour cases there was no diurnal rhythm.

Urinary 17-oxogenic steroids and 17-oxosteroids. The increase in plasma cortisol concentration in the latter half of the day would be expected to lead to increased excretion of cortisol metabolites. These are mostly 17-OGS, only a small fraction being excreted as 17-OS. Increased

Adrenocortical Function Tests

TABLE 3,3

Excretion of 17-Oxogenic Steroids and 17-Oxosteroids in Cushing's Syndrome of Differing Aetiology

Aetiology	17-OGS (upper) and 17-OS (lower)*									Total no.
	0	17.5	35	52.5	70	87.5	105	122.5	140 μmol/24 h	
	0	5	10	15	20	25	30	35	40+ mg/24 h	
Adrenal hyperplasia I			4	5	8	5	4	2	5⎫	33
	6	10	15		2				⎭	
hyperplasia II				3	4	3	2	1	1⎫	14
			1	4	2	3	2		2⎭	
Adrenal adenoma			2	1	2	2		1		8
	2	4	2							
Adrenal carcinoma									2⎫	2
									2⎭	
Ectopic ACTH syndrome				1			1		6⎫	8
	1		5		2				⎭	

* The figures refer to the number of patients whose 17-OGS and 17-OS excretion fell within different ranges.

Ranges are indicated by the figures at the head of each column: 0-17.4; 17.5-34.9; 35-52.4 μmol/24 h, etc; 0 = 0-4.9; 5 = 5-9.9 mg/24 h, etc.

production of adrenal C_{19} steroids results in a corresponding increase in 17-OS but 17-OGS are unaffected. Table 3,3 shows the distribution of excretion of these two groups of steroids in 65 of our patients (56 females and 9 males) with Cushing's syndrome of varying cause and severity. The diagnosis of hyperplasia or adenoma was made at operation in all cases. Diagnosis in the other cases relied on biopsy or autopsy findings. Only 6 patients had no increase in daily 17-OGS excretion above the upper limit of normal of 52 μmol (15 mg) for females and 70 μmol (20 mg) for males. In contrast, using the same criteria for 17-OS, only 19 patients excreted abnormal amounts, a situation quite different from that in CAH (p. 93). This increase was most apparent in adrenal carcinoma and in certain patients with hyperplasia segregated as group II in Table 3,3 and presumably arises from the variable relative activity of the cortisol and C_{19}-steroid synthetic pathways. The pattern of 17-OGS excretion is very similar in the two groups of patients with hyperplastic adrenals. Although 17-OS excretion differs there was no clinical difference between the two groups, suggesting that the C_{19}-steroids are only weakly androgenic.

Additional information comes in some cases from the ratio of 17-OGS to 17-OS excretion. This varies from 0.8 to 1.2 in normal persons but is increased after administration of ACTH or cortisol, often to over 4.5, and also rises in stress, for example after surgery, during physical illness and even, temporarily, after admission to hospital. All these increases revert to

98   *Practical Clinical Biochemistry*

normal after the treatment or the stress ceases. In Cushing's syndrome, however, the relative increase of 17-OGS over 17-OS seen in the majority of cases results in a sustained rise in the ratio, 17-OGS/17-OS. The distribution of its values is shown in Table 3,4. Normal ratios are seen in patients with adrenal hyperplasia in Group II and in patients with adrenal carcinoma but in all these the 17-OGS excretion was unequivocally increased. In the six patients with daily 17-OGS excretion less than 52 μmol (15 mg), the ratio was abnormal in five. The exception was a 3-year-old girl with a proven adrenal adenoma. In practice therefore a sustained increase in the 17-OGS/17-OS ratio *or* the 17-OGS excretion is highly suggestive of Cushing's syndrome and often both will be increased. It is apparent from Tables 3,3 and 3,4 that the results of 17-OGS and 17-OS determinations do not enable the cause of Cushing's syndrome in an individual patient to be determined, and further investigation is necessary.

TABLE 3.4

Ratio of Excretion of 17-Oxogenic Steroids to 17-Oxosteroids in Cushing's Syndrome of Differing Aetiology

Aetiology	17-OGS/17-OS ratio							
	0.5-0.9	1.0-1.4	1.5-1.9	2.0-2.9	3.0-3.9	4.0-4.9	5+	Total no.
Adrenal hyperplasia I			6	12	9	4	2	33
hyperplasia II	7	7						14
Adrenal adenoma	1			2	3	1	1	8
Adrenal carcinoma	1	1						2
Ectopic ACTH syndrome				1	3	3	1	8

Other base line investigations. Urinary free cortisol (Mattingly *et al.,* 1964) is derived from plasma cortisol not bound to protein and is thus correlated with biologically active cortisol. One of our patients excreted 30 μmol/24 h (11 mg/24 h) of cortisol out of a total 17-OGS output of approximately 140 μmol/24 h (40 mg/24 h). In the majority of cases of Cushing's syndrome, further partition of the products after the borohydride-metaperiodate sequence is unhelpful as most of the steroids are 11-hydroxylated so that the oxygenation index is normal to low. If GLC separation is used additional information can be obtained regarding the proportion of the 5α to normal 5β product but this does not, at the moment, appear to be of any additional value. A different situation arises in those adrenal tumours which release large amounts of cortisol precursors (p. 94).

Adrenocortical Function Tests 99

The use of the dexamethasone and metopirone tests in the further investigation of Cushing's syndrome. If a normal diurnal cortisol rhythm is obtained the diagnosis of Cushing's syndrome is unlikely but if clinical suspicion is high a suppression test with dexamethasone 2 mg/day is carried out measuring urinary 17-OS and total 17-OGS. Failure to suppress suggests Cushing's syndrome. If the plasma cortisol diurnal rhythm is lost and urinary 17-OS and 17-OGS outputs or ratio suggest Cushing's syndrome, the dexamethasone suppression test using 8 mg/day should be used instead. With this dose the 17-OGS output on the third day of dexamethasone expressed as a percentage value clearly differentiates hyperplasia from tumour with few exceptions; the former show an average fall to 26 per cent, whereas the latter have a mean figure of 106 per cent (Table 3,5). Higher doses of dexamethasone may suppress but carry an

TABLE 3,5

Dexamethasone Suppression Test (8 mg/day) in Cushing's Syndrome

Aetiology	No.	Mean (range) 17-OGS excretion A = μmol/24 h B = mg/24 h				100 x b/a
		Control day (a)		3rd day of dexamethasone (b)		
		A	B	A	B	
Hyperplasia	18	100 (69-178)	29.1 (20-52)	26 (9-50)	7.5 (2.5-14.5)	25.9 (7-48)
Hyperplasia (atypical)	1	112	32.5	112	32.5	100
Adrenal adenoma	8 ⎫	109 (34-252)	31.7 (10-73)	117 (48-336)	34 (14-98)	105.6 (83-144)
Adrenal carcinoma	2 ⎭					

unacceptable risk. Failure to suppress with 8 mg/day dexamethasone should be followed by an ACTH stimulation test. Although an adenoma will not usually respond, prolonged stimulation can stimulate the unaffected atrophied adrenal on the other side with misleading results. When an adrenal adenoma is of very recent onset even the short Synacthen test can give a normal response. The metopirone test is best reserved for such cases. There is no response if the patient has an adenoma but most cases of hyperplasia respond adequately. Table 3,6 shows the results in 17 patients. 17-OGS output on the day after metopirone is expressed as a percentage of the control value. Ten out of 11 patients with hyperplasia show an average threefold increase whereas in 6 patients with tumour there is a mean fall to 74 per cent. Table 3,7 shows the response for selected patients. Patients 1 to 4 with proven adrenal hyperplasia show the characteristic fall after dexamethasone and increase after metopirone, both

Practical Clinical Biochemistry

TABLE 3,6

Metopirone Stimulation Test in Cushing's Syndrome

Aetiology	No.	Mean (range) 17-OGS excretion A = μmol/24 h B = mg/24 h				
		Control day (a)		Day after metopirone (b)		100 x b/a
		A	B	A	B	
Hyperplasia	10	105 (79-138)	30.4 (23-40)	325 (195-645)	95 (57-187)	308 (204-550)
Hyperplasia (atypical)	1	180	52	163	47.5	90
Adrenal adenoma	5 ⎫	113	33	81	23.4	74
Adrenal carcinoma	1 ⎬	(38-235)	(11-68)	(15-205)	(4.5-59)	(16-164)

17-OS and total 17-OGS being affected. Patients 5 and 6, found to have adrenal hyperplasia at operation, are those showing atypical responses in Tables 3,5 and 3,6; they indicate that it is not sufficient to rely on one function test only. In the adenoma group, patient 7 was given metopirone after dexamethasone. 17-OGS excretion was unaffected after dexamethasone but fell markedly after metopirone when the patient became very ill, thus showing the danger of this test. In patient 8, 17-OS and total 17-OGS outputs were initially normal and metopirone was given before dexamethasone. Over the 16 days of the investigation steroid output increased steadily without reference to the substance administered. In patient 9 who had an adrenal carcinoma there is no response to both agents but 17-OS and 17-OGS are markedly increased.

Summary of Findings in Cushing's Syndrome

Although useful generalisations can be made about the features of the different causes of Cushing's syndrome an individual patient may show peculiarities.

Adrenocortical hyperplasia has highest incidence in women aged between 20 and 50. Onset is insidious with amenorrhoea an early symptom. At this stage the 0900 h plasma cortisol may still be normal but diurnal rhythm is lost. 17-OS excretion is usually normal but total 17-OGS are increased; less often both are increased similarly. Steroid excretion is suppressed more than 50 per cent by 8 mg/day dexamethasone and is at least doubled after administration of metopirone. The circulating ACTH level will be high normal or high and the plasma potassium decreased but not less than 3.5 mmol/l. Some patients show very marked fluctuations in steroid output and in clinical severity.

Adrenal adenoma has similar onset, age and sex distribution to hyperplasia but the plasma cortisol may be a little higher; excretion of

Response to Dexamethasone and Metopirone Tests of Selected Patients with Cushing's Syndrome of Differing Aetiology

Excretion of 17-OGS (upper) and 17-OS (lower)

A = μmol/24 h   B = mg/24 h

| | Control days | | | | Day of dexamethasone dose | | | | | | Metopirone test | | | |
| | 1 | | 2 | | 1 | | 2 | | 3 | | Day of dose | | Day after | |
	A	B	A	B	A	B	A	B	A	B	A	B	A	B
Adrenal hyperplasia														
1	95	27.5	74	21.5			32	9.3	21	6.2			325	94
	38	11.0	47	13.5			34	9.8	22	6.5			97	28
2	110	32	80	26			38	11	11	3.2			296	85
	76	22	69	20			41	12	29	8.4			155	45
3	117	34	117	34			69	20	45	13			285	82
	114	33	96	28			48	14	38	11			165	48
4	69	20	96	28			19	5.5	3	1.0			220	63
	21	6.0	22	6.5			5	1.5	7	2.0			41	12
5*	116	33.5	112	32.5	150	43	114	33	112	32.5			295	85.5
	22	6.5	21	6.0	21	6.0	19	5.5	22	6.5			50	14.5
6*	180	52	215	62	106	30	74	21.5	50	14.5			121	35
	48	14	96	28	62	18	38	11	29	8.5			41	12
Adrenal adenoma														
7	97	28	117	34	107	31	81	23.5	97	28	55	16	16	4.5
	35	10	38	11	47	13.5	48	14	48	14	24	7	7	2.0
8	38	11	41	12	83	24	86	25	100	29	52	15	62	18
	12	3.5	12	3.5	14	4.0	17	5.0	19	5.5	21	6.0	24	7.0
Adrenal carcinoma														
9	235	68	275	80	340	98	220	63	260	76	210	61	205	59
	138	40	120	35	145	42	135	39	170	50	145	42	83	24

* Patient 5 is the atypical one from Table 3,5 and patient 6 is the atypical one from Table 3,6.

102   *Practical Clinical Biochemistry*

17-OS is normal or low with normal or raised total 17-OGS. The ratio 17-OGS/17-OS is high. No response is obtained using 8 mg/day dexamethasone, and metopirone may lead to a dangerous fall in steroid output. Plasma ACTH is undetectable and the patient may show signs of failure of other pituitary functions if the suppression has been present for some time.

Adrenal carcinoma usually has a much more rapid onset and may occur in either sex at any age. Plasma cortisol is often much increased as are both 17-OS and 17-OGS excretions. In women and children, hirsutism and virilisation are usually more severe than in other types of Cushing's syndrome. There is no response to dexamethasone or metopirone and ACTH is undetectable. Electrolyte and carbohydrate disturbances may be marked.

"Ectopic ACTH syndrome". The commonest ACTH-secreting tumour is the oat-cell bronchial carcinoma occurring most commonly in middle aged or elderly men. It is one of the few types of Cushing's syndrome in which males predominate. Ectopic ACTH production has also been reported with carcinoma thymus or cervix and the carcinoid syndrome. Onset is often rapid and severe. As the subject is usually emaciated and pigmented rather than obese and florid, electrolyte and metabolic disturbances may be investigated first. Serum potassium is usually below 2.5 mmol/l and is not increased by potassium supplements. Severe alkalosis with blood pH about 7.50 and base excess about 15 mmol/l with glycosuria is also present. Plasma cortisol usually exceeds 1 400 μmol/l (500 μg/l) and may exceed 2 800 nmol/l (1 000 μg/l). 17-OS and 17-OGS excretions are very high with the proportion of free cortisol greater than is usually seen in Cushing's syndrome. There is no response to dexamethasone or metopirone and the plasma ACTH is extremely high.

Adrenocortical Hypofunction

Adequate secretion of cortisol can only be maintained if the HPA axis is intact. Adrenocortical insufficiency may arise from disease of the adrenal itself, as in Addison's disease, referred to as primary failure, whereas lack of ACTH production leads to secondary failure. They differ in that primary failure involves loss of aldosterone production whereas secretion of this hormone is relatively independent of ACTH and is little affected in secondary failure. In both cases secretion of glucocorticoids and adrenal androgens is impaired.

Primary adrenocortical failure, Addison's disease. This uncommon condition, usually of insidious onset, follows destruction of the adrenal either by tuberculosis or more often now, by an autoimmune process. The reduction in cortisol production increases pituitary stimulation by CRH through the negative feed-back control resulting in excess ACTH secretion. ACTH has some melanocyte stimulating activity so that pigmentation occurs in addition to symptoms of adrenocortical deficiency

Adrenocortical Function Tests

103

involving all three classes of activity. Thus there is often hypoglycaemia with a flat glucose tolerance curve; a tendency to lose sodium leading to dehydration and shock, with potassium retention; protein catabolism with wasting. These features result from cortisol, aldosterone and androgen deficiency respectively.

The prolonged excessive stimulation with ACTH may maintain normal basal cortisol secretion from the adrenal remnant. However, there is no reserve of response even to mild stress; this can lead to an "Addisonian crisis". It is this deficient response which must be demonstrated before the diagnosis is established. A diagnosis of Addison's disease implies lifelong replacement therapy and is a matter of grave importance.

Secondary adrenocortical failure. Failure of ACTH production due to hypothalamic or pituitary disease leads to partial adrenal atrophy. Symptoms of adrenal origin are less severe than in Addison's disease as aldosterone production is relatively well preserved. However, loss of other pituitary hormones may result in symptoms referable to hypofunction of the thyroid or gonads.

Investigation of Patients with Adrenocortical Deficiency

The diagnostic problem is to differentiate between primary and secondary adrenal failure. Also, chronically ill patients, especially those with malabsorptive states, may show some of the clinical features of Addison's disease and require recognition.

Determination of urinary 17-OS and 17-OGS is unhelpful in discriminating between these conditions. Chronically ill patients often show daily excretions of each below 17 μmol (5 mg), whereas proven cases of Addison's disease on the verge of adrenal failure may excrete 28 to 35 μmol (8 to 10 mg). The diagnostic tests based on plasma cortisol determinations are much to be preferred.

Initially carry out a diurnal rhythm study combined with a short Synacthen test as follows:

0000 h Plasma cortisol specimen.
0900 h Plasma cortisol specimen, followed by injection of 250 μg Synacthen.
0930 h Further plasma cortisol specimen.
1000 h Optional plasma cortisol specimen (p. 88).

Chronically ill patients without adrenal disease usually show some increase in plasma cortisol and an exaggerated response to Synacthen. A normal rhythm and adequate response to Synacthen, shows that the symptoms are not of primary adrenal origin. When the response is impaired further investigation is needed to differentiate primary and secondary failure. If hypopituitarism is of recent onset the adrenal may still be sufficiently sensitive to ACTH to give a normal or only a slightly reduced response 30 min after Synacthen. In such cases determination of plasma ACTH, growth hormone and gonadotrophins may be more satisfactory. An

104 *Practical Clinical Biochemistry*

insulin stimulation test may also be helpful. If pituitary failure is of longer duration plasma cortisol levels are minimal, usually lower than in Addison's disease and more prolonged stimulation is necessary before cortical responsiveness can be properly assessed.

The 5 h Synacthen test using the Depot preparation may show an adequate rise in plasma cortisol in some cases of secondary failure but if doubt remains then it is better to carry out a 3-day Synacthen test. Total lack of response clinches the diagnosis of Addison's disease. A definite but impaired response indicates secondary failure. Where secondary failure is clearly established it is desirable to carry out further tests to assess thyroid and gonadal function. If determination of ACTH is possible, it is very helpful. In cases of adrenal insufficiency, under basal conditions plasma ACTH is markedly increased in Addison's disease and CAH. Low or undetectable levels indicate dysfunction of the pituitary or the hypothalamus.

In those cases where the 5 h or 3-day Synacthen tests give a normal response further investigation of the HPA axis is suggested. The metopirone test has been used but although a normal response indicates that the feed-back mechanism is operative it gives little information concerning the patient's responsiveness to stress. This is better assessed using the insulin stimulation test. The order of increasing sensitivity of response to this stimulus is blood glucose, plasma cortisol, plasma ACTH and plasma growth hormone (see p. 85).

Patients with absent or reduced response to the 3-day Synacthen test should not be subjected to the insulin stimulation test. It can produce severe sustained hypoglycaemia.

For further, and extended, discussion of these investigations see Cope (1972).

REFERENCES

Bush, I. E. and Mahesh, V. B. (1959), *J. Endocrinol.*, **18**, 1.

Cope, C. L. (1972), *Adrenal Steroids and Disease*, 2nd edition, Pitman Medical Publishing Co., London.

Fotherby, K. (1959), *Biochem. J.*, **73**, 339.

Gold, E. M., Diraimond, V. C. and Forsham, D. H. (1960), *Metabolism*, **9**, 3.

Hill, E. (1961). In *"The Adrenal Cortex"*, editors G. K. McGowan and M. Sandler, Pitman Medical Publishing Co. Ltd., London, p. 193.

James, V. H. T. and Landon, J. (1971), *Hypothalamic-Pituitary-Adrenal Function Tests*. A Working Guide for Clinicians and Laboratory Staff, CIBA Laboratories Ltd., Horsham, Sussex.

Landon, J., James, V. H. T., Cryer, R. J., Wynn, V. and Frankland, A. W. (1964), *J. clin. Endocrinol. and Metab.*, **24**, 1206.

Liddle, G. W., Eslep, H. L., Kendall, J. W. Jr., Williams, W. C. Jr. and Townes, A. W. (1959), *J. clin. Endocrinol. and Metab.*, **19**, 875.

Mattingly, D., Dennis, P. M., Pearson, J. and Cope, C. L. (1964), *Lancet*, **2**, 585.

Pavlatos, F. Ch., Smilo, R. P. and Forsham, P. H. (1965). *J. Amer. med. Assoc.*, **193**, 96.

Whigham, W. R. (1968), *Clin. Chem.*, **14**, 675.

Wood, J. B., Frankland, A. W., James, V. H. T. and Landon, J. (1965), *Lancet*, **1**, 243.

CHAPTER 4

OESTROGENS AND PROGESTOGENS. TESTS OF GONADAL FUNCTION. FETO-PLACENTAL FUNCTION TESTS IN PREGNANCY

TWO groups of steroids, the oestrogens and progestogens, are produced in varying degree in the adrenal cortex, testis, ovary and placenta. Many of the pathways of steroid metabolism are identical for these tissues and some have already been discussed in Chapter 2. The amounts of oestrogens and progestogens secreted are greater in the female and are mainly produced by the mature ovary. The amounts secreted vary during the normal menstrual cycle. Before puberty the secretory rate is low, as it is in the adult male, and the production of both hormones diminishes about the time of the menopause. Determination of these hormones is used to give information about ovarian function.

In pregnancy there is a markedly increased production of oestrogens and progestogens. The progressive changes allow the normal development of pregnancy to be followed and the determination of these hormones is used to detect pathological changes in the fetus or placenta. A variety of other tests of fetal or placental function has been used. These are complementary and have therefore been included in this chapter.

Some disorders of male gonadal function are also included here as some of the tests are based on similar physiological principles to those used for female gonadal dysfunction.

Oestrogens

The three main oestrogens are oestrone (V), oestradiol-17β (VI) and oestriol-16α,17β (VII) (p. 46). Figure 4.1 shows their biosynthesis from androstenedione (XX) and testosterone (XXI) through the intermediate, 19-hydroxyandrostenedione (LIII). The formation of the two starting materials from cholesterol follows the pathway already described for the adrenal cortex in Fig. 2,1 in Chapter 2 and is also present in the testis. The two latter organs also produce small quantities of oestrogens. In the ovary the formation of oestriol from oestrone or oestradiol is only a minor pathway but in pregnancy an additional route for oestriol synthesis becomes available (p. 113) and this steroid becomes the major oestrogen produced.

The site of production in the ovary in the non-pregnant state is the Graafian follicle, the development of which is stimulated after puberty by follicle-stimulating hormone (FSH) secreted by the anterior pituitary. Increasing size of a particular follicle is followed by its rupture with release of the ovum. The ruptured follicle is converted into a corpus luteum

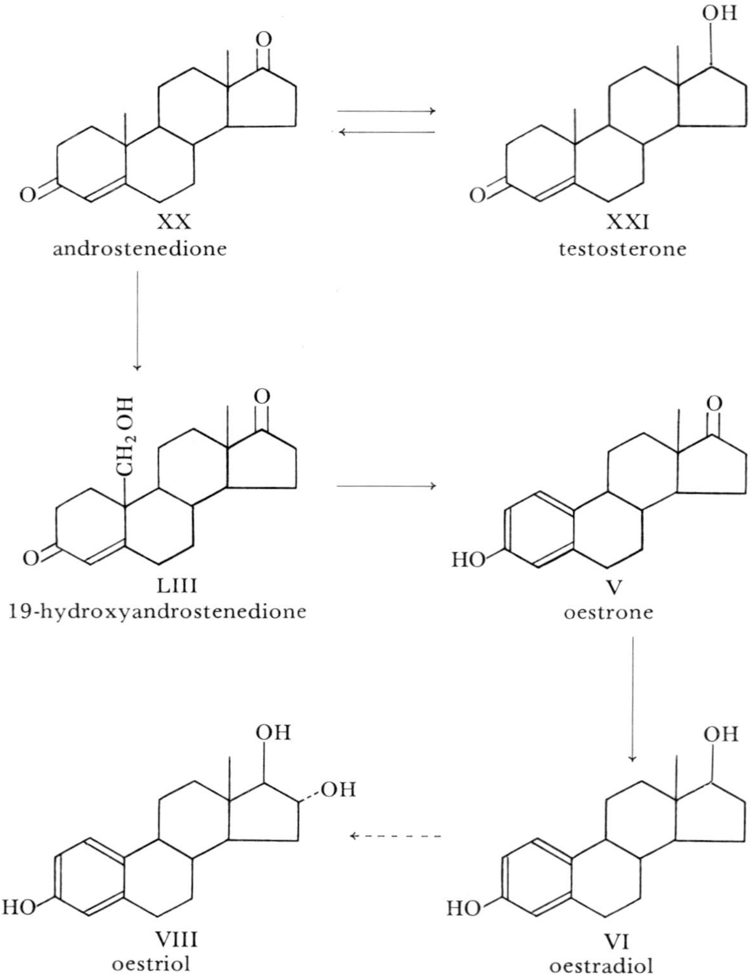

Fig. 4,1. Biosynthesis of the Oestrogens.

(yellow body), the further development of which is controlled by the anterior pituitary product, luteinising hormone (LH). The corpus luteum also secretes oestrogens.

Of the three classical oestrogens, oestradiol is biologically the most potent and accounts for most of the oestrogenic activity in the non-pregnant woman. The plasma oestrogens are mainly present in protein-bound form, probably less than 5 per cent being in the free form. Normal plasma contains all three oestrogens and oestrone is also present as its sulphate. Oestriol sulphate is present during pregnancy. Some oestradiol is converted into oestrone and oestriol during metabolism and all are excreted as conjugates, mainly glucosiduronates with some sulphates, in the urine.

Oestrogens and Progestogens   107

The relative proportion of oestriol, oestrone and oestradiol conjugates in urine is approximately 3/2/1.

The fate of radioactive oestradiol in the human female has been investigated. About 65 per cent of the radioactivity appears in the urine, 10 per cent in the faeces; the fate of the remainder is uncertain. The three main oestrogens in urine account for a third of the radioactive products excreted by this route. Urine also contains a number of other metabolites several of which are present in quantities similar to oestradiol. A wide range of oestrogen metabolites has also been isolated from normal pregnancy urine (Table 4,1). These arise by oxidation at various positions on the

TABLE 4,1
Minor Oestrogens Present in Urine

a. Modified *oestrone* molecules:

>   2-hydroxy- and 2-methoxy-
> 6α- and 6β-hydroxy-
> 11β-hydroxy-
> 15α- and 15β-hydroxy-
> 16α- and 16β-hydroxy-
>   16-oxo-
>   18-hydroxy-

b. Modified *oestradiol* -17β molecules:

>   2-methoxy-
> 6α-hydroxy-
> 15α- and 15β-hydroxy-
>   16-oxo-
>   11-dehydro-oestradiol-17α

c. Modified *oestriol* -16α, 17β molecules

>   2-methoxy-
> 15α-hydroxy-
>   oestriol-16α, 17α
>   oestriol-16β, 17α and -16β, 17β

steroid nucleus. These substances are usually less potent than the main oestrogens but 16α-hydroxyoestrone (LVIII, Fig. 4,3) is as potent as oestriol. The various oestrogen metabolites may be included in some of the extraction procedures used for urinary oestrogen determinations (p. 121) and contribute in varying degree to the "total oestrogens" figure.

Progestogens

A progestogen is a substance which brings about changes in the endometrium of the uterus after this has been under oestrogen influence. The changes are such as to favour the implantation of a fertilised ovum and its subsequent gestation. The only naturally-occurring progestogen is

108   *Practical Clinical Biochemistry*

progesterone (IX) but a number of synthetic progestogens are used therapeutically and possess some of the biological actions of progesterone with variable oestrogenic or androgenic activity in some cases. These, substances, usually in combination with a synthetic oestrogen, are widely prescribed as oral contraceptives.

The formation of progesterone in the adrenal cortex is shown in Fig. 2,1 in Chapter 2. Progesterone is a precursor of adrenocortical steroids, the androgens and oestrogens. The production and further metabolism of progesterone follows similar pathways in the adrenal cortex, testis and ovary. A small amount of progesterone may be secreted into the circulation by the adrenal cortex but the major site of secretion is from the corpus luteum of the ovary and, in pregnancy, from the placenta.

Progesterone occurs in the plasma bound to protein for the most part and is rapidly metabolised by the liver. The main change is the reduction of the unsaturated ketone grouping in ring A and of the C-20 ketone group. About 20 per cent of metabolised progesterone is excreted as pregnanediol (XXIX).

IX
progesterone

XXIX
pregnanediol

There are smaller quantities of pregnanolone (XXVIII), allopregnanolone (XXX) and allopregnanediol (XXXI) the formulae of which are given earlier (pp. 48, 49). Urinary "pregnanediol" as determined in the usual colorimetric methods may contain up to eight isomers due to stereoisomerism at positions 3, 5 and 20 but the 3α, 5β, 20α, isomer (XXIX) predominates. The fate of more than three quarters of the progesterone secreted is uncertain. Also "pregnanediol" may be derived from adrenal progesterone and from other steroids such as Δ^5-pregnenolone (VIII) (Fig. 2,1). Despite these limitations pregnanediol excretion has been used as an index of ovarian and placental production of progesterone.

Other Hormones Concerned with Gonadal Function

The role of the pituitary gonadotrophins, FSH and LH in stimulating ovarian function has already been mentioned. The same hormones are involved in the maintenance of the secretion of testosterone from the post-pubertal testis. Like other anterior pituitary hormones, their release is

Oestrogens and Progestogens

under the control of the hypothalamus and is subject to negative feed-back by the secretory products of the gonad.

A single decapeptide is produced in the hypothalamus and acts as the releasing hormone (RH) for both FSH and LH when it reaches the anterior pituitary by passing along the hypothalamic-hypophyseal portal system. The release of FSH and LH occurs within a few minutes of the arrival of LH/FSH-RH. The relative proportion of LH to FSH is probably influenced by the local balance of ovarian hormones in the anterior pituitary circulation.

Before puberty the production of the pituitary gonadotrophins is low but an early sign of the onset of puberty is a fluctuating but sub-threshold secretion of FSH and LH. Once more marked and sustained secretion occurs there is gonadal growth in both males and females and their secretion initiates development of the secondary sexual characters and, in the normal female, the onset of menstruation. The sex hormones exert a negative feed-back on the hypothalamic and anterior pituitary function in secreting FSH and LH. The more complex situation in the menstrual cycle is described below.

In the female the dwindling ovarian function at the menopause is associated with an increased release of FSH and LH as the negative feed-back control becomes less effective. The situation in the male is less abrupt but older men have higher outputs of pituitary gonadotrophins on average. Active gonadotrophins are excreted in the urine of the post-menopausal woman and may be partially purified and used therapeutically under the name of human menopausal gonadotrophin (HMG).

An additional source of gonadotrophin is present in pregnancy and is secreted by the chorionic membrane produced at the earliest stages of fetal development. The product, referred to as human chorionic gonadotrophin (HCG), is responsible for maintaining the corpus luteum in the early stages of pregnancy and hence for ensuring the continued and increasing secretion of progesterone before the placenta is formed and is able to take over this function. HCG is excreted in the urine and its detection affords a method for the early diagnosis of pregnancy. It is also produced by abnormal chorionic tissue, such as hydatidiform mole and chorion carcinoma, and is used for detection of such states.

Hormonal Changes during the Normal Menstrual Cycle

Cyclical changes occur in oestrogens, progesterone, FSH, LH and hypothalamic activity during the menstrual cycle. The changes are well documented but the details of control are still not fully understood (Fig. 4,2).

The average length of the cycle is 28 days, the first day being the day of onset of the menstrual flow. Ovulation occurs on average on the 14th day. The period up to ovulation is the proliferative phase and the remainder of the cycle is the luteal phase. During the proliferative phase a Graafian

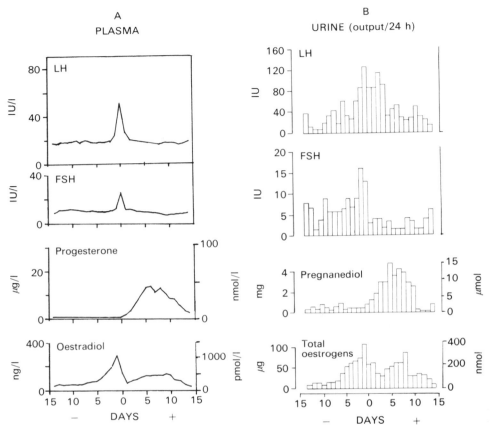

Fig. 4,2. Hormonal Changes During the Normal Menstrual Cycle.
A — Plasma median concentrations (after Kletzky et al., 1975).
B — Urinary mean excretion (after G. D. Searle Ltd.).
Day 0 represents the day of the LH peak.

follicle enlarges and eventually ruptures and in the same phase the endometrium undergoes changes. Initially the superficial layer is shed during the menstrual flow but then proliferation occurs and the endometrium thickens. Following ovulation, the luteal phase is characterised by the formation of the corpus luteum and the further thickening and glandular development of the endometrium to prepare it for the implantation of an ovum which has been fertilised and undergone early development during its passage down the Fallopian tube.

At the start of the cycle the circulating level of oestrogens and progesterone is low and the anterior pituitary releases increasing quantities of FSH and LH. These, but especially FSH, stimulate the development of several follicles but usually only one is selected for eventual rupture. The developing follicle produces an increasing output of oestrogen with some

Oestrogens and Progestogens 111

depression of FSH and LH output. Towards the end of the follicular phase the rapidly growing follicle produces an exponential rise in oestrogen production. This triggers by positive feed-back an abrupt release of LH/FSH-RH from the hypothalamus and an abrupt pituitary release of LH and FSH. A final growth spurt of the follicle results with rupture and ovulation about 30 hours later. The pre-ovulatory peak of oestrogens is followed by a fall. LH activity assists in the formation and early maintenance of the corpus luteum in the luteal phase. Progesterone, which has been present in low concentration in the plasma during the follicular phase, now appears in increasing quantities over the next 4 or 5 days reaching a peak shortly after the middle of the luteal phase. A second peak of oestrogens occurs around this time. This is probably secreted by the corpus luteum but some may come from follicles which were stimulated but did not rupture. This increasing output of oestrogens and progesterone suppresses FSH and LH release and the corpus luteum which relies on LH for its support starts to decay. As it does so there is a rapid fall in the levels of oestrogens and progesterone. This is associated with spasm of the arterioles supplying the superficial layers of the thickened endometrium leading to their sloughing with haemorrhage as the cycle ends.

Hormonal and Structural Changes during Normal Pregnancy

The endometrial changes brought about by progesterone secreted by the corpus luteum provide a suitable structure in which the blastocyst derived from the fertilised ovum can be embedded. The process is aided by the trophoblastic layer of the chorion derived from the embryo which invades the endometrium.

This layer secretes HCG which is detectable by the time of the first missed period and is instrumental in preserving the corpus luteum and its secretions. As the pregnancy progresses the placenta is formed for the proper nutrition of the developing fetus. This structure has maternal and fetal components. The latter, the chorionic villi, are derived from the chorion. The fetus develops within the amniotic sac, the wall of which is derived from fetal ectoderm. As the sac expands this cellular wall comes to be in close contact with the chorion to form the fetal membrane within which lies the amniotic fluid. The volume is about 60 ml at the 12th week, 200 ml at the 16th week but increases to an average of about one litre at term.

This fluid is constantly being secreted and removed. In the first half of pregnancy its volume is closely correlated with fetal size. Its composition in so far as electrolytes and small diffusable molecules is concerned, is very similar to that of fetal extracellular fluid from which it is separated only by the fetal skin. It is thought to be derived by diffusion through the fetal surface which is freely permeable at this stage (Lind, 1975). There is a small contribution from the fetal urine. In the second half of pregnancy, the fetal skin becomes thickened and impermeable, so that the amniotic fluid is

112 *Practical Clinical Biochemistry*

isolated from the fetal body fluids. Its composition changes towards that of fetal urine which is excreted into the fluid. It also receives materials from the fetal lungs and stomach. Cells of fetal origin, probably mainly from the skin, can be recovered from the amniotic fluid. The daily turnover of fluid is of the order of 25 to 30 per cent of its total volume. Some fluid is swallowed by the fetus, some passes through the wall of the amniotic sac into the maternal circulation. Amniocentesis, the collection of a sample of amniotic fluid by puncturing the sac, can give information about biochemical changes in the fetus as discussed later for amniotic fluid bilirubin, phospholipids and α-fetoprotein. The fetal cells recovered from the fluid may permit the detection of fetal sex and certain genetic defects of chromosomal structure or biochemical function. Some serious genetic disorders are detectable at a stage early enough for the termination of pregnancy to be performed if ethically justified.

The hormonal changes in pregnancy vary with the stage to which this has progressed. The changes involve maternal, placental, ovarian and pituitary function but the fetal chorion and the fetal adrenal and liver also play a role.

HCG secretion increases steadily to reach a maximum at the 8th to 9th week and then falls steadily to about a tenth of the maximal concentration by the 17th week when it remains relatively constant to term. This reflects the developing function of the placenta and the dwindling importance of the corpus luteum once placental production of hormones is established. Pituitary gonadotrophins, particularly LH, also continue to increase in the maternal circulation in pregnancy reaching a maximum about the 12th week and then falling.

Progesterone secretion in the late luteal phase of the cycle in which conception occurs does not fall but remains at the peak value or slightly increases further until the 12th week, when it starts to rise reaching a maximum at 36 to 38 weeks and falls before the onset of labour. Very little progesterone is detectable one week post-partum. The production is mainly from the corpus luteum during the first 12 weeks after which the placenta is progressively the major source eventually secreting about 250 mg daily.

Oestrogens also remain at the luteal peak until the 5th week when they start to rise with increasing rapidity up to the 20th week and then rise slowly to term. There is a rapid fall to non-pregnant levels within 5 days post-partum. The magnitude of the total rise is considerable and near term oestrogen excretion may be 1 000 times that in the non-pregnant state. The major part of this increase is due to oestriol, the formation of which requires both maternal and fetal tissues as indicated in Fig. 4,3. 17α-Hydroxypregnenolone (XIII) is formed from the progesterone precursor, pregnenolone (VIII, Fig. 2,1), in the placenta and is transported to the fetus where it is converted in the fetal adrenal to DHA sulphate (LIV) by loss of the groups at C-17 and sulphation. The fetal liver is able to convert (LIV) to its 16α-hydroxy-derivative (LV). Both these sulphated 17-oxosteroids when transported back to the placenta are hydrolysed by

Oestrogens and Progestogens

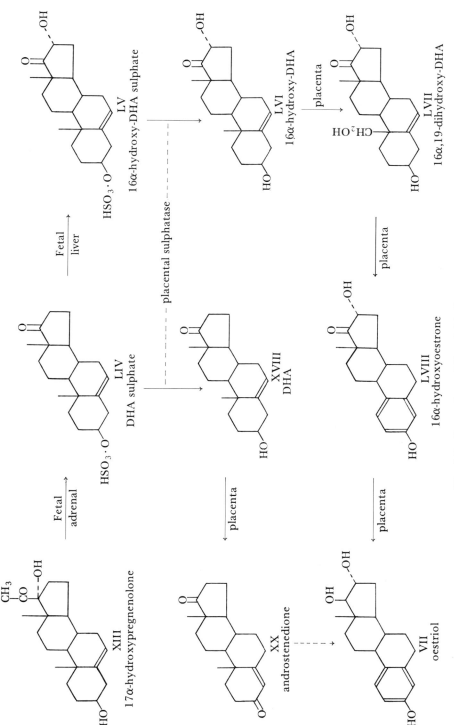

Fig. 4.3. Formation of Oestriol in Pregnancy.

114 *Practical Clinical Biochemistry*

placental sulphatase to DHA (XVIII) and 16α-hydroxy-DHA (LVI) respectively. The DHA is converted into androstenedione (XX) in the placenta and thence to oestrone and oestradiol as outlined in Fig. 4,1. The major route is, however, from 16α-hydroxy-DHA which is converted in the placenta into oestriol (VII) in several steps indicated in Fig. 4,3. The enormous increase in oestriol synthesis thus requires normal functioning of the placenta and of the fetal pituitary, adrenal cortex and liver.

Oestriol is excreted in the maternal urine as the glucosiduronate and, to a lesser extent, as the sulphate. Oestriol is also present in the fetal circulation mainly as the sulphate (85 per cent) with traces (1 per cent) of the glucosiduronate. Amniotic fluid contains oestriol glucosiduronate (50 per cent), unconjugated oestriol (35 per cent) and oestriol sulphate (15 per cent). Much is derived from fetal urine which contains a much higher proportion of glucosiduronate than does fetal blood. This diffuses only slowly from the amniotic fluid but the sulphate is hydrolysed to free oestriol by sulphatases in the fetal membranes.

TESTS OF GONADAL FUNCTION

It is convenient to consider tests of function of both male and female gonads together as a number of clinical problems are similar in both sexes as are the principles of the methods used to investigate gonadal function. In the female however, the final products of ovarian secretion are oestrogens and progesterone while testosterone is the product in the male.

Clinical Problems Associated with Disordered Gonadal Function

These are discussed in outline here and the results of the various function tests are described later after the practical details of the methods have been recorded.

In the Female

These are mainly disorders of puberty, disorders of menstruation and infertility.

Puberty is a process extending over a few years. The first sign is usually breast development, commencing in this country between the ages of 8.5 and 13 years. This is followed by the growth of pubic and then axillary hair with a growth spurt in body height and weight. Usually these features precede the first menstruation, the menarche, which occurs in the majority of girls by the age of 16. The pubertal process including the menarche may occur at a much earlier age, *precocious puberty*. In contrast, all the pubertal changes may be delayed long beyond the usual time, *delayed puberty*. In these cases menstruation never commences, *primary*

Gonadal Function Tests 115

amenorrhoea, although sometimes pubertal changes seem to be developing in a normal fashion but the menarche does not occur. The normal process involves the orderly development of hypothalamic, anterior pituitary and ovarian functions. The various glands may be anatomically abnormal and fail to produce their characteristic secretion or they may be exposed to abnormal influences from other parts of the body. Gonadal function tests help to define the origin of the disorder.

Disorders of the menstrual cycle and menstrual flow include alterations in the length or regularity of the cycle and the volume of the menses, normally 30 to 180 ml. Disorders include failure of ovulation also. *Anovular cycles* which are otherwise apparently normal occur with varying frequency. Often the length of an anovular cycle is shortened to 20 to 24 days but menstrual flow is normal. An abnormally long cycle often lasting 6 to 8 weeks, *oligomenorrhoea,* is associated with a prolonged follicular phase, ovulation and a normal luteal phase. In severe oligomenorrhoea, menstruation may occur only three times a year and ovulation is unusual. This condition merges into *secondary amenorrhoea,* a cessation of periods for more than six months. Disorders of the menstrual cycle involving profuse loss with alterations in length of cycle may arise from obvious organic disease but when this cannot be demonstrated it is usually classed as *dysfunctional uterine haemorrhage.*

The disorder of *female infertility* can have a number of causes. After the husband has been shown to have adequate production of sperm and anatomical abnormalities in the female have been excluded, tests of gonadal function are important in assessing whether ovulation is occurring and in controlling the use of potent drugs used to try to initiate ovulation.

In the Male

As in the female, the process of puberty is extended over a period of time. The earliest signs are usually an increase in the size of the testes and scrotum, followed by penile growth, the development of pubic hair with a male distribution and of axillary hair. The somatic growth spurt in males is usually later than in females. There is no sudden change to correspond to the menarche but an increasing ability to produce an ejaculate containing viable spermatozoa.

As in the female there may be *precocious puberty* or *delayed puberty.* Failure to produce a sufficient number of normal spermatozoa is seen in *male infertility.* Some cases are due to anatomical abnormalities but in others disordered function of the pituitary or testis may be involved. A further disorder, not necessarily related to infertility is *impotence.* In some patients, breast tissue may undergo development due to various tumours or disorders of function of other organs leading to *gynaecomastia.* The various gonadal function tests are of assistance in the investigation of these conditions in the male.

Practical Clinical Biochemistry

Principles Involved in Gonadal Function Tests

As is the case with adrenocortical function (Chap. 3), a proper assessment of the hypothalamic — anterior pituitary — gonadal axis may involve the stimulation of the different organs involved and the determination of their secretions or the consequences of such secretions.

In the case of the ovary the two different products, the oestrogens and progesterone may either be determined as such in plasma, or the excretion of their metabolites in urine may be assessed. Progesterone production is indicative of ovulation and the formation of a corpus luteum. In the male, the primary hormone, testosterone, is best measured in the plasma. Although it is metabolised and excreted in the urine as a 17-oxosteroid (17-OS), the contribution of adrenal androgens to total 17-OS excretion is greater than the testicular one (Chap. 2). Fractionation of the 17-OS fraction is also not helpful as testosterone and adrenal androgens produce common metabolites.

In cases where gonadal secretion is inadequate, a differentiation between primary gonadal failure and failure to secrete gonadotrophins leading to secondary gonadal failure, has to be made. This is sometimes possible by measuring FSH and/or LH in the plasma. Reduced secretion as a consequence of anterior pituitary or hypothalamic disease may be difficult to differentiate from low normal values with some present methods but abnormally high figures are seen with a normal hypothalamus and pituitary released from negative feed-back suppression by primary gonadal failure. This is the normal state of affairs in women after the menopause but the situation is more variable in older males. The gonad may also be directly stimulated for diagnostic purposes or in the treatment of infertility where there is the potential for normal gonadal function. Although FSH has been used for diagnostic methods, the clinical use in the induction of ovulation has usually employed other gonadotrophins. Maturation of the follicle is achieved using a preparation of HMG (Pergonal) and final rupture with ovulation requires a much larger dose of HCG.

Such dynamic tests of ovarian function can be extended to test hypothalamic and anterior pituitary function. Now that LH/FSH-RH is available it can be administered and the ability of the pituitary to release FSH and LH can be assessed by direct measurement of these hormones in plasma. Differentiation between hypothalamic and anterior pituitary disorders is not always possible by this method but stimulation of the hypothalamus can be achieved using the triarylethylene product clomiphene citrate (Clomid)

$$C_2H_5\diagdown N\text{-}CH_2 . CH_2 . O\text{—}\langle\text{—}\rangle\text{—}C\text{=}C . C_6H_5$$
$$C_2H_5\diagup \qquad \qquad Cl | \qquad C_6H_5$$

clomiphene

Gonadal Function Tests

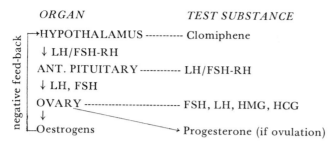

Fig. 4,4. Dynamic Tests of Ovarian Function.

This substance is thought to interfere with the suppression of the hypothalamic release of LH/FSH-RH by oestrogens. It therefore allows the hypothalamic-pituitary connection to be tested by measuring the release of FSH and LH, or in some cases, the amount of circulating oestrogen or testosterone. Clomiphene is also used in the treatment of some cases of infertility.

The various steps in the control and investigation of ovarian function are shown in Fig. 4,4.

Analytical Methods for Basal Secretion Studies

The main methods involve the determination of the gonadal hormones themselves and the pituitary gonadotrophins, LH and FSH. These substances are measured either in plasma or in urine where they are often present as metabolites. In many cases, the basal secretion of these hormones gives sufficient information, but if necessary, these studies can be supplemented by dynamic studies (p. 139).

Determination of Oestrogens in Plasma

Whereas the determination of urinary oestrogens is well-established, the low concentrations in plasma have required the development of highly sensitive and specific techniques. Much of the literature has therefore been concerned with investigations using urine.

Oestrogens occur in plasma in low concentrations and in several different forms. The three major oestrogens, oestrone (E1), oestradiol (E2) and oestriol (E3) occur also as conjugates. The unconjugated steroids circulate bound to plasma proteins. In particular, E2 is bound to sex-hormone binding globulin (SHBG) which also binds other 17β-hydroxysteroids, especially testosterone. Methods for plasma oestrogen determination may measure several compounds together or concentrate on one oestrogen only, usually E2 in studies in non-pregnant patients. A similar situation exists for oestrogen measurements in urine (pp. 122, 158).

The first suitable analytical methods used fluorimetry, isotope dilution, or gas-liquid chromatography (see Loraine and Bell, 1971). They were

118   *Practical Clinical Biochemistry*

relatively complex and insensitive and have been almost entirely superseded by competitive protein binding (CPB) and radioimmunoassay (RIA) techniques (Chap. 5, Vol. 1). Most methods employ a preliminary extraction of plasma with an organic solvent. This breaks the weak binding to plasma proteins but conjugates are not extracted into non-polar solvents. Further chromatographic purification of the extract may be required depending on the specificity of the antiserum or other protein used in the assay. Onikki and Adlercreutz (1973) selectively precipitated hormones bound to SHBG before making an extract from this.

The CPB technique for E2 was used first and has been gradually modified (Murphy, 1968; Shutt, 1969; Corker *et al.*, 1970; Korenman *et al.*, 1970; Ahmed and Mester, 1973; Pratt *et al.*, 1974). Most authors use a rabbit uterine cytosol as the binding protein for E2. The binding affinity is greater for this protein than for artificially raised antisera but other substances, including clomiphene, can also bind. Tritium-labelled E2 has usually been used as the competing labelled molecule. Since their initial introduction (Jaing and Ryan, 1969; Abraham *et al.*, 1970; Mikhail *et al.*, 1970) the RIA methods have been improved by developing more specific antisera. The oestrogens themselves are not antigenic but become so when covalently linked to a protein, usually bovine serum albumin (BSA). The position on the steroid nucleus at which the linkage is made is important. If a characteristic group is employed to create the linkage it is only poorly recognised by the antiserum and hence discrimination between steroids differing in respect of the characteristic group may be poor. Thus E2 possesses two characteristic hydroxyl groups at C-3 and C-17β. If either of these is converted to the hemisuccinate and then linked to BSA, some specificity is lost. Thus E2-17β-succinyl-BSA produces antibodies which cross react with E1 (71 per cent), E2-17α (42 per cent) and E3 (12 per cent) making a chromatographic separation step essential (Schiller and Brammall, 1974). Such lack of specificity may be employed to measure a group of oestrogens including metabolites in a crude methanolic plasma extract as "plasma E2 equivalent" (Wu *et al.*, 1973).

More specific antisera have used steroid antigens linked at C-6 or C-11 thus leaving the determinants in rings A and D intact. Kuss and Goebel (1972) prepared the 6-carboxymethoximes of E1, E2 and E3 and used these to form an amide link to the lysine amino groups in BSA. Antisera to E2-6-carboxymethoxime-BSA are highly specific and only cross react significantly with C-6 substituted-E2. (Doerr *et al.*, 1973; Exley and Moore, 1973; Loriaux *et al.*, 1973.) Although such steroids occur in urine (Table 4,1) they are probably not present in significant amounts in plasma. Linkage to BSA using a succinyl group linked at C-11 has been used for 11α-hydroxy-E2 (Onikki and Adlercreutz, 1973) and for 11β-hydroxy-E2 (England *et al.*, 1974). The antiserum to the 11β variant seems to have the higher specificity. The most specific antisera can be used on simple benzene extracts of plasma without further purification.

While many workers have used tritiated E2 for the assay, it is possible to use radio-iodine labelled products which are easier to count (Chap. 8,

Gonadal Function Tests

Vol. 1). Thus England *et al.* (1974) conjugated the hemisuccinate of 11β-hydroxy-E2 with tyrosine methyl ester and then radio-iodinated the tyrosine group. Lindberg and Edqvist (1974) found that iodination of ring A of the oestrogen could lead to loss of immunoreactivity and preferred to conjugate E2-6-carboxymethyloxime with ^{125}I-tyramine.

The practical details for performing these assays are outside the scope of this book. They vary with each author and with the particular antiserum used. The original papers should be consulted.

Normal Ranges. Only ranges in males and in the normal menstrual cycle of adult ovulating women are discussed here. Ranges at other ages and in pathological states are amalgamated with other hormonal findings later.

Table 4,2 shows the wide variation in E2 levels seen in apparently normal females. Each author reports a relatively wide range at any stage of the menstrual cycle and there is some disagreement between authors. In part this may be due to the use of different antisera but most figures are based on relatively few cycles. Also Kletzky *et al.* (1975) have shown that the E2 figures at any stage of the cycle are not distributed in a Gaussian fashion but are better represented as a "log normal" distribution (Chap. 9, Vol. 1). They give the 95 per cent ranges and median figures for each day in 22 women. For comparison with Table 4,2 they find these figures to be: early follicular, 41 to 470 (median 137) pmol/l (11 to 128 (37) ng/l); late follicular, 74 to 1 000 (median 270) pmol/l (20 to 270 (74) ng/l). In general the lowest figures occur at the very end and beginning of the cycle with a progressive increase after day 6 to the ovulatory peak. The wide variation of peak level is partly due to its relatively short duration and the true peak may be missed if samples are only collected every 24 h. Thorneycroft *et al.* (1974) record 4 hourly readings for E2 and other hormones in 4 normal women around the period of ovulation. In all cases the E2 peak preceded that of LH which is believed to be followed very quickly by ovulation. In two cases the E2 figures were declining by the time the LH surge commenced; this LH peak lasts on average 48 h. Abraham *et al.* (1972), measuring plasma concentrations daily, reported that the E2 peak preceded the LH peak by one day in 6 cases, by 2 days in one and occurred on the same day in two. These relationships are of importance in assessing the period when conception is most likely.

Few figures for other oestrogens are available in the normal cycle. E1 shows similar changes to E2 but they are less marked. In the early follicular phase, the figures are: 193 ± 19 (SE) pmol/l (52 ± 5 ng/l) (DeVane *et al.,* 1975) 148 ± 15 pmol/l (40 ± 4 ng/l) (Loraine and Bell, 1971), 108 ± 19 pmol/l (29 ±5 ng/l) (Kim *et al.,* 1974). The last-named authors also quote mean figures for the mid-cycle and mid-luteal phase peaks of 300 pmol/l (81 ng/l) with SE's of 33 and 70 pmol/l (9 and 19 ng/l) respectively. Loraine and Bell (1971) quote mid-cycle values of 630 (SE 48) pmol/l (170 (SE 13) ng/l). Wu *et al.* (1973) measured several oestrogens together as "plasma E2 equivalent" recording mean figures on days 11 and 27 of the cycle of 405 pmol/l (110 ng/l) which are within the ranges quoted for E2 alone.

TABLE 4,2

Plasma Oestradiol Concentrations during the Normal Menstrual Cycle

(figures are in pmol/l with ng/l in parentheses)

Phase						
Early follicular (Day 1 to 5)	37-210[7] (10-57)	44-370[3] (12-100)	115, SE = 11[4] (31, SE = 3)	115, SD = 40[6] (31, SD = 11)	110-185[1] (30-50)	230, SE = 30[2] (63, SE = 8)
Late follicular (Day 6 to day before ovulatory peak)	175-220[7] (47-60)	265, SD = 100[6] (72, SD = 27)	185-1 880[3] (50-510)			
Ovulatory peak	480-1 470[1] (130-400)	480-1 750[5] (130-475)	560-1 360[7] (153-370)	1 610, SD = 490[6] (436, SD = 132)	2 140-2 660[3] (580-720)	
Early luteal (up to 3 days after peak)	295[1] (80)	110-420[7] (30-114)	405-1 440[3] (110-390)			
Mid luteal (4 to 10 days after peak)	92-1 000[7] (25-273)	120-960[5] (33-260)	300, SE = 70[4] (81, SE = 19)	370-1 120[3] (100-310)	440[1] (120)	920, SD = 290[6] (249, SD = 79)

References: [1] Abraham *et al.*, 1972; [2] DeVane *et al.*, 1975; [3] England *et al.*, 1974; [4] Kim *et al.*, 1974; [5] Onikki and Adlercreutz, 1973; [6] Pratt *et al.*, 1974; [7] Shaaban and Klopper, 1973.

Gonadal Function Tests 121

In normal males, E2 figures are lower, as expected, and have been given as 75-250 pmol/l (20 to 68 ng/l) by Onikki and Adlercreutz (1973), 45 to 130 pmol/l (12 to 35 ng/l) by Doerr *et al.* (1973) and 124 ± 13 (SE) pmol/l (46 ± 4.9 ng/l) by Wu *et al.* (1973). The method of Doerr *et al.* was the most specific.

The plasma clearance of E2 has been estimated as 1 200 (SE 97) litres/24 h (Fraser and Baird, 1974). Multiplication by the plasma concentration gives the rate of release into the plasma at any time. Thus a mid-cycle concentration of 1.1 nmol/l (300 ng/l) would correspond to the production of 1.3 μmol (360 μg) in 24 h.

Although the characteristic E2 pattern is abolished by oral contraceptives through hypothalamic-pituitary suppression (England *et al.*, 1974) the adrenal cortex does not seem to be important in E2 production in women in their reproductive phase as indicated by the unchanged E2 levels following dexamethasone suppression of the hypothalamic-pituitary-adrenal axis (Abraham, 1974; Kim *et al.*, 1974).

The Determination of Oestrogens in Urine

The separate determination of oestrone, oestradiol and oestriol in urine in the non-pregnant state (Brown, 1955a) is laborious and for many purposes the determination of the "total oestrogens" in extracts of urine is adequate. Not all the derivatives of the three main oestrogens (Table 4,1) withstand hydrolytic conditions and some are not extracted by the standard procedures. The phrase, total oestrogens, has been used for many years, and is used here also, in the more limited sense as the mixture of oestrogens present in the extract analysed. The proportion of the different oestrogens in urine varies and oestriol greatly predominates in pregnancy urines. It is important therefore to use reaction conditions and primary standards which give similar reactions with the different oestrogens.

The oestrogens are excreted as sulphates and glucosiduronates and require hydrolysis, except where direct reactions are carried out as indicated below. Hydrolysis, using approximately 100 ml/l hydrochloric acid, presents few problems with oestrone, oestradiol and oestriol but such derivatives as 2-hydroxyoestrone and 16α-hydroxyoestrone are destroyed. Except at high dilution, glucose interferes with the hydrolysis and in diabetic pregnancy the unstable oestrogens have been shown to form a greater part of the oestrogens excreted than in normal pregnancy.

After hydrolysis and extraction of the products, further purification of the extracts presents greater problems than for neutral steroids. The oestrogens are weak acids extractable into wash reagents above a pH of about 11. Certain contaminating substances are conveniently oxidised in alkaline solution so that rather complex wash procedures have been evolved. In that of Brown (1955a), the ether extract is shaken with dilute sodium hydroxide solution into which the oestrogens pass. Then bicarbonate is added to bring the pH to about 10.5 permitting the oestrogens to be re-extracted into fresh ether.

122   *Practical Clinical Biochemistry*

Oestrone and oestradiol can be separated from the more polar oestriol by partition between a mixture of equal volumes of benzene and light petroleum (b.p. 40 to 60°C) containing 20 ml/l ethanol, firstly with water which removes oestriol and then dilute alkali which extracts oestrone and oestradiol.

Originally colour reactions were applied to such partially purified extracts. Oestrogens react with reducing phenols in the presence of sulphuric acid (600 to 750 ml/l) to give yellow complexes with a green fluorescence. Dilution of the product followed by reheating results in the formation of pink coloured compounds, a reaction originally introduced by Köber (1931) who used phenol. Brown (1952) used quinol in a technique which was thoroughly investigated by Bauld (1954). He concluded that more reliable results could be obtained for the first stage of the reaction if fresh reagents were used, or reagents to which quinol had been added immediately prior to the reaction. The concentration of acid used was important. It was later found that preliminary hydrolysis and extraction could be avoided when Ittrich (1958) showed that the product formed by direct reaction of conjugates with the reagent could be extracted into chlorinated hydrocarbons containing *p*-nitrophenol or trichloracetic acid. Depending on the level of oestrogen present, the final estimation could be made colorimetrically or fluorimetrically (Hobkirk and Metcalf-Gibson, 1963; Brown *et al.*, 1968a). Greater sensitivity and less interference from opalescence is obtained if tetrachlorethane or tetrabromethane replaces chloroform but these solvents are extremely toxic (see Chap. 1, Vol. 1) and are probably best avoided in the routine laboratory. This extraction procedure, a purification stage, enables direct fluorimetric estimations to be made at very high dilution on urine samples obtained during pregnancy.

Although the methods for determination of total oestrogens, mainly oestriol, in pregnancy urine are given later (p. 158) the various factors which are of importance in the determination of oestrogens are discussed here. Some of them have been investigated using pregnancy urine but the findings are relevant to all urinary oestrogen determinations.

Acid concentration in the Köber reagent. In their original methods for the determination of oestrogens, Brown (1952) and Bauld (1954) paid particular attention to the reaction conditions especially the preparation of the Köber reagent and the optimal concentration of the sulphuric acid for the different oestrogens. As the latter is critical it is important for it to be unambiguously defined. When sulphuric acid and water are mixed at the concentrations usually employed there is approximately 10 per cent reduction of the final volume. The description "60 per cent v/v" may be interpreted as *either* 60 ml sulphuric acid diluted with water and made up to 100 ml (equivalent to 600 ml/l) *or* 60 ml sulphuric acid mixed with 40 ml water, the final volume being unspecified. The latter interpretation is implied even if not stated. Campbell and Gardner (1971) mix 1 000 ml sulphuric acid and 1 000 ml water and refer to it as 50 per cent (v/v) sulphuric acid. The final volume however, will be somewhat less than 2

Gonadal Function Tests

litres and the actual concentration of the order of 55 per cent. Oakey *et al.* (1967), Hainsworth and Hall (1971) and Lever *et al.* (1973) give their sulphuric acid reagent details as volume of acid plus volume of water, with no strength implied which is certainly clearer. This point is important as the final acid concentration affects the relative response of the various oestrogens. The relative fluorescence for oestrone and oestradiol is much greater with the more dilute acids (50-60 per cent, exact preparation uncertain) than for oestriol. If the latter is used as the standard, overestimation of "total oestrogens" will occur, the actual amount depending upon the relative amounts of the other oestrogens present. With acid strengths increased to 65 to 80 per cent, the contribution of the other oestrogens is much reduced relative to oestriol.

Temperature of reaction. This also affects the relative fluorescence obtained for different oestrogens. Lever *et al.* (1973) found that when the reaction is carried out at 95°C much higher responses are obtained for oestrone and oestradiol than for oestriol. This can be corrected for by increasing the acid concentration of the Köber reagent to 85 per cent. Simkins and Worth (1975) also found marked increase in fluorescence of oestrone and oestradiol relative to oestriol at the lower temperatures. This results in marked overestimation in pregnancy urines compared with results obtained at higher reaction temperatures if oestriol is used as the standard.

Standard used. Simkins and Worth (1975) after investigating the use of various standards for calibration of the method, recommend the use of oestriol-16β-D-glucosiduronate as a water-soluble derivative which is probably the most abundant oestriol conjugate in pregnancy, or free oestriol dissolved in carbonate-sodium hydroxide buffer (pH 10.8, 50 mmol/l). Lever *et al.* (1973) used a mixture of sulphonated and sulphated derivatives dissolved in acid on the ground that free oestrogens react with the softer plastic pump tubes in the automated methods but Hainsworth and Hall (1971) and, more recently, Little *et al.* (1975) used aqueous ethanolic standards of free oestriol. The methods given here have been standardised using oestriol in aqueous ethanol.

Fluorimetric Determination of Total Oestrogens. Method of Brown *et al.* (1968a)

The oestrogen conjugates in diluted urine samples are hydrolysed by heating with dilute hydrochloric acid. The oestrogens are extracted and purified by solvent partition. From the dried extract, Köber chromogens are formed and extracted into Ittrich reagent before being assessed fluorimetrically. A correction formula is applied for non-oestrogen contaminants.

Reagents. 1. Concentrated hydrochloric acid.
2. Solid sodium chloride.
3. Diethyl ether, technical grade redistilled.

124   *Practical Clinical Biochemistry*

4. Carbonate solution, pH 10.5. Dissolve 21 g sodium hydroxide and 70 g sodium bicarbonate in 1 litre distilled water.

5. Light petroleum, b.p. 40 to 60°C, AR grade redistilled.

6. Sodium hydroxide solution, 1 mol/l.

7. Solid sodium bicarbonate.

8. Quinol solution, 20 g/l in ethanol.

9. Köber reagent. Disolve 20 g quinol in 1 litre sulphuric acid 660 ml/l.

10. Ittrich reagent. Disolve 2 g *p*-nitrophenol in 1 ml ethanol and add 100 ml *sym*-tetrachloroethane. Prepare in a fume hood and use an automatic pipette when adding to reaction mixtures.

11. Standard oestriol solution. Prepare a stock solution in ethanol, 4 mmol/l (115 mg/100 ml). Dilute the stock solution 1 vol to 10 vol with ethanol. Further dilute this 1 in 100 to give 4 μmol/l (1.15 mg/l).

Optional Equipment. Brown *et al.,* used an automatic extractor holding 12 extraction tubes, supplied by Paton Industries Ltd., 35 Henry Street, Stepney, S. Australia. They also employed combined extraction and fluorimeter tubes as used in the determination of cortisol (p. 75) and first described by Brown *et al.* (1968b). These comprise a glass fluorimeter tube fused to the lower end of a glass extraction tube fitted with a stopper.

Technique. *Hydrolysis and extraction.* Pipette 1/2 000-1/10 000 th. of the 24 h urine volume into a 150 × 15 mm test tube graduated at 6 ml. Dilute the urine sample to 6 ml with water and add 0.9 ml hydrochloric acid. Mix and add an alundum granule, place the tubes in a tray of water and heat in a steam pressure steriliser for 15 min at 120°C. Release the pressure slowly and cool, transfer to the extractor or proceed manually. Add approximately 1 g sodium chloride to improve the extraction of oestriol, shake gently until dissolved, and add 6 ml ether. Shake, allow the layers to separate and discard the urine layer. Add 2 ml carbonate solution and shake to remove the acid fraction, then discard the aqueous lower layer. Add 6 ml light petroleum to improve the extraction of oestrone, mix and add 6 ml sodium hydroxide solution. Shake and discard the upper ether — light petroleum layer which contains the neutral fraction. Add approximately 0.8 g sodium bicarbonate and shake until solution is complete to bring the pH of the solution to about 10.5. Add 6 ml ether and shake to extract the oestrogens; discard the lower carbonate layer.

Fluorimetry. Transfer the ether extract to a suitable tube, add 50 μl quinol solution and evaporate to dryness in a warm water bath in the fume cupboard. Prepare standard tubes in triplicate each containing 100 μl standard and also a blank and to each tube add 6 ml ether and 50 μl quinol solution before evaporating. To the dry residues add 1 ml Köber reagent and heat in a boiling water bath until the quinol has dissolved. Stopper and heat at 120°C for 10 min and cool in an ice bath. Dispense 0.75 ml Ittrich reagent into each fluorimeter tube and cool to below 0°C. Add 1.5 ml iced water to the Köber tubes, mix and again immerse in iced water for several minutes. Pour each diluted Köber solution into the corresponding prepared

Gonadal Function Tests

fluorimeter tube and shake 100 times to extract the fluorescent product. Centrifuge at 2 000 rpm for 3 min at $-5°C$. Allow to stand at room temperature until misting of the lower optical section no longer persists. Wipe carefully and read in the fluorimeter. The steps from dilution with water to the measurement of the fluorescence should be completed in less than 20 to 25 min. Read at 2 wavelength combinations (a) excitation 546 nm, emission 565 nm and (b) excitation 490 nm, emission 520 nm.

$$\text{Corrected fluorescence (Fc)} = F_{546/565} - 2\, F_{490/520}$$

Calculation. Urinary total oestrogens (μmol/24 h) =

$$\frac{\text{Fc of unknown}}{\text{Fc of standard}} \times \frac{0.4}{1\,000} \times \text{dilution factor}$$

Notes. 1. Oestrogens measured by the method are oestradiol, oestriol and oestrone together with minor Köber-chromogenic and alkali-stable oestrogens. The contribution of 2-hydroxy and 2-methoxy oestrogens is negligible.

2. Fluorimetry is the method of choice when measuring less than 3.5 μmol/24 h (1 mg/24 h).

3. Glucose in the urine may cause destruction of oestrogens unless the glucose is removed (p. 168).

4. The average amount of impurity eliminated by the fluorimetric correction is 20 nmol/24 h (6 μg/24 h).

Fluorimetric Determination of Total Oestrogens. Method of Outch *et al.* (1972).

In this method hydrolysis of the oestrogen conjugates is avoided by extracting them into ethyl acetate after saturating the urine with ammonium sulphate and adding pyridinium sulphate. The conjugates are then estimated directly by fluorimetry using the Köber reaction and Ittrich extraction.

Reagents. 1. Ammonium sulphate, solid.

2. Aqueous pyridine, 2 mol/l. Dilute 16 ml pyridine to 100 ml with water.

3. Sulphuric acid, 2 mol/l. Carefully add 10.6 ml concentrated sulphuric acid to about 80 ml water, cool and make up to 100 ml with water.

4. Pyridinium sulphate. Prepare fresh daily by mixing equal volumes of reagents 2 and 3.

5. Ethyl acetate.

6. Köber reagent. Dissolve 2 g quinol in 150 ml concentrated sulphuric acid.

7. Ittrich reagent. Dissolve 2 g p-nitrophenol in 100 ml chloroform.

8. Stock oestriol solution, 400 μmol/l (115 mg/l). Dissolve 11.5 mg oestriol in 100 ml methanol. Prepare a sub-stock standard containing 4 μmol/l (1.15 mg/l) by diluting the stock standard 1 to 100 with methanol. Store at 4° C.

126   *Practical Clinical Biochemistry*

9. Oestriol working standard, 400 nmol/l (115 μg/l). Prepare daily by diluting the sub-stock standard 1 to 10 with methanol.

Technique. Carry out the analysis in duplicate. Dilute 1 ml urine with 9 ml water in a 50 ml glass stoppered tube. To each tube add 15 g ammonium sulphate using a graduated scoop followed by 10 ml pyridinium solution. Stopper and shake vigorously by hand for 30 s to dissolve the solid. To each tube add 25 ml ethyl acetate, re-stopper and shake for 1 min before filtering the ethyl acetate through phase-separating paper (Whatman IPS, 11 cm). Transfer a 15 ml aliquot of the filtrate to a clean 50 ml tube. At the same time set up a blank and 200, 400 and 600 pmol standards (57.5, 115 and 230 ng) using 0.5, 1 and 2 ml of the oestriol working standard and transfer all the tubes to an 80°C water bath. Evaporate to dryness using an adaptor and gentle suction from a water pump. To the dry tubes add 3.4 ml water and 6.6 ml Köber reagent, mix well, cap with aluminium foil and heat at 120°C in a steam steriliser. Remove from steriliser, add 10 ml water to each tube, mix thoroughly and place in an ice bath. When cool add 10 ml *p*-nitrophenol in chloroform to each tube, stopper and shake for 1 min. Aspirate the upper aqueous phase and discard. Pour the lower phase into 15 ml centrifuge tubes and centrifuge at 2 000 rpm for 1 min then aspirate the residual aqueous phase before returning the tubes to the ice bath. Use semi-automatic dispensers for pipetting solutions wherever possible.

Read at 540/560 and 490/520 nm as described for the method of Brown *et al.* (1968a) above, making all readings within 25 min of extraction into the Ittrich reagent.

$$\text{Corrected fluorescence (Fc)} = F_{540/560} - 2\,F_{490/520}$$

Calculation. Urinary total oestrogens (μmol/24 h) =

$$\frac{\text{Fc of unknown}}{\text{Fc of standard}} \times \frac{25}{15} \times \text{urine volume (ml)}.$$

Normal Ranges. For both methods, total oestrogen excretion is converted into μg/24 h, expressed as E3, by multiplying μmol/24 h by 0.288. The figures for the separate oestrogens shown in Table 4,3 indicate that E3 is usually the major oestrogen and that E2 is excreted in the smallest amounts at all stages of the cycle. There is, however, a wide variation and the distribution of results is probably non-Gaussian. More detailed figures are given by Brown and Matthew (1962).

With the total oestrogen methods given above, in our experience the daily excretion (expressed as E3) during the follicular phase is usually 24 to 122 nmol (7 to 35 μg) but rises to a mid-cycle maximum of 174 to 347 nmol (50-100 μg), then falls and reaches a second maximum in the luteal phase of the same order.

TABLE 4,3
Urinary Oestrogen Excretion in the Normal Menstrual Cycle
(Figures are nmol/24 h with µg/24 h in parentheses)

	E1	E2	E3
Onset of menstruation	15-26, mean 19[1] (4-7, mean 5) 15.6 ± 7.4 (SD)[2] (4.2 ± 2.0)	0-11, mean 7[1] (0-3, mean 2) 7.7 ± 6.6 (SD)[2] (2.1 ± 1.8)	0-52, mean 21[1] (0-15, mean 6) 19.4 ± 9.0 (SD)[2] (5.6 ± 2.6)
Follicular phase	23.0 ± 11.1 (SD)[2] (6.2 ± 3.0)	9.9 ± 7.7 (SD)[2] (2.7 ± 2.1)	27.4 ± 17.4 (SD)[2] (7.9 ± 5.0)
Ovulatory peak	41-115, mean 74[1] (11-31, mean 20) 49.6 ± 20.0 (SD)[2] (13.4 ± 5.4)	15-52, mean 33[1] (4-14, mean 9) 21.3 ± 11.8 (SD)[2] (5.8 ± 3.2)	45-188, mean 94[1] (13-54, mean 27) 65.6 ± 39.9 (SD)[2] (18.9 ± 11.5)
Luteal phase	*37-85, mean 52[1] (10-23, mean 14) 38.5 ± 18.5 (SD)[2] (10.4 ± 5.0)	*15-37, mean 26[1] (4-10, mean 7) 15.4 ± 9.9 (SD)[2] (4.2 ± 2.7)	*28-250, mean 76[1] (8-72, mean 22) 56.6 ± 9.4 (SD)[2] (16.3 ± 2.7)

References: [1] Brown (1955c); [2] Loraine and Bell (1971)
* Peak values

128   *Practical Clinical Biochemistry*

In men, Brown (1955b) quotes daily total oestrogen excretions of 21 to 62, mean 36 nmol (6.0 to 17.8, mean 10.3 μg) but the pattern of the different oestrogens is somewhat different; E1, 11 to 30, mean 20 nmol (3.0 to 8.2, mean 5.4 μg): E2, 0 to 23, mean 5.5 nmol (0 to 6.3, mean 1.5 μg): E3, 3 to 38, mean 12 nmol (0.8 to 11.0, mean 3.5 μg).

Determination of Progesterone in Plasma

As with the oestrogens, the first studies were done on urine in which the chief metabolite of progesterone is pregnanediol glucosiduronate. The development of methods for measuring circulating progesterone in plasma was much later. There are problems in that the proportion of secreted progesterone which is excreted as pregnanediol is very variable (Klopper and Billewicz, 1963) so that it is difficult when comparing results between patients to infer that differences in progesterone production exist.

Earlier methods for the determination of plasma progesterone (see Loraine and Bell, 1971; Klopper, 1971) have been replaced by CPB or RIA techniques. Most CPB methods use transcortin as the binding protein (Yoshimi and Lipsett, 1968; Johansson *et al.*, 1968; Hagerman and Williams, 1969; Johansson, 1969; Lurie and Patterson, 1970; Martin *et al.*, 1970). The method requires extraction of the plasma with an organic solvent usually light petroleum. Tritiated progesterone is used as the isotopic marker. Some cross reaction occurs with other steroids, particularly 17α-hydroxyprogesterone, 20α-hydroxyprogesterone and the corticoids: deoxycorticosterone, corticosterone, 11-deoxycortisol and cortisol. Some of these are relatively poorly extracted but many workers use a further chromatographic or solvent partition separation of the crude extract. With a light petroleum extract alone, Demetriou and Austin (1971) found the following steroids to be partly measured as progesterone, the figures indicating the percentage of the total steroid interfering in this way: 20α-hydroxyprogesterone (22), 17α-hydroxyprogesterone (21), deoxy-corticosterone (17), testosterone (2), others (1 or less). A more specific binding protein is present in guinea pig serum (Swain, 1972) allowing simple light petroleum extracts to be assayed with interference from other individual steroids of 4 per cent or less.

RIA methods for progesterone have been developed and as with oestradiol the specificity of the antiserum depends on the nature of the steroid linkage to BSA. Antisera raised to progesterone linked to BSA through position 20 (Midgley and Niswender, 1970) or position 3 (Furuyama and Nugent, 1971) show cross reaction with related steroids and a chromatographic separation is required. The same need is apparent using 11-deoxycortisol linked to BSA through position 21 as there is well marked cross reaction with deoxycorticosterone and 17α-hydroxy-progesterone (Abraham *et al.*, 1971). Greater specificity is shown by antisera raised to progesterone linked to BSA by the 11α-hemisuccinate group (Midgley and Niswender, 1970; Furr, 1973). Appreciable cross

Gonadal Function Tests

reaction occurs with epimers of 11-hydroxyprogesterone but these are very poorly extracted into light petroleum. Some cross reaction occurs with 5α-dihydroprogesterone (10 per cent) and 5β-dihydroprogesterone (5.1 per cent). While these substances are extracted into light petroleum they do not appear to be present in plasma (Furr). Interference from other steroids in the extract is likely to be less than 1 per cent.

Practical details of these techniques vary with the particular antiserum used and are not given here. The original sources should be consulted.

Normal Ranges. The progesterone pattern in the normal menstrual cycle is simpler than that for E2 and concentrations at peak levels are some 25 times greater than those at maximal E2 secretion. Figures are low during the follicular phase and rise after the E2 and LH peaks if ovulation has occurred with formation of a corpus luteum. Some representative figures appear in Table 4,4. Kletzky *et al.* (1975) find that the figures show a log

TABLE 4,4

Plasma Progesterone Concentrations during the Normal Menstrual Cycle

(figures are in nmol/l with µg/l in parentheses)

Phase	
Early follicular	2.5 (0.8)[2], < 3.2 (< 1)[4]
Mid follicular	1.75, SD = 0.32 (0.545, SD = 0.103)[1], 1.0-1.3 (0.3-0.4)[2], <3.2 (<1)[4]
Late follicular (2 to 5 days before LH peak)	4.2-6.7 (1.3-2.1)[4], occasionally
Early luteal (0 to 2 days after LH peak)	3.2-6.4 (1-2)[2]
Mid luteal (4 to 9 days after LH peak)	27.4, SD = 14.9 (8.56, SD = 4.66)[1], 32-64 (10-20)[2], 9-99, median = 30.4 (2.8-31, median = 9.5)[3], mean 35.6 (11.2) with individual maxima 25-74 (7.8-23)[4]

References: [1] Abraham *et al.*, 1971; [2] Abraham *et al.*, 1972; [3] Kletzky *et al.*, 1975; [4] Shaaban and Klopper, 1973.

normal distribution and give detailed values for each day of the cycle. It is generally agreed that progesterone concentrations fall rapidly in the last 2 to 6 days of the luteal phase. The timing of the progesterone peak is later than that for LH. Significant increases occur on the day after the LH peak and ovulatory levels are reached in 36 to 62 h (Kletzky *et al.*, 1975; Thorneycroft *et al.*, 1974).

Plateau levels are seen during the period 4 to 9 days after the LH peak. It is of some importance to decide on the biochemical criteria for ovulation and establishment of a corpus luteum. Shaaban and Klopper (1973) suggested that a plasma progesterone figure of more than 16 nmol/l (5 µg/l) indicates ovulation and that normal luteal function is shown by figures of more than 22 nmol/l (7 µg/l) persisting for at least 7 days. Abraham *et al.*

130 *Practical Clinical Biochemistry*

(1974) preferred not to rely on a single reading as an index of ovulation and suggested that the sum of any three results on different days should be greater than 48 nmol/l (15 µg/l) even if one of them was as low as 9.5 nmol/l (3 µg/l).

In males, the concentration of progesterone in plasma is low. Abraham *et al.* (1971) give a range of 0.75 ± 0.20 (SD) nmol/l (0.233 ± 0.064 µg/l) and similar figures are quoted by Swain (1972).

Little progesterone is derived from adrenal sources in normal menstruating women as judged by the failure of dexamethasone to alter its plasma concentration (Abraham, 1974; Kim *et al.,* 1974). The fate of the progesterone secreted from the ovary is variable so that between 15 and 77 per cent may be excreted in the urine where about half of it is in the form of pregnanediol (Abraham *et al.,* 1974).

Determination of the Urinary Metabolites of Progesterone

Metabolism of progesterone involves reduction of the double bond in ring A, and of one or both ketone groups at C-3 and C-20. The products are the pregnanolones and pregnanediols. Of the various isomers only two are of clinical interest namely, 5β-pregnan-3α-ol-20-one and 5β-pregnane-3α, 20-diol. While methods for the former are available (Klopper, 1971) most use has been made of pregnanediol determinations and only these are considered here.

Pregnanediol methods involve hydrolysis of the conjugate and extraction into an organic solvent. Two main types of technique are currently in use, colorimetric and gas-liquid chromatographic (GLC). The former relies on the yellow colour given by pregnanediol with concentrated sulphuric acid and an early method of this type (Sommerville *et al.,* 1948) required 100 ml of urine. Klopper *et al.* (1955) made a careful study of the specificity of several methods and concluded that a chromatographic step was necessary to remove interfering impurities satisfactorily. Their method is given below and has been used as a reference method against which other colorimetric procedures have been compared (Loraine and Bell, 1971). Various GLC procedures were reviewed by Klopper (1971). Enzymic hydrolysis of the urine gives simpler extracts for analysis than does acid hydrolysis and some further purification steps other than simple washing of the extract with acid and alkali, may be needed with such extracts. Most workers have made derivatives of pregnanediol before GLC on a variety of liquid phases. In more recent methods, attempts have been made to simplify the procedure and to obtain simultaneous measurements of pregnanetriol and the different 17-oxosteroids and their 11-oxygenated derivatives. Holub (1971) gives details of various extraction and hydrolytic procedures. He prefers precipitation of the conjugates, hydrolysis with glucuronidase and sulphatase, and separation of the trimethylsilyl (TMS) derivatives isothermally on a column of SE-30 and neopentyl glycol succinate (NPGS). Slob and Winkel (1973) used acid hydrolysis, conversion

Gonadal Function Tests 131

to the heptafluorobutyrates and isothermal separation on a NPGS column. Chevins *et al.* (1974) used enzymic hydrolysis, conversion to TMS derivatives and isothermal separation on OV225 while Moore and Cooper (1974) partitioned the extract after glucuronidase hydrolysis between isopentane and saline before acetylation and isothermal separation on OV101. Sanghvi *et al.* (1974) avoided derivative formation by using two internal standards to measure precise retention times following glucuronidase and sulphatase hydrolysis and isothermal separation on OV17.

The following GLC procedure is an amalgamation of several procedures and has been used in our laboratories by our colleague Dr. Audrey Axon for some time with satisfactory performance.

Determination of Pregnanediol by Gas-liquid Chromatography

Conjugates are hydrolysed with acid and the washed extract of urine is used to form TMS derivatives which are separated on a Carbowax column.

Reagents. 1. Hydrochloric acid, 50 per cent. Mix equal volumes of concentrated acid and water.

2. Sodium hydroxide solution, 1 mol/l.

3. Pyridine, redistilled.

4. NO-(Bis-trimethylsilyl) acetamide, BDH Ltd or Phase-Sep Ltd.

5. Trimethylchlorosilane, BDH Ltd or Phase-Sep Ltd.

6. TMS reagent. Mix 40 drops pyridine with 20 drops of reagent 4 and 1 drop of reagent 5. Use fresh.

7. Toluene, redistilled.

8. Benzene, redistilled.

9. Acetone, pure.

10. Sodium sulphate, anhydrous.

11. Pregnanediol standard in ethanol. Dissolve 25.6 mg in 100 ml. This contains 0.2 μmol in 0.25 ml.

Equipment. A Pye Series 101 Gas Chromatograph is used with a glass column, 1 m long, filled with 3 per cent Carbowax on Chromosorb W. The oven temperature is 235-240°C and the carrier gas is nitrogen at a flow rate of 50 ml/min. A flame isonisation detector is used.

Technique. To 5 ml of a 24 h collection of urine in a glass stoppered tube (150 × 20 mm) add 2 ml toluene and 1 ml hydrochloric acid. Stopper and heat in a boiling water bath for 20 min. Cool quickly in cold water, add 20 ml benzene and shake mechanically for 5 min. Remove the aqueous layer by suction and shake the solvent with 4 ml sodium hydroxide 100 times on the shaker before discarding the lower phase. Repeat twice with 4 ml portions of water. Dry the organic layer with 1 g sodium sulphate and filter through a Whatman No. 1 paper. Transfer 6 ml filtrate to a glass

132 *Practical Clinical Biochemistry*

stoppered tube (100 × 15 mm) and evaporate to dryness at 70°C under nitrogen after adding an anti-bumping granule. Add 6 drops TMS reagent, stopper the tube and keep at 37°C for 1 h or at room temperature overnight. Evaporate to dryness under nitrogen at 70°C. Dissolve the residue in 100 μl acetone. Inject 4 μl onto the GLC column. Prepare standards in duplicate by evaporating 0.25 ml of the pregnanediol standard solution to dryness in the 100 × 15 mm tubes and proceed as for the urine extracts except that the final solution is in 1 ml acetone. Inject 4 μl as before. Measure the peak heights of the standards and the unknowns.

Calculation. Urinary pregnanediol (μmol/24 h) =

$$\frac{\text{Peak height of unknown}}{\text{Mean standard peak height}} \times \frac{0.2}{5} \times 24 \text{ h volume (ml)}$$

To convert μmol/24 h to mg/24 h multiply by 0.32

Determination of Pregnanediol. Colorimetric Method of Klopper *et al.* (1955)

Conjugates are hydrolysed with acid. The crude extract in toluene is oxidised with permanganate to remove pregnanetriol and unsaturated substances produced during acid hydrolysis. Chromatographic separation on alumina is followed by acetylation of the pregnanediol fraction and further alumina chromatography. The amount of pregnanediol diacetate in the final eluate is determined by the yellow colour developed with sulphuric acid.

Reagents 1. Toluene redistilled.

2. Hydrochloric acid, concentrated, analytical reagent grade.

3. Alkaline sodium chloride solution. Make 250 g NaCl to 1 litre with 1 mol/l sodium hydroxide solution.

4. Potassium permanganate solution, 40 g made to 1 litre with 1 mol/l sodium hydroxide solution. Prepare freshly before use.

5. Deactivated alumina. Deactivate Camag MFC alumina (100-200 mesh, alkaline, Brockmann activity 2, Hopkin and Williams Ltd) by adding 1 ml of water to every 100 g and mixing thoroughly by repeated inversion.

6. Benzene, redistilled, water saturated.

7. Silver sand, 40-100 mesh, acid washed, BDH Ltd.

8. Ethanol—benzene. Make 8 ml ethanol to 1 litre with benzene. Use analytical reagent grade solvents.

9. Ethanol—benzene. Make 30 ml ethanol to 1 litre with benzene.

10. Acetyl chloride, BDH Ltd, AnalaR.

11. Light petroleum, b.p. 40° to 60°, redistilled, water saturated.

12. Sodium bicarbonate solution, 80 g/l.

13. Sodium sulphite, solid.

14. Sulphuric acid, concentrated, analytical reagent grade.

Gonadal Function Tests

15. Standard pregnanediol solution, 3 mmol/l in ethanol. Dissolve 96.2 mg in 100 ml ethanol.

Technique. Collect a 24 h specimen without preservative and store at 4° C. Measure one-twentieth of the total volume into a 500 ml round-bottomed flask and dilute to 150 ml with water. Add 50 ml toluene and heat to boiling under a reflux condenser, adding an anti-bumping granule. Add 15 ml hydrochloric acid through the condenser and boil for 10 min. Cool the flask rapidly under running water and transfer the contents to a separating funnel. Remove the urine layer and re-extract with a further 50 ml toluene. Combine the toluene extracts, discard any urine which settles out and shake with 25 ml alkaline saline. Discard the aqueous layer including the curdy precipitate at the interface and shake the toluene layer for 10 min with 50 ml potassium permanganate. Discard the permanganate layer and wash the toluene layer four or five times with successive 50 ml amounts of water to remove all the permanganate colour. Then filter the toluene through a Whatman No. 1 filter paper into a 250 ml flask pouring from the separating funnel so as to leave behind a few drops of emulsion. Distil to a volume of approximately 10 ml and cool to room temperature.

First chromatography. Use a Pyrex 12 x 1 cm tube containing a sealed-in sintered glass disc, porosity grade 1, to the top of which tube a 40 ml reservoir has been joined. Occlude the bottom end of the tube, fill the narrow part with benzene and pour in 3 g alumina. Allow the column to settle and add a protective 5 mm layer of sand. Apply the toluene extract to the column, rinsing the distillation flask with a few ml benzene and adding this to the column. When all the extract has percolated through, add 25 ml reagent 8. Discard this eluate, which contains some pigments and faster running steroids. Then add 12 ml reagent 9 collecting the eluate, which contains all the pregnanediol, in a 150 x 25 mm tube. These reagent volumes depend on the activity of the alumina and should be adjusted by ascertaining how pure pregnanediol behaves on a similar column. Allow adequate safety margins. Since variable losses can occur when the solvent is evaporated, do this carefully under reduced pressure.

Acetylation and second chromatography. While still warm dissolve the residue of pregnanediol from the first chromatography in 2 ml dry benzene and add 2 ml acetyl chloride. Loosely stopper the tube and leave at room temperature for 1 h. Add 25 ml light petroleum, transfer to a separating funnel and wash, once with 50 ml water, once with 25 ml sodium bicarbonate and twice with 25 ml water. Carefully run off the last drop of water, then pour the light petroleum on to an alumina column prepared as above except that light petroleum is used instead of benzene. When the solution has percolated through, elute the pregnanediol diacetate with 15 ml benzene into a 150 x 25 mm stoppered tube. Again the volume of benzene used depends on the activity of the alumina. Evaporate the solvent to dryness as before and place for at least an hour over calcium chloride in a desiccator. At the same time put up a standard as follows. Evaporate 0.2 ml pregnanediol solution (0.6 μmol), dissolve in 2 ml benzene, add 2 ml

134 *Practical Clinical Biochemistry*

acetyl chloride, loosely stopper the tube, leave at room temperature for about an hour, add 25 ml light petroleum, transfer to a separating funnel and wash as above. It is not necessary to chromatograph this except when checking the alumina. This should be done whenever a fresh batch of alumina is introduced. Evaporate off the light petroleum and dry over calcium chloride.

Colorimetry. Add approximately 10 mg sodium sulphite to the residue in each tube, then 10 ml concentrated sulphuric acid. Stopper, shake well and place in a water bath at 25°C for 17 h. Read against a sulphuric acid blank at 430 nm.

Calculation. Urinary pregnanediol (μmol/24 h) =

$$\frac{\text{Reading of unknown}}{\text{Reading of standard}} \times 20 \times 0.6$$

To convert μmol/24 h to mg/24 h multiply by 0.32. It is advisable to check whether Beer's Law is obeyed over the range intended to be covered.

Normal Ranges. The excretion of pregnanediol during the menstrual cycle reflects the changes in plasma progesterone described above and an increased excretion is characteristic of the luteal phase and indicates that ovulation has occurred. The changes are less rapid and less marked than for plasma progesterone (Fig. 4,2). Klopper *et al.* (1955) found during the follicular phase a mean daily excretion of 3.5 (range 2.4 to 4.7) μmol or 1.12 (0.78 to 1.50) mg. In the luteal phase the figures rise to 10.3 (6.6 to 13.1) μmol or 3.3 (2.1 to 4.2) mg. Similar mean figures are recorded by Loraine and Bell (1971), namely; follicular phase, 4.1 μmol (1.3 mg); luteal phase 10.0 μmol (3.2 mg). However, the normal range is quite wide and daily variations in excretion occur. These changes may be related to varying metabolism of progesterone. It follows that it is often difficult to be certain whether ovulation is occurring unless a series of measurements is made allowing a definite rise to be established. Peak values in our experience using the GLC method vary from 7.3 to 29 μmol/24 h (2.3 to 9.3 mg/24 h). In the last few days of the cycle, pregnanediol excretion drops rapidly towards follicular levels. The drop does not happen if fertilisation has occurred.

In the male, pregnanediol excretion is similar to that in the follicular phase. Klopper *et al.* (1955) give a mean daily excretion of 2.9 (1.2 to 4.4) μmol or 0.92 (0.38 to 1.42) mg.

Determination of Testosterone and its Metabolites

Testosterone is the most potent of the androgens and is produced in largest amount from the testis. Small quantities are released from the adrenal cortex and from the ovary. Interest in androgen production arises in the investigation of hirsute women and of infertile or eunuchoid males.

Testosterone is present in the circulation mainly bound to SHBG and a small portion is excreted as its glucosiduronate. This product is formed in

Gonadal Function Tests 135

part from adrenal androgens of weaker potency, particularly andro-stenedione and DHA. In comparison with the estimates of testosterone secretion rate mentioned below, the excretion of testosterone glucosiduronate accounts for only about 2 per cent of the total metabolism. Testosterone and such adrenal androgens are also metabolised to the group of 17-oxosteroids discussed in Chap. 2. The determination of 17-OS is a poor index of true androgen production and is not usually helpful in the study of gonadal dysfunction. Plasma testosterone is probably the method of choice.

Determination of Plasma Testosterone

As with other steroid hormones, the plasma methods in current use employ either CPB or RIA techniques and have replaced the earlier gas chromatographic and isotopic methods (see Loraine and Bell, 1971).

The CPB methods use SHBG as the specific binding protein. The plasma is made alkaline and extracted using an organic solvent. Oestradiol is not extracted but other 17β-hydroxysteroids also bind. These are mainly dihydrotestosterone, Δ^4-androstenediol and Δ^5-androstenediol, all reduction products of testosterone. Accordingly some further purification of the extract is usually performed (Hollberg *et al.*, 1968; Kato and Horton, 1968; Mayes and Nugent, 1968; August *et al.*, 1969; Rosenfield *et al.*, 1969). Assay of the crude extract gives a measure of plasma "androgens" (Horton *et al.*, 1967; Murphy, 1969).

RIA methods have used antisera prepared against BSA linked to testosterone 3-oxime (Furuyama *et al.*, 1970) or testosterone 17-hemisuccinate (Thorneycroft *et al.*, 1973) thereby blocking one of the characteristic groups in testosterone. Most antisera cross react appreciably with dihydrotestosterone, androstenedione, Δ^4- and Δ^5-androstenediols. Solvent extracts have therefore often been purified further by solvent partition (Furuyama *et al.*, 1970) or by chromatography (Dufau *et al.*, 1972; Thorneycroft *et al.*, 1973; Pirke and Doerr, 1975). Others have used relatively crude extracts to measure plasma "androgens" (Chen *et al.*, 1971; Ismail *et al.*, 1972; Pohlman *et al.*, 1971; Andre and James, 1974).

Normal Ranges. The figures for males remain relatively constant over the age range 18 to 50 years, but decline somewhat later. Pirke and Doerr (1975) found median concentrations of 20.3 nmol/l (5.85 µg/l) at age 22 to 61 and 14.7 nmol/l (4.25 µg/l) at age 69 to 93 years. The corresponding ranges were 10.9 to 33.4 nmol/l (3.15 to 9.65 µg/l) and 6.8 to 23.0 nmol/l (1.95 to 6.65 µg/l). The figures of other authors are similar. There is, however, quite marked fluctuation in plasma testosterone concentrations with several broad peaks during the 24 h period. Lowest levels occur at 0100 and 1500 h with highest concentration at 0500 h, up to twice that at the nadir (Pirke and Doerr, 1975). There are also slow cyclical variations with mean periodicity of 3 weeks with an amplitude of 9-28 per cent (mean 17) around the individual average figure (Doering *et al.*, 1975).

136 *Practical Clinical Biochemistry*

Much lower figures are seen in pre-pubertal boys. Lee *et al.* (1974) found that the testosterone increase followed the increase in LH and the start of gonadal growth and was followed by growth of the penis and pubic hair. The mean figures for successive years from ages 10 to 17 inclusive were 1.4, 3.0, 7.5, 11.7, 13.2, 17.3, 18.7 and 31.2 nmol/l corresponding to 0.41, 0.86, 2.16, 3.37, 3.81, 4.97, 5.39 and 8.94 µg/l.

In the normal menstruating female the testosterone concentration is much lower with mean figures ranging from 1.1 to 2.8 nmol/l (0.33 to 0.82 µg/l) (DeVane *et al.*, 1975; Dufau *et al.*, 1972; Easterling *et al.*, 1974; Ismail *et al.*, 1972; Kim *et al.*, 1974). It increases slightly at mid-cycle (Kim *et al.*) and is doubled on oral contraceptive regimes due to an increase in SHBG (Easterling *et al.*). The fraction of testosterone not bound to SHBG is greater in males (1.71 per cent) than in females (1.02 per cent) according to Fisher *et al.* (1974). Approximately half the circulating testosterone in the menstruating female orginates from the adrenal cortex (Abraham, 1974; Kim *et al.*, 1974) but Oake *et al.* (1974) believe that the adrenal is the major source whereas such adrenal contribution is absent in the male.

Testosterone is converted in male target organs to dihydrotestosterone which is biologically active. It is present in plasma in normal males at a concentration about 10 per cent that of testosterone and responds in parallel to testosterone during the day and following stimulation or suppression tests (Pirke and Doerr, 1975). Much lower levels occur in normal menstruating females and the adrenal cortex contributes approximately half (Abraham, 1974).

The plasma metabolic clearance rate of testosterone is approximately 1 000 litres/24 h (Loraine and Bell, 1971). At the average plasma levels of testosterone this would correspond to a daily secretion into the plasma of 24 µmol (7.0 mg) in males and 1.7 µmol (0.5 mg) in females. These figures are similar to those calculated from isotope dilution studies on the excretion of urinary testosterone glucosiduronate. Although some of this is derived from androstenedione and DHA in the liver leading to a possible overestimate of daily testosterone secretion the figures for males are 12 to 41 µmol (3.5 to 11.8 mg) and for females 1.4 to 10 µmol (0.4-2.9 mg).

Determination of Urinary Testosterone

Following hydrolysis of the glucosiduronate and extraction of the testosterone this may be purified and determined by colorimetric, fluorimetric, GLC or CPB methods (see Loraine and Bell, 1971). More recently, RIA methods have been employed.

Normal Ranges. Earlier methods gave a mean daily excretion, expressed as testosterone, of 430 (104-1 220) nmol or 124 (20 to 352) µg in males. Much lower figures are seen in pre-menopausal females, namely 24 (10-42) nmol or 7.0 (2.9 to 12.1) µg (Bishop and Sommerville, 1970); similar figures of 30 ± 3.5 nmol or 8.6 ± 1.0 µg have been reported for an

Gonadal Function Tests

immunological technique by Leigh *et al.* (1974). In comparison with the estimates of testosterone secretion rate mentioned above, the excretion of testosterone glucosiduronate accounts for only about 2 per cent of the total metabolism.

The 17α-epimer of testosterone, epitestosterone, is also excreted as its glucosiduronate in comparable amounts. It is probably derived by reduction of androstenedione. Whereas the excretion of testosterone is relatively constant during the menstrual cycle, that of epitestosterone increases in mid-cycle and luteal phases (Bishop and Sommerville, 1970) as does plasma androstenedione (*v. infra*). The adrenal origin of much of the testosterone excreted in the female is shown by its increase following ACTH and suppression by dexamethasone (Leigh *et al.*, 1974).

Related Plasma Steroids

RIA methods have been employed to study the biological roles of the progesterone derivative, 17-hydroxyprogesterone and of dehydroepian-drosterone (DHA) and androstenedione, precursors of testosterone and the oestrogens (Figs. 4,1 and 4,3).

17α-Hydroxyprogesterone (XIV, Fig. 2,1) which is excreted as its metabolite, pregnanetriol (XXXIII, Fig. 2,2) appears to be of ovarian origin as judged by the failure of dexamethasone to alter its plasma concentration (Abraham, 1974). This changes during the menstrual cycle in a similar way to that of E2 rising from 0.6 to 1.5 nmol/l (0.2 to 0.5 μg/l) in the early follicular phase to 6 nmol/l (2.0 μg/l) at the ovulatory peak, then falling and increasing again in the mid-luteal phase to 3 to 6 nmol/l (1 to 2 μg/l) before falling prior to menstruation. Pregnanetriol excretion follows a similar pattern.

DHA and its sulphate are present in female plasma, do not change greatly during the menstrual cycle and are very largely of adrenal origin. The concentrations are: DHA 7.0 ± 1.3 μmol/l (2.0 ± 0.37 mg/l), DHA sulphate 20.3 ± 3.3 μmol/l (7.5 ± 1.2 mg/l) (Abraham, 1974; DeVane *et al.*, 1975).

Androstenedione changes during the menstrual cycle like E2 rising from 4.20 ± 0.94 (SE) nmol/l (1.21 ± 0.27 μg/l) in the early follicular phase to an ovulatory peak of 6.9 ± 2.0 nmol/l (1.97 ± 0.57 μg/l), subsiding to a mid-luteal plateau of 5.03 ± 0.97 nmol/l (1.45 ± 0.28 μg/l) and falling premenstrually. (DeVane *et al.*, 1975; Kim *et al.*, 1974.) The figures in males are 4.03 ± 1.22 nmol/l (1.15 ± 0.35 μg/l) (Thorneycroft *et al.*, 1973). It is of ovarian and adrenal origin, both organs contributing similar amounts in the early follicular phase with a rise in ovarian production later in the cycle (Thorneycroft *et al.*, 1973; Abraham, 1974; Kim *et al.*, 1974). Its metabolic plasma clearance rate, of 2 400 litres/24 h (Loraine and Bell, 1971), is much greater than that of testosterone and corresponds to the daily secretion into the plasma of about 4.9 μmol (1.4 mg) in males and 11.8 μmol (3.4 mg) in females.

Gonadotrophins

The pituitary gonadotrophins, LH and FSH are glycoproteins released from the anterior lobe by LH/FSH-RH. The chorionic gonadotrophin, HCG, shows well marked luteinising activity which is important in maintaining the corpus luteum in early pregnancy. Gonadotrophins present in the urine of post-menopausal women, HMG, have both luteinising and follicle stimulating activity. A purified preparation of this is used as a reference material. This Second International Reference Preparation (2nd-IRP-HMG) is supplied by the Medical Research Council (MRC) in ampoules of an assigned potency of 40 IU of LH and 40 IU of FSH activity. Results of LH and FSH assays are either reported in such IU or in terms of weight of a defined purified pituitary preparation such as LER 907 (National Institutes of Health, USA) or various MRC materials.

For many years bio-assays were used to measure FSH and LH usually in urine. Such assays (reviewed by Loraine and Bell, 1971) were laborious and often did not discriminate clearly between the two types of activity. Some assays, in fact, measure total pituitary gonadotrophins. With the development of immunological methods using antisera reacting differently with FSH and LH, specificity was improved. The earlier agglutination — inhibition methods were rather insensitive making extraction and concentration steps necessary for normal levels of the gonadotrophins. Considerable improvement in sensitivity came with the development of RIA techniques for the determination of LH (Midgley, 1966) and FSH (Foreman and Ryan, 1967; Midgley, 1967). A variety of methods have now been published (see Loraine and Bell, 1971).

While practical details for such assays are beyond the scope of this book, a few general comments are appropriate in understanding the place of these determinations in clinical practice. Antisera to LH show marked cross reaction with HCG and vice versa. Different workers have therefore used either of these substances to raise antibodies, for radio-iodination to prepare the labelled hormone, and as pure hormone for constructing the standard curve. The antisera show less but varying cross reaction with FSH. Antisera raised against different FSH preparations react to varying degree with LH and HCG. It is probable that common antigenic determinants are present in each molecule but produce antibodies to different degrees in different animals. Relatively monospecific antisera for FSH are now available allowing reasonably satisfactory quantitation of this hormone.

Agreement between RIA methods for the steroid hormones is fairly good but is less satisfactory for peptide hormones including LH and FSH. Variations in the relative activity of different antisera to different parts of the hormone molecule and the use of different standards contribute to the difficulties. Hence "normal ranges" vary from one laboratory to another.

The various studies on LH agree that there is a mid-cycle peak of plasma LH. When results for different cycles and different women are combined by superimposition of the peaks, the mean values show a clearly defined peak

Gonadal Function Tests

of relatively short duration, about 48 h on average (Thorneycroft *et al.*, 1974). The results for an individual cycle can be less clear cut and fluctuating levels around the period of ovulation may give the appearance of a broader peak or of several peaks. Fluctuations of plasma LH activity are also seen during the 24 h period in males suggesting that episodic release of the hormone may be common (Boyer *et al.*, 1972). These peaks, including the ovulatory peak can be of only a few hours duration in the individual. These factors sometimes make it difficult to be sure when or whether ovulation has occurred on the basis of plasma LH measurements alone. In the case of urine brief peaks of activity have less effect on overall 24 h excretion. The ovulatory peak is less marked and requires the analysis of a series of 24 h urines for its proper definition (Fig. 4,2). The demonstration of ovulation can thus only be retrospective.

In the case of FSH there is general agreement that there is an ovulatory peak of plasma concentration which is relatively transient and usually less marked than that of LH. Urinary FSH measurements give results similar to those for LH but less marked. Authors vary in their findings regarding changes in FSH at other parts of the menstrual cycle. Part of the difference of opinion may arise from variations in cross reaction with LH.

According to Kletzky *et al.* (1975) the distribution of LH and FSH values is log normal at all stages of the cycle. They quote for LH the following 95 per cent ranges (and median) in IU/l related to 2nd IRP-HMG: follicular, 10.0 to 31.5 (18.0); ovulatory peak (day 0), 30.0 to 86 (50.0); days −1 and +1, 15.0 to 36.0 (23.0); luteal, 9.8 to 29.0 (17.0). For FSH, the figures in the same units are lower: follicular, 6.0 to 17.0 (10.0); ovulatory peak (day 0), 17.0 to 40.0 (26.0); days −1 and +1, 6.2 to 22.5 (12.0); luteal, 4.3 to 15.0 (8.0).

Investigations using Dynamic Methods

The availability of clomiphene and LH/FSH-RH offer the possibility of testing hypothalamic and anterior pituitary function in relation to the control of gonadal activity and of differentiating disordered function at the two intra-cranial sites. The tests are similar in principle to the TRH test used in the investigation of thyroid function (p. 24) and to the dexamethasone, metopirone and insulin tests for adrenocortical hormone studies (Chap. 3).

The Use of LH/FSH Releasing Hormone

Besser *et al.* (1972) found that after an intravenous dose of 100 µg of synthetic LH/FSH-RH, plasma LH rose significantly reaching peak levels in 20 to 30 min. Plasma FSH responses were slower and smaller often not moving outside the normal basal range. The mean responses were similar for males and for females in the early follicular phase of the cycle but there

140 *Practical Clinical Biochemistry*

were marked individual variations. Similar results are reported by others and occur also with higher doses (Crosignani *et al.*, 1974). The responses are relatively constant for the individual and bigger LH increases are associated with a definite FSH response (Shahmanesh *et al.*, 1975). The release of gonadotrophins might be expected to be followed by an increase in gonadal hormone output. In the male the plasma testosterone response is variable and may not be helpful, but in the female, plasma E2 increases to a maximum about 6 h after stimulation and the response has been used as a test by Katz and Carr (1974).

The gonadotrophin increase is greatest in females near the time of ovulation, diminishes during the luteal phase and is least in the follicular phase. Also the greater increases are accompanied by an increase in LH/FSH ratio. (Yen *et al.*, 1972.) In the male at least, the response varies at different times of the day being maximal at 0600 h and 1800 h and minimal at 1200 h (Schwarzstein *et al.*, 1975).

The protocol for the test varies somewhat between authors but a typical one might be as follows (Marshall, 1975). Collect 2 basal samples of plasma at 10.00 and 10.15 h and then give 100 μg LH/FSH-RH in a small volume of saline intravenously and rapidly. Collect further samples at 20, 60 and 120 min later. Analyse the samples for LH and FSH. The analytical method used affects the absolute values for the basal readings and increments. In males, the average LH increase over basal levels is 2.5 fold and is usually at 20 min. The average FSH increase is 2 fold but 15 per cent of cases show no rise. The maximal response is usually at 60 min. Greater responses are seen over the age of 40 when basal levels are also higher.

Variations in responses in various clinical states are discussed later. Unfortunately the test does not distinguish between primary hypothalamic and primary pituitary failure (Mortimer *et al.*, 1973; Jacobs, 1975) unlike the situation with TRH. It appears that an adequate store of gonadotrophins in the anterior pituitary, released during the test, requires the tonic effect of the releasing hormone and is also affected by the steroid milieu. Repeated stimulation with releasing hormone eventually results in a normal response if the pituitary is intact.

The Use of Clomiphene

Clomiphene citrate is given orally and the tempo of response is much slower. It is believed to act by initiating the hypothalamic release of LH/FSH-RH, possibly by modifying the feed-back control of circulating oestrogens or testosterone. The action is made use of in the treatment of infertility (p. 151), when a variety of dose schedules may be employed. The usual dose for dynamic studies is 50 mg twice daily for 5 to 7 days. Plasma samples are collected at intervals which vary with different workers. After collecting basal samples, the frequency of plasma sampling is not greater than once daily at various times between the 3rd and 19th day. Once again the response of LH is more marked than that of FSH. The former is therefore the more useful determination.

Gonadal Function Tests

Most studies of normal responses have been made in adult males. Following administration of 100 mg daily for 7 days, plasma LH activity increases on average to 180-200 per cent of the basal figures, this maximal level occurring about the 7th day (Bardin *et al.*, 1967; Boyer *et al.*, 1973). Responses are greater on a 200 mg daily dose for 10 days, namely 172-345 per cent (Marshall, 1975). Single readings may be misleading however as marked fluctuations in LH occur in both basal and stimulated states. Boyer *et al.* (1973) found that the mean figures throughout the 24 h period rose to 135 to 245 per cent of mean basal levels but at times during the day the LH figures were not increased above basal levels. The number and size of the peaks of LH activity were increased after clomiphene stimulation. The plasma testosterone also increases to about 180 per cent of basal level on the 7th day (Bardin *et al.*, 1967) or 140-320 per cent on the 10th day (Marshall, 1975).

Figures for normal females are not available but experience with non-ovulating women indicates that those who respond to clomiphene show a peak response of similar degree and timing to that in males but that this is followed 13-14 days after starting clomiphene by a second, ovulatory, peak of LH and FSH. Thus Jacobsen *et al.* (1968) found that after 100-200 mg doses for 5 days the mean figures expressed as a percentage of basal levels (and mean time in brackets) were: clomiphene peak, FSH 165 (4.1 days), LH 215 (6.6 days); follicular nadir, FSH 57 (12.4 days), LH 98 (11.0 days); ovulatory peak, FSH 125 (14.1 days), LH 331 (13.3 days). Further discussion of responses to clomiphene treatment of infertility is deferred to p. 151.

The Use of Human Chorionic Gonadotrophin

HCG is used in females in the therapeutic induction of ovulation (p. 152) to simulate the pre-ovulatory surge of LH. In males it has been employed to demonstrate the presence of testicular tissue when this is in doubt, to assess the Leydig cell reserve in the testis in disorders of that organ and to assess its possible therapeutic use in hypogonadotrophic states. The dose used varies considerably, 1 000 to 5 000 IU daily for 1-4 days. Marshall (1975) uses a dose of 2 000 IU i.m. on days 0 and 3 and collects plasma for testosterone on days 0, 3 and 5. The normal response is a rise to 150-300 per cent of the basal level on either day 3. or day 5. The peak value is usually greater than 35 nmol/l (10 μg/l). Dihydrotestosterone shows smaller increases (Pirke and Doerr, 1975).

Interpretation of Gonadal Function Tests in Various Clinical Conditions

In this section are collected the results of applying the above function tests to normal persons at times other than normal sexual maturity and to patients with disordered gonadal function. In many cases measurements in

142   *Practical Clinical Biochemistry*

the basal state are sufficient but where equivocal results are obtained or if
further discrimination is needed, then stimulation tests are helpful. The use
of stimulating agents for the treatment of disordered gonadal function
requires laboratory control of hormone measurements and is therefore
included here. Although most emphasis is on the female, related tests in
males are conveniently considered here also. For a general review of earlier
work in this field see Loraine and Bell (1971).

Puberty

Normal puberty (p. 114) is associated with hormonal changes. In the
pre-pubertal *female,* the plasma and urinary FSH and LH concentrations
are very low and there is an increased ratio of FSH/LH. In the early stages
of puberty these hormones increase as the negative feed-back at the
hypothalamus by oestrogens lessens. Eventually the marked cyclic
variations characteristic of the mature menstrual cycle appear. This starts
with the pulsatile release of LH during sleep. The pituitary develops
increased responsiveness to FSH/LH-RH particularly in relation to the
formation of LH (Roth *et al.,* 1972). The consequent increased circulation
of gonadotrophins produces an increased circulation of oestrogens and
there is gradual development of the positive feed-back response with
eventual mid-cycle peaks of LH and FSH release as the cyclical pattern is
established.

The gonadal and adrenal hormones also change. Initially plasma E2
values are very low but increase to 37-63 pmol/l (10-17 ng/l) at the onset of
puberty and rise further during the progress of puberty to reach adult levels
at the end. Plasma testosterone also increases but relatively much less than
E2. Urinary oestrogen excretion, mainly E1 and E3, similarly increases
from very low levels, 10 nmol/24 h (3 μg/24 h) starting at 8 to 11 years.
Cyclical variations in output precede the menarche by one to two years.
Pregnanediol excretion, initially less than 90 μmol/24 h (0.3 mg/24 h) also
increases but may not reach the levels characteristic of formation of a
proper corpus luteum until after the menarche. The incidence of anovular
cycles is about 60 per cent in girls aged 12 to 14 and 43 per cent at age 15
to 17 (Doring, 1969). The adrenal products DHA, DHA sulphate and
androstenedione show several-fold increased plasma concentrations with
the onset of puberty and the urinary excretion of DHA and androsterone as
well as total 17-OS also increases. Less marked increases in plasma and
urinary testosterone are probably a consequence of peripheral conversion
of androstenedione to testosterone. This adrenarche appears to be due to
increased sensitivity to ACTH and is suppressable by dexamethasone.

In *normal male puberty* there is a general increase in FSH and LH
activity. Initially the ratio FSH/LH is high but falls to adult levels later as
LH secretion increases preferentially. The changes are accompanied by an
increase in plasma and urinary testosterone (p. 136). Plasma levels of

Gonadal Function Tests

androstenedione, androstenediol, androstanediol and dihydrotestosterone all increase. Peripheral conversion of some of these results in a smaller increase of plasma oestrogens, particularly E1 rather than E2, and these reach adult male values by age 13 on average. Thus the ratio of E1 or E2 to testosterone which is similar in both sexes in the prepubertal state increases in females and falls in males with the progress of puberty. The urinary excretion of oestrogens also increases from prepubertal figures to those of the normal adult male. The urinary excretion of 17-OS and the various fractions thereof also rises with greater adrenal and testicular activity.

Precocious puberty can occur in both sexes and is usually constitutional or familial. Pathological causes include tumours of the hypothalamus, adrenal or gonad, and a group of tumours secreting material similar to HCG — chorionepithelioma of testis, ovary or non-gonadal teratoma, or an hepatoblastoma or bronchial carcinoma. In the constitutional and hypothalamic types, isosexual precocious pubertal changes are accompanied by increases in FSH, LH, testosterone and E2 well above those expected for the chronological age but consistent with the stage of puberty achieved. Ovarian or testicular tumours producing isosexual precocity are distinguished by the low levels of FSH and LH, the gonadal hormones being released in excessive amounts by the tumour. Such tumours and some arising in the adrenal can also produce predominantly the hormone characteristic of the opposite sex with heterosexual abnormal development. These cases have to be differentiated from congenital adrenal hyperplasia (see Chap. 3). Increases in testosterone, E2 and HCG are characteristic of HCG-secreting tumours. Depending on the assay system used the HCG may be measured as LH or, less often, as FSH activity.

Delayed puberty occurs in both sexes and is again usually constitutional in origin with related delay in somatic growth and skeletal ossification. Some cases are associated with generalised disease or malnutrition and a minority result from hypothalamic or pituitary failure, or from primary gonadal failure which may be co-existent with a genetic disorder.

In the *male* the *constitutional type* is associated with basal levels of LH, FSH, E2 and testosterone which are low for the chronological age but appropriate for the stage of puberty achieved. As similar findings occur in other conditions, stimulation tests are helpful. With the LH/FSH-RH test, normal prepubertal boys respond, mainly by a rise in FSH but the LH response increases with the progressive steps of normal puberty. In constitutional delayed puberty responses are appropriate to the stage of puberty reached. A negative test is against the diagnosis. The clomiphene test is usually negative until the later stages of puberty but may be helpful if pubertal changes are arrested after partial development. The HCG test is often negative in prepubertal boys unless the hormone is given over a few weeks, when responses appear.

Hypothalamic or pituitary disorders have low to normal basal levels of FSH, LH, E2 and testosterone. Panhypopituitarism is associated with hypofunction of the adrenals and thyroid but pituitary tumours affect the

144   *Practical Clinical Biochemistry*

various pituitary hormones to different degrees. Isolated gonadotrophin deficiency occurs, probably due to deficient formation of LH/FSH-RH. It may be accompanied by anosmia, mid-line facial abnormalities, deafness and colour blindness as Kallman's syndrome. The various stimulation tests help to differentiate these conditions. In panhypopituitarism the clomiphene and LH/FSH-RH tests usually give no response while the response to HCG is normal or only slightly depressed if the lesion is recent but diminishes with time. With less complete pituitary insufficiency and with pituitary tumours some response to clomiphene may be seen in proportion to the basal FSH and LH secretion. The LH/FSH-RH test gives variable results from absent to apparently normal with greater preservation of FSH responses. It can be useful however in assessing pituitary responsiveness for therapeutic purposes. In isolated gonadotrophin deficiency the diagnosis may be difficult to establish before the age of 20 when constitutional delay is no longer likely. The clomiphene test is negative, the LH/FSH-RH test response varies from nil to apparently normal depending on the level of endogenous releasing hormone. Depressed responses can be restored to normal on repeated therapeutic administration of LH/FSH-RH. The HCG test responses resemble those of early puberty but increase if HCG is administered over a period of time. The response is a useful test of Leydig cell reserve function.

Primary testicular disorders include primary testicular failure, absent gonad or anorchia as in pure gonadal dysgenesis (p. 149), cryptorchidism when the testes are not in the scrotum, and Klinefelter's syndrome. In the latter there is a genetic abnormality in the form of an extra X chromosome so that the sex chromosome composition is XXY. This is detectable as the "chromatin body" in cells from the buccal mucosa, a feature of normal females. Usually the height is normal but muscular and facial hair development is poor. Some penile growth occurs, the voice deepens but the testes become very small. Excessive breast development, gynaecomastia, often a temporary feature of normal male puberty may persist. In some cases the genetic constitution is XXXY or even XXXXY when mental retardation and skeletal abnormalities occur also. In primary testicular failure many of the features of Klinefelter's syndrome are present but the cells are chromatin-negative. In primary failure testosterone levels are low, E2 may be normal or low and the lack of circulating testosterone leads to increased concentrations of LH and FSH. The clomiphene test usually fails to produce any further increase. The LH/FSH-RH response is usually increased proportionally to the increase in basal gonadotrophin secretion. The HCG test is helpful in assessing whether any functional testicular tissue remains. In Klinefelter's syndrome the basal changes are less marked. FSH is usually increased, LH may be increased or normal. The testosterone values are on average low but in a quarter or a third of cases are in the low normal range. E2 figures are normal or increased. The failure of ACTH or dexamethasone to alter the testosterone concentration suggests that it is not of adrenal origin (Smals *et al.,* 1975). Clomiphene gives no consistent

Gonadal Function Tests

response. The LH/FSH-RH test sometimes gives normal LH and exaggerated FSH responses, commensurate with the basal levels of these hormones. Administration of HCG occasionally produces a slight rise in testosterone. In cryptorchidism, basal levels are frequently normal but in some cases FSH is increased. Where doubt exists as to the presence of testicular tissue, it can be demonstrated by the testosterone response to HCG.

Delayed puberty in the female of constitutional type is the commonest form. Where the disorder is due to hypothalamic or pituitary causes the findings and methods of investigation are similar to those used in boys with the emphasis on E2 rather than testosterone where appropriate. The delay in sexual maturation is discussed further under the heading of primary amenorrhoea.

For reviews of the hormonal changes associated with normal and abnormal puberty see Bierich (1975), Marshall (1975), Swerdloff and Odell (1975).

The Menopause and Post-Menopausal Period

The term, *menopausal*, refers to absence of menstruation for three months following some menstrual cycles in the preceding year. The *post-menopausal* female has had no periods for twelve months. Before these stages many cycles may be anovular and Doring (1969) records an incidence of 12 per cent in women aged 41 to 45.

LH and FSH patterns during the menstrual cycle are often atypical in pre-menopausal women with high readings at the beginning and end of the cycle and absent peaks at mid-cycle. Post-menopausally both plasma and urinary FSH and LH are present in increased and relatively constant amount usually exceeding that seen in most of the normal menstrual cycle and sometimes even exceeding ovulatory peak concentrations. This increase is still apparent 25 years later but there is a tendency for the levels to decline with increasing age.

The increased gonadotrophin secretion is a consequence of ovarian follicular failure as demonstrated by the reduced oestrogen and progesterone output. The mean plasma E2 figure of 53.5 pmol/l (14.6 ng/l) reported by Judd et al. (1974) is similar to the average results of 24 to 54.5 pmol/l (6.5 to 14.8 ng/l) reported by others and is less than that seen in the normal early follicular phase (Table 4,2). Plasma E1 figures (Judd *et al.*) are higher at 112 pmol/l (30.3 ng/l) but are lower than in the normal follicular phase (p. 119). Total urinary oestrogen excretion is reduced to 11 to 39 nmol/l (3.2 to 11.2 μg/24 h) according to Loraine and Bell (1971) who also give figures for individual oestrogens. These are again lower than in the early part of the menstrual cycle and tend to fall with age with the exception of E3 which may increase. Plasma progesterone values are reduced to 0.575 ± 0.201 (SD) nmol/l (0.180 ± 0.063 μg/l) which are much lower than the follicular levels given in Table 4,4 (Abraham *et al.*, 1971).

146   *Practical Clinical Biochemistry*

Pregnanediol excretion is also low at 1.2 to 2.7 μmol/24 h (0.38 to 0.86 mg/24 h).

The ovary responds to the high gonadotrophin level by secreting testosterone and androstenedione (Judd *et al.*, 1974) and these may be the source of the small quantities of oestrogen. The mean plasma levels of testosterone, 0.69 nmol/l (0.20 μg/l) and androstenedione, 2.6 nmol/l (0.75 μg/l) are however still lower than in the female during reproductive life and the urinary 17-OS excretion and that of its subfractions is also diminished. Androstenedione is still lower at 2.3 nmol/l (0.67 μg/l) in the menopause produced by ovariectomy but is reduced to very low levels, 0.5 nmol/l (0.14 μg/l) if adrenalectomy is also performed (Thorneycroft *et al.*, 1973) indicating that the adrenal cortex is an important source. These findings are relevant to the ablation of the pituitary, ovary or adrenal in the treatment of oestrogen-sensitive tumours.

In the male there is no abrupt cessation of testicular function and testosterone secretion, production of viable spermatozoa and sexual potency may continue into old age. There is however, some reduction in testosterone secretion (p. 135) in older males and the FSH and LH figures are rather higher.

Hirsutism in the Female

Hirsutism in association with adrenal tumours, Cushing's syndrome and congenital adrenal hyperplasia is discussed in Chap. 3. Two conditions are considered here, namely simple hirsutism and the polycystic ovary (Stein-Leventhal) syndrome.

Simple hirsutism usually occurs with normal menstruation and normal urinary oestrogen and pregnanediol excretion. The increased hair growth is a response to the increased circulation of androgens. No single androgen is consistently increased above the normal range although the mean figures for testosterone, androstenedione, androstenediol and total 17β-hydroxy-androgens in plasma are significantly different from the normal mean; dihydrotestosterone is not significantly raised (Andre and James, 1974). The same authors noted that androstenedione gave the best discrimination and was poorly correlated in individuals with the testosterone figures whereas good correlation exists in normal subjects. There is altered binding of testosterone to SHBG with the percentage of free hormone increasing from 1.02 in normal women to 1.68 in hirsutism, a similar figure to that of 1.71 for normal males (Fisher *et al.*, 1974).

Urinary excretion of testosterone and epitestosterone is also increased on average but there is still overlap with normal females. The difference is greater if menstrual irregularity is a feature. The production rate of testosterone as judged by dilution methods using urinary testosterone glucosiduronate (p. 136) is in the upper normal or high ranges. Leigh *et al.* (1974) found that testosterone excretion increased after ACTH and fell after dexamethasone in hirsute women as a group but there were individual

Gonadal Function Tests 147

variations unrelated to the clinical severity. This suggests an adrenal origin for the androgens and this is confirmed by direct analysis of venous blood leaving the ovary and adrenal (Oake *et al.*, 1974).

Some hirsute women have menstrual irregularities and may develop amenorrhoea when the condition merges with the polycystic ovary syndrome.

The *polycystic ovary syndrome* is probably a mixed group of related conditions. In its full form there is hirsutism, amenorrhoea, infertility and ovarian abnormalities in the form of follicular cysts and a thickened capsule preventing ovulation. The condition may be discovered during investigations for infertility (see later). Breast development is usually normal but endometrial proliferation varies from the unstimulated state to hyperplasia.

The cyst fluid is rich in androstenedione but progesterone and E2 content is low. This differs from normal follicular fluid which is rich in progesterone and E2 but has a low concentration of androstenedione. DeVane *et al.* (1975) in a detailed study of plasma changes find increased mean concentrations of LH, E1, testosterone, androstenedione and DHA sulphate but no significant increase in FSH, E2, or DHA. This suggests both ovarian and adrenal involvement and the possible peripheral formation of E1 from androstenedione. These findings and an increased ovarian venous testosterone concentration are similar to simple hirsutism. In patients in whom plasma testosterone is not increased the SHBG levels are low and free testosterone is increased. The contraceptive pill increases SHBG concentration in normal women and in the polycystic ovary syndrome resulting in a fall in free testosterone to normal levels in the latter group but no change in the former (Easterling *et al.*, 1974).

In the urine there is some increase in 17-OS excretion, especially in the 11-deoxy fraction but not all cases show a definitely abnormal result. Testosterone excretion is increased as is that of LH and, sometimes, that of pregnanetriolone but pregnanetriol excretion remains in the follicular range. Some cases may therefore have 21-hydroxylase insufficiency. Oestrogen excretion varies being consistently at follicular levels in some but showing cyclical fluctuations in others. A feature of many cases is a marked variation in all hormone levels in urine and plasma at different times. Various forms of treatment have been employed. Wedge resection of the ovarian capsule is often followed by ovulation with its accompanying biochemical features but the hirsutism is unaltered. Clomiphene induces ovulatory cycles in some and adrenal suppression with prednisolone may result in improvement in others. The contraceptive pill can improve the hirsutism if pregnancy is not the aim.

Gynaecomastia in the Male

Breast enlargement at puberty is not uncommon but when it persists and the testes do not develop, Klinefelter's syndrome (p. 144) should be

148   *Practical Clinical Biochemistry*

considered. Some familial cases are associated with deficiency of 17β-hydroxysteroid reductase, the enzyme which converts androstenedione to testosterone. The former accumulates in the plasma where concentrations above 10 nmol/l (3 μg/l) are suggestive of this condition (Bierich, 1975). Some pubertal boys with temporary gynaecomastia have transient low levels of testosterone with some increase in E2. In others hypogonadism is present in sufficient degree to cause an increase in FSH and LH.

Gynaecomastia may occur at other periods of life in association with hepatic, renal or pulmonary disease and hormonal studies are often unhelpful. Certain oestrogen-secreting tumours of the adrenal or testis are accompanied by an increase in E2 with low levels of FSH and LH. Some teratomas producing an HCG-like peptide can cause gynaecomastia and are suggested by an apparent rise in LH due to cross-reaction in the assay but FSH is suppressed. A positive pregnancy test occurs in the urine. Occasionally breast enlargement and milk secretion is found in patients with pituitary tumours which secrete prolactin.

Normal breast development in an apparent female with a male chromosomal pattern, 46 XY, is seen in the "testicular feminisation syndrome" (see below).

Infertility in the Female

This discussion excludes structural abnormalities in the mature female genital tract, local factors hostile to sperm and sub-fertility in the male partner. Most of the problems then centre on the absence of ovulation in association with varying disturbance of the menstrual cycle. In primary amenorrhoea the menarche has yet to occur, in secondary amenorrhoea, periods have ceased for 6 months or longer. This may be preceded by oligomenorrhoea or this may persist with associated infertility problems. Also apparently normal menstrual cycles may be anovular. These are common at the beginning and end of menstrual life but reduce to a minimum of about 5 per cent of cycles at 26 to 30 years of age (Doring, 1969).

In *primary amenorrhoea* the age of the patient and the extent of development of secondary sex characters as part of the normal pubertal process is important. Constitutional delayed menarche is suggested by a normal sequence of pubertal development but with delayed onset. Delayed menstruation two years after full breast development and attainment of female body contour may be associated with an imperforate hymen or vaginal atresia and is a surgical rather than a biochemical problem. A rare condition, the *testicular feminisation syndrome,* also characterised by little or no pubic hair, arises in persons with a male chromosomal structure, 46 XY, with end organ insensitivity to the testosterone produced in near normal amounts by the testes. This leads to development of a female body habitus with absent uterus and a short blind vagina. It may be familial and

Gonadal Function Tests

is recognised by buccal smear and chromosome studies. No further biochemical investigations are required unless it is desired to check that testicular removal, desirable as there is a risk of malignant change, is complete.

Absent secondary sexual development suggests gonadal or pituitary failure. Ovarian failure (gonadal dysgenesis) with stunting of growth to less than 60 in (152 cm) is seen in *Turner's syndrome* with a variable number of other skeletal changes. This genetic abnormality can be recognised by buccal smear and chromosome studies. The common type lacks one X chromosome, 45X karyotype, and is chromatin-negative but mosaic forms are known. Ovulation will not occur and further hormonal investigations are not warranted. In *pure gonadal dysgenesis* growth is normal and the patient may be tall due to late closure of epiphyses. The gonad is reduced to a streak of fibrous tissue in an undeveloped "female" body. Chromosome analysis may reveal a true female karyotype, 46 XX, or a male karyotype, 46 XY i.e. anorchia. No further hormonal investigation is required; the potentially malignant male streak gonad is usually removed. In the absence of such genetic disorders the patient is investigated for pituitary insufficiency, tumour, or hypothalamic disorder (p. 143) and may be a candidate for hormone therapy. Some patients have primary amenorrhoea in association with severe generalised disease.

A few patients have evidence of some heterosexual development. These include cases of congenital adrenal hyperplasia and adrenal tumours which secrete androgens (Chap. 3). Occasionally an ovarian tumour secreting testosterone may be present and plasma testosterone determinations help in the diagnosis. Some patients are genetically male, 46 XY, with sufficient rudimentary testicular tissue to secrete some testosterone.

Secondary amenorrhoea. Cessation of menstrual periods may result from many causes including pregnancy, with its characteristic biochemical and clinical changes. A major group arises from hypothalamic malfunction in association with physical or mental stress, with psychoses, or in severe malnutrition, sometimes self-induced (anorexia nervosa). Thus amenorrhoea is a feature of severe generalised disease and of sudden changes in personal circumstances. Another common finding is a previous history of oligomenorrhoea or very irregular cycles. In some of these there is ovarian failure or the development of a premature menopause. A further group occurs after taking the contraceptive pill or as a continuation of the temporary amenorrhoea in the puerperium. Some of the latter may represent impaired pituitary function and this factor is present in other cases also. Pituitary tumour, varying degrees of selective pituitary failure up to panhypopituitarism, and structural changes in the hypothalamus are all associated with secondary amenorrhoea. Obesity is sometimes present with hypothalamic lesions while hypothyroidism, with or without obesity, is also a cause (Akande, 1975). Some cases are associated with hirsutism (see p. 146).

The investigation of secondary amenorrhoea may include the assessment

150 *Practical Clinical Biochemistry*

of thyroid function (Chap. 1), of secondary adrenocortical hypofunction (Chap. 3) and of hirsutism (p. 146) where appropriate. Important information is obtained from the basal state of LH, FSH and oestrogen activity. Several samples should be taken for LH and FSH to allow for fluctuating concentrations. Oestrogen investigations are often worth continuing for a longer period. FSH is usually more discriminating than LH (Jacobs, 1975). High levels in association with low oestrogen figures indicate an early menopause. High LH, E1 and testosterone figures suggest the polycystic ovary syndrome. Normal FSH results may be seen with low oestrogens but with normal oestrogen figures suggest the possibility of spontaneous return of menstruation. Many patients have low LH and FSH levels in association with low or, less often, normal oestrogen figures. Longer study of basal oestrogen excretion may reveal either continuous readings characteristic of the follicular phase or fluctuations not unlike those of anovular cycles. Where premature menopause has been excluded, dynamic tests of hypothalamic and pituitary function help to decide the likely site of the failure and the appropriate therapy. Most patients show a positive response to the LH/FSH-RH test but the FSH response may be more marked than that of LH (Crosignani *et al.*, 1974). The few cases of hypopituitarism give no response. As this test does not discriminate between hypothalamic and pituitary abnormalities, the clomiphene test can give valuable information (Ginsburg *et al.*, 1975). A positive test is less common when basal gonadotrophins are low in our experience and that of Dignam *et al.* (1969). A positive response to clomiphene suggests disordered cyclical gonadotrophin release and the probability that clomiphene treatment of infertility will be successful. A negative response is seen in hypothalamic defect, isolated gonadotrophin deficiency and anorexia nervosa. Infertility in these patients responds better to gonadotrophins.

Other tests used to assess clomiphene responsiveness involve the administration of large doses of progesterone or E2. After progesterone a rise in LH followed by endometrial bleeding suggests that ovulation can be induced by clomiphene (see review by Jacobs, 1975). Shaw *et al.* (1975) investigated the ability of a large dose of E2 to produce a sharp release of LH and sometimes of FSH by positive feed-back and found responders to ovulate when treated with clomiphene.

Oligomenorrhoea and irregular menstruation is often accompanied by ovulation and some degree of fertility but the chances of conception are reduced. Some patients with oligomenorrhoea when investigated by the usual basal hormone measurements can be shown to have a prolonged follicular phase with a relatively normal luteal phase in their extended cycle. In many of these women earlier ovulation can be induced with clomiphene. When oligomenorrhoea is severe so that menstruation only occurs two or three times a year, spontaneous ovulation is unlikely and their investigation and management becomes that of secondary amenorrhoea.

Gonadal Function Tests 151

Anovular cycles occur at times in many women but if frequent, are a cause of infertility. Although menstrual bleeding is present the cycle length is reduced to 20 to 24 days. The basal hormonal investigations may show either follicular phase levels of oestrogens throughout with an absent LH peak or in a few cases, some cyclical variation of oestrogens with an inadequate progesterone response. The latter group may ovulate but the corpus luteum is inadequate. Many patients with anovular cycles respond to clomiphene.

Biochemical Investigations in the Control of Ovulation Induction

The previous discussion indicates that defective ovulation might be corrected by suitable stimulation of the hypothalamus, pituitary or ovary. Clomiphene acts at the hypothalamus and has the advantage of oral administration and relatively low costs. At present it is too early to assess the use of synthetic releasing hormone to stimulate the pituitary. A well established procedure is ovarian stimulation by gonadotrophins. Follicular maturation is achieved by the repeated intramuscular administration of HMG which has FSH and LH activity. This is available as Pergonal (Searle). The pre-ovulatory surge of LH activity is then stimulated by giving a large dose of HCG. Ovulation should then follow. This form of treatment is expensive.

There is a markedly different individual sensitivity to the dose used and the response of one patient can vary appreciably from one course to another. Inadequate stimulation fails to produce follicular ripening and ovulation is unlikely even if HCG is given. Overstimulation produces multiple follicular maturation and a strong possibility of multiple pregnancy if HCG is given. Even if this is withheld, the hyperstimulation syndrome produces detectable ovarian enlargement and abdominal pain. Particularly when HCG is given, follicular rupture can lead to ascites, pleural effusion, bleeding from the ovary and hypovolaemic shock.

Clomiphene is usually given on 5 successive days. If menstruation is occurring, treatment starts on the 5th or 6th day of the cycle. Initial daily doses are 50 mg increasing in successive courses to 200 mg as judged by the response. When ovulation occurs it does so 7 to 10 days after the last dose and can be assessed either by finding an increase in pregnanediol excretion to consistently more than 6.3 μmol/24 h (2 mg/24 h) or a plasma progesterone of 32 to 160 nmol/l (10 to 50 μg/l) (Kellie, 1973). The urinary total oestrogen excretion usually increases to more than 175 nmol/24 h (40 μg/24 h) with a secondary and similar peak if ovulation occurs. With too big a dose the follicle grows too quickly and produces inadequate amounts of oestrogen. Kellie (1973) found plasma E2 levels of 1.9 to 7.4 nmol/l (500 to 2 000 ng/l) at the peak. Jones *et al.* (1970) reported a high incidence of impaired luteal function in clomiphene-treated patients leading to poor conception rates or early abortion if the pregnanediol excretion was less than 12.5 μmol/24 h (4 mg/24 h) on the

152   *Practical Clinical Biochemistry*

seventh luteal day. This suggests that gonadotrophin requirements differ for adequate function of the corpus luteum and for follicular rupture. Some clinicians therefore give HCG three days after the last dose of clomiphene if luteal function is poor.

Pergonal may be given in two different ways: repeated daily injections starting on the third day of the cycle if menstruation is occurring and continuing until an adequate response is obtained followed two days later by 10 000 units of HCG; or Pergonal injections on days 1, 3 and 5 followed by 10 000 units of HCG on day 8 if an adequate response occurs. The response is judged by the increase in plasma or urinary oestrogens and the dose is adjusted accordingly.

With daily injections the suppliers of Pergonal, G.D. Searle & Co. recommend achieving a minimal urinary total oestrogen excretion of 175 nmol/24 h (50 μg/24 h), or for E1, 74 nmol/24 h (20 μg/24 h) and E3, 87 nmol/24 h (25 μg/24 h) immediately before HCG is given. Tredway *et al.* (1974) measuring plasma "immunoreactive oestrogen" as E2 found ovulation to be unlikely if this figure was below 1 040 pmol/l (300 ng/l) by the time Pergonal was stopped and preferred figures in the range 1 740 to 3 480 pmol/l (500 to 1 000 ng/l). Higher levels were associated with a risk of the hyperstimulation syndrome and HCG was withheld.

With the three injections schedule, Searle recommend measuring urinary oestrogen excretion on days 1 and 6 and using the difference between these to define an adequate response for total oestrogens as 108 to 435 nmol/24 h (31 to 125 μg/24 h); or for E1 as 48 to 186 nmol/24 h (13 to 50 μg/24 h); or for E3 as 54.5 to 226 nmol/24 h (16 to 65 μg/24 h). HCG can then be given on day 8 provided the response is adequate and the absolute values on day 6 do not exceed 488 nmol/24 h (140 μg/24 h) for total oestrogens, 222 nmol/24 h (60 μg/24 h) for E1, or 244 nmol/24 h (70 μg/24 h) for E3. Others have preferred to study the rate of increase of several urinary total oestrogen measurements. Hyperstimulation is likely if this is more than 50 per cent per day. Kellie (1973) measured plasma E2 and found ovulation unlikely if this was less than 1 100 pmol/l (300 ng/l) on day 7 but gave HCG with plasma E2 in the range 1 100 to 4 400 pmol/l (300 to 1 200 ng/l).

Infertility in the Male

This may be due to impotence or a reduced content of spermatozoa in the ejaculate, oligospermia, or absence of spermatozoa — azospermia. Testicular failure, either primary or secondary to reduction in pituitary gonadotrophin output, affects testosterone secretion from the Leydig cells and maturation of the germinal cells.

A number of structural abnormalities of the genital tract affect fertility and psychogenic factors are an important factor in impotence. Hormone investigations are not usually indicated in these cases. Varicocele, a varicosity of the venous plexus draining the testis is sometimes relevant.

Gonadal Function Tests 153

Primary testicular failure raises the possibility of Klinefelter's syndrome and has been discussed earlier (p. 144). In oligospermia or azospermia with maintained potency, germinal cell damage is suggested by increased basal secretion of FSH with relatively normal levels of LH, E2 and testosterone. Stimulation tests usually give normal responses. In many cases of varicocele, hormone investigations are normal but Comhaire and Vermeulen (1975) found some patients with sexual inadequacy, abnormal ejaculates and low testosterone secretion whose abnormalities recovered after surgical removal of the varicocele. They found no testosterone suppression in cases of psychogenic impotence. Gonadotrophin deficiency leading to secondary testicular failure occurs with hypothalamic and pituitary disease and to a lesser degree with advancing years. The basal secretion of FSH, LH, testosterone and E2 is low. Clomiphene usually gives no response, neither does LH/FSH-RH unless continued for a period, in isolated gonadotrophin deficiency. HCG responses vary with the duration of pituitary hypofunction but testicular responsiveness can be demonstrated by repeated administration. The selection of clomiphene or gonadotrophins for therapeutic correction of the defect may be made by assessing the testosterone response to longer courses of treatment.

For a review of male infertility problems see Marshall (1975).

Dysfunctional Uterine Haemorrhage

This condition (DUH) is usually diagnosed when clinical investigation fails to reveal any cause for recurrent excessive menstrual bleeding sometimes with alteration in the length or regularity of the cycle. The incidence is highest in premenopausal women over the age of 40 (Beazley, 1972). Hormonal disorders may be involved but the situation is complex; many factors may be responsible and differ in individual cases. General disorders such as cirrhosis of the liver, or iron deficiency produce DUH as does hypothyroidism and disordered adrenocortical function. Abnormalities in the plasma or urinary concentrations of LH, FSH, oestrogens and progesterone throughout the cycle are common especially near the menopause and anovular cycles often occur.

Fraser and Baird (1974) studied E2 secretion using isotopic methods and found normal E2 clearance and conversion to E1. However, many cases had evidence of significant E2 secretion by both ovaries with bilateral formation of mature follicles and eventually of corpora lutea. They suggest that DUH in at least some cases arises from inappropriate E2 secretion from multiple follicles arising from the abnormal function of gonadotrophins. Some cases had high blood production rates of E2 especially when the endometrium showed cystic hyperplasia.

In general, however, the role of hormone investigations in DUH is not properly established.

FETO-PLACENTAL FUNCTION TESTS IN PREGNANCY

Many tests have been used in an attempt to assess the function and development of the fetus and the placenta. Some tests are mainly directed at the fetus itself; others give information mainly about the placenta, much of which is of fetal origin. The fetus receives its nutrition through the placenta and in a normal pregnancy both develop harmoniously. Consequently it is best to consider the feto-placental unit as the important element. Tests are available to investigate different aspects of this unit. They are usually performed on maternal fluids, urine or plasma, or on amniotic fluid which is mainly of fetal origin (p. 111). Fetal blood is only sampled rarely.

Substances used to assess *placental* development and function include: progesterone or its metabolites; the maternal serum peptide hormones, HCG and human placental lactogen (HPL); the maternal serum enzymes, heat-stable alkaline phosphatase, diamine oxidase and cystine aminopeptidase (oxytocinase). In order to assess placental function, the substance used should be produced by the placenta alone, the maternal contribution being restricted to excretion. Circadian variations should be minimal and the half life should be short enough to allow changes in production to be recognised without delay using simple measurement methods. Most of the placental tests are estimates of its synthetic power which is assumed to be related to its important transfer functions which are difficult to assess directly.

The *fetal* component, often assessed by examination of the amniotic fluid, includes: α-fetoprotein, produced maximally by the fetal liver during the second trimester and appearing in excessive quantities in neural tube defects; surfactants containing lecithin, secreted by the relatively mature fetal lung; bilirubin, used as an index of Rhesus sensitisation; various electrolytes and excretory products, for example, creatinine, used to assess renal development and general maturity of the fetus. Various genetic abnormalities may be detected by examination of fetal cells in the amniotic fluid.

The only commonly used tests of the function of the *whole feto-placental unit* concern the production or excretion of oestriol (E3).

The fluid chosen for the investigation depends on its aim and will be influenced by the stage of the pregnancy and of fetal development, the concentration of the substance under consideration and the relative ease of the determination. Amniotic fluid, essential when detection of serious fetal abnormalities is sought with the possibility of termination of the pregnancy, may be obtained by amniocentesis but collection before the 20th week is a skilled procedure not without hazard to the fetus. Sometimes maternal serum may be used to define those cases in which amniocentesis is justified, for example, the determination of α-fetoprotein to detect spina bifida. Later in pregnancy, amniotic fluid is more easily obtainable with less, but still finite, risk. At this stage, its examination for

Feto-Placental Function Tests

lecithin to assess fetal lung maturity, for bilirubin in pregnancy complicated by Rhesus incompatibility and for other assessments of fetal function is well established. These examinations are for substances unsuitable for determination in maternal serum where either the concentration is too low or the contribution from maternal sources is too great.

Many fetal or placental products enter the maternal circulation and their concentration may be measured there. This will be determined by the rates of entry into and clearance from the plasma. The sample analysed will give information about conditions only at the time of sampling and these may change at different times of the day. The volume of sample is limited and sensitive methods may be required for some substances. In compensation, the substances may be present in relatively unchanged form, metabolites often being cleared quickly by the kidney, and there is no delay in obtaining the sample as occurs with a 24 h collection of urine. Where the analytical method is also rapid, as with some enzymes, clinically important information can be available with minimal delay but in some cases the measurement of a substance in plasma may be technically more demanding than in urine making for analytical delay.

The maternal urine is the fluid used for most steroid investigations. Variations in excretion during the day require collection over at least 24 h and 48 h is the optimal period (Klopper *et al.,* 1969). Often metabolites have to be analysed and several may be present in varying proportions. Urinary investigations generally give the average production of the substance in question over a period of time and the amount of material available for analysis is not a limiting factor. They avoid repeated venepunctures but inevitably impose a delay between initiating the investigation and obtaining a result on which to base clinical decisions. Also there are often errors in making a complete urine collection over a 24 h period.

These biochemical tests of feto-placental function are additional to the regular and proper clinical assessment of the pregnant patient and are only part of the full range of investigations which are available to the obstetrician. In addition to haematological and bacteriological tests, such procedures as fetal heart monitoring, radiology and assessment of fetal maturity by ultrasound are employed.

For a review of feto-placental function tests see Wilde and Oakey (1975).

Oestrogens

The use of oestrogen analyses for monitoring the progress of a pregnancy is well established for the urinary excretion of total oestrogens or of E3 by the mother. Most of the oestrogens, and especially E3, arise in the feto-placental unit (p. 112). E3 in amniotic fluid has been investigated as it enters this liquid in the fetal urine. Plasma oestrogen determinations were less often used because of the lack of suitable rapid and highly sensitive analytical methods but this situation is now changing.

156   *Practical Clinical Biochemistry*

Experience of amniotic fluid oestrogen determinations is rather limited but suggests that it is often unhelpful and offers little advantage over the other methods.

The Use of Maternal Plasma Oestrogen Determinations

The oestrogen concentration in the plasma at the moment of sampling depends on the balance of three factors — the rate of release from the sites of formation, the volume of the maternal distribution space, and the rate of removal from the circulation particularly by the kidney. There is, as yet, no agreement as to which oestrogen gives the best indication of feto-placental function. All three main oestrogens, E1, E2 and E3 are present in conjugated and unconjugated forms, E1 predominating. There is an increase in all fractions as pregnancy progresses, particularly during the last trimester.

The oestrogen present in highest concentration in unconjugated form is E2 with E1 and E3 in varying proportions as pregnancy progresses. The main conjugated oestrogens are E1-3-sulphate, E3-3-sulphate, E3-3 and 16-glucosiduronates and E3-3-sulphate-16-glucosiduronate. The rate of removal of the different forms of E3 by the kidney varies considerably. Thus, while unconjugated E3 has a very low clearance, that of E3-3-sulphate is similar to the glomerular filtration rate and the combined glucosiduronates have a high clearance as they are actively secreted by the tubules (Swapp *et al.*, 1975).

The earlier GLC and fluorimetric methods for plasma oestrogens have largely been replaced by the more sensitive CPB and RIA methods. Various extraction methods, further chromatographic separation and the possibility of hydrolysing conjugates have allowed different oestrogen fractions to be determined. Similar problems exist in regard to cross reactions between related steroids as for E2 (p. 118). Unconjugated E2 is measured by the methods previously described for non-pregnant patients. Unconjugated E3 is readily extracted from plasma without the need for hydrolytic procedures. Following chromatographic separation from other unconjugated oestrogens it may be measured by CPB methods (Tulchinsky *et al.*, 1971) or by RIA techniques using relatively non-specific antisera to E2-17β-hemisuccinyl-BSA (Tulchinsky *et al.*, 1972; Patten *et al.*, 1973; Cleary and Young, 1974; Cohen and Cohen, 1974). Antisera to E3-16, 17-dihemisuccinyl-BSA also require a chromatographic separation step (Youssefnejadian and Sommerville, 1973) but antisera raised to BSA linked to the 6-oxime of E3 show little cross-reaction with other unconjugated oestrogens, E3-16-glucosiduronate or E3-3-sulphate-16-glucosiduronate but some reactivity against E3-3-sulphate or glucosiduronate (Katagiri *et al.*, 1974). This selective action has been used to measure unconjugated E3 following its absorption onto Sephadex (Christner and Fetter, 1974) and could be used on untreated plasma to measure "immunoreactive E3". Less selective antisera can be used for similar determinations of mixtures of E3

Feto-Placental Function Tests

and some of its conjugates using crude extracts of plasma (Podoba *et al.,* 1973). A different approach is to measure total plasma E3 by acid hydrolysis of the conjugates, extraction and separation of the unconjugated E3 before its measurement by a CPB method (Corker and Naftolin, 1971) or using RIA (Masson, 1973; Wilson, 1973).

Details of these techniques are beyond the scope of this book as they depend on the particular antisera used. The original sources should be consulted.

INTERPRETATION

Plasma E2 concentrations are much higher than in the non-pregnant state (Table 4,2) especially during the last trimester when they increase steadily. Cohen and Cohen (1974) give figures in nmol/l (μg/l) at 16 weeks of 4 to 19 (1 to 5), at 28 weeks of 44 to 70 (12 to 19) and at 39 weeks of 37 to 144 (10 to 39), while Ahmed and Mester (1973) give mean figures of 63 (17) at 30 to 36 weeks increasing to 92 (25) at 40 weeks and Patten *et al.* (1973) give a mean figure of 73 (19.8) at term with standard error 7.4 (2.0). The concentration of unconjugated E3 is generally lower but the relative increase in the last trimester is greater (Table 4,5). The same table indicates that at all stages, unconjugated E3 is only a minor component of total E3. For each measurement the normal range is wide. It is not established whether there is a significant diurnal rhythmn for the various oestrogens as reports are conflicting (Wilde and Oakey, 1975). Goebel and Kuss (1974) report average variations for unconjugated E3 of 31 per cent during different times of the day. Any such effect might increase the day-to-day variation for an individual patient and Klopper (1975) found an average coefficient of variation of 13.2 per cent for plasma total E3 while that for unconjugated E3 was 30.9 per cent. The corresponding figure for E3 in 24 h urine collections is 17.9 per cent.

At present the clinical usefulness of plasma oestrogen determinations is not defined. Both total E3 and unconjugated E3 levels are low after fetal death *in utero* or in the case of an anencephalic fetus in which the absent pituitary leads to poor adrenal function. In general, toxaemia reduces the total E3 level compared with the average for the gestation period. Several measurements show a reduced rate of increase in the milder cases and a failure to rise after 33 to 34 weeks in the more severe case. A similar pattern is seen in other causes of placental insufficiency with a "small for dates" fetus, depending on the severity of the impairment. The average figures in diabetic pregnancy are also low with a tendency to be more markedly affected when the fetal hazard is greater. High levels of total E3 are seen in the nephrotic type of toxaemia. The wide normal range requires repeated measurement to follow the course of an indivdual pregnancy. The criteria for recognising the fetus in serious difficulties are not yet defined. Indeed, Dubin *et al.* (1973), comparing plasma total E3 with urinary oestrogen excretion in high risk pregnancies preferred the latter, while

158   *Practical Clinical Biochemistry*

TABLE 4,5

Plasma Concentration of Oestriol and its Conjugates at Various
Stages of Pregnancy

(figures are in nmol/l with µg/l in parentheses)

Gestation (weeks)	Unconjugated E3	Total E3 (or immunoreactive E3*)
16	< 3.5 (< 1)[2]	
16-20	2.4-19 (0.7-5.4)[6]	
20	3.5-28 (1-8)[1]	
20-24	4.2-28 (1.2-8.2)[6]	
24-28	21-52 (6.1-15)[6]	
30	10-21 (3-6)[2]	*69 (20)[5]
28-32	21-111 (6-32)[6]	
29-32	15-48 (4.3-13.8)[3]	310; SD 100 (90; 30)[4]
33		350; SD 100 (100; 30)[4]
33-36	17-53.5 (4.8-15.4)[3]	
32-40	18-230 (5.3-66)[6]	
34		380; SD 100 (110; 30)[4]
35		415; SD 140 (120; 40)[4]
36		435; SD 140 (125; 40)[4]
37		470; SD 175 (135; 50)[4]
37-40	37.5-92.5 (10.8-26.7)[3]	
38		575; SD 210 (165; 60)[4]
39	30-56 (8.5-16)	660; SD 210 (190; 60)[4]
40	21-78 (6-25)[1]	⎰ 695; SD 210 (200; 60)[4] ⎱ *555 (160)[5]

References: [1]Cleary and Young (1974); [2]Cohen and Cohen (1974);
[3]Katagiri *et al.* (1974); [4]Masson (1973); [5]Poboda *et al.* (1973);
[6]Youssefnejadian and Sommerville (1973).

Townsley *et al.* (1973) found plasma unconjugated E2 determinations
similarly unsatisfactory. Several workers have found plasma oestrogen
measurements to be unhelpful in the management of Rhesus immunisation.

Determination of Maternal Urinary Oestrogen

Although conjugated forms of E1, E2 and E3 are excreted in the urine of
pregnant women, those of E3, particularly E3-16-glucosiduronate, account
for most of the total urinary oestrogens. The clinical usefulness of urinary
oestrogen determinations depends on rapid availability of results. As the
fractionation of oestrogens increases the time spent on the analysis, most
workers prefer to measure "total oestrogens" in the urine. The earlier
methods involved hydrolysis of the conjugates, glucosiduronates and some
sulphates, before extraction and determination by colorimetry or
fluorimetry. For such hydrolysis, heating in acid solution is quick and the
major oestrogens are relatively unaffected by the procedure. Enzymic
hydrolysis, preferably using a mixture of glucuronidase and sulphatase, is
milder but takes longer and is more expensive.

Feto-Placental Function Tests

Prior hydrolysis of the conjugates is avoided in methods whereby the Köber reaction is carried out on diluted urine. This is followed by extraction into chloroform containing trichloracetic acid or p-nitrophenol in order to develop highly fluorescent products—the Ittrich reaction. Such direct procedures have allowed the development of automated versions. Examples of the various techniques are given below.

Colorimetric Method of Brown *et al.* (1968a)

The fluorimetric version of this method (p. 123) is suitable for urine collected up to the 16th to 20th week of pregnancy provided the smaller volumes of urine are used. Thereafter further dilution of the urine will be needed and the less sensitive colorimetric method may be more convenient. The colour developed in the Köber reaction is read at three wavelengths to allow for the effect of non-specific chromogens.

Reagents. 1 to 8 as on pp. 123, 124.

9. Köber reagent. Dissolve 20 g quinol in 1 litre sulphuric acid, 700 ml/l, with gentle heating.

10. Standard oestriol solution. Prepare a stock solution in ethanol, 4 mmol/l (115 mg in 100 ml). Dilute this for use 1 vol to 10 vol with ethanol giving a concentration of 400 μmol/l.

Technique. *Hydrolysis and extraction.* Depending on the period of gestation, pipette 1/500th to 1/4 000th of the 24 h specimen into a 150 × 15 mm test tube graduated at 6 ml and proceed as for the fluorimetric method (p. 124).

Colorimetry. Transfer the ether extract to a glass tube which can be stoppered and add 0.2 ml quinol solution. Place the tubes in a warm water bath in a fume cupboard and evaporate to dryness. To ensure complete dryness, which is essential, apply suction to the hot tube as soon as the ether has evaporated. Reduce the suction and reapply. At the same time pipette 100 μl standard containing 40 nmol (11.5 μg) oestriol into a similar tube, add 6 ml ether and 0.2 ml quinol and evaporate to dryness. Prepare a blank similarly using 6 ml ether and 0.2 ml quinol. To the dry residues add 3 ml Köber reagent, place in a boiling water bath until the quinol has dissolved, then stopper and heat at 120° C for 5 min to develop the colour. Cool, add 0.75 ml water and reheat at 120° C for another 5 min. Cool in a cold water bath for about 10 min and read against the reagent blank at 480, 518 and 556 nm. Calculate the corrected extinction at 518 nm using the Allen formula:

$$E \text{ corr }_{518} = 2E_{518} - (E_{480} + E_{556})$$

Calculation. Urinary total oestrogens (μmol/24 h) =

$$\frac{E \text{ corr of unknown}}{E \text{ corr of standard}} \times \frac{40}{1\ 000} \times \text{dilution factor}$$

Notes. 1. In the absence of facilities for heating at 120° C develop at 100° C as in the method of Brown (1955a). Add 3 ml Köber reagent to

160   *Practical Clinical Biochemistry*

each tube and heat for 20 min in a boiling water bath shaking the tubes twice during the first 6 min of heating. Cool in a bath of cold water, add 0.75 ml water, shake and reheat in a boiling water bath for a further 10 min.

2. See notes for fluorimetric method (p. 125).

3. The average percentage recovery of radioactive unconjugated E3 added to urine is: in initial ether extract (92); after carbonate wash (88); in sodium hydroxide extract (75).

4. The method gives linear calibration curves up to 174 μmol/l (50 mg/l) of E3. The coefficient of variation at 49 μmol/l (14 mg/l) is about 12 per cent.

Colorimetric Method of Oakey *et al.* (1967)

The conjugates are hydrolysed by heating with acid and the free steroids are extracted into ether. After removal of acidic contaminants with sodium carbonate, the crude mixture of oestrogens is subjected to the Köber reaction. The colour developed is read at three wavelengths to correct for the effect of non-specific chromogens. An internal standard is used to correct for losses.

Reagents. 1. Concentrated hydrochloric acid.

2. Diethyl ether, technical grade redistilled.

3. Carbonate solution, pH 10.5. Dissolve 80 g sodium bicarbonate in 1 litre water and add 150 ml 5 mol/l sodium hydroxide.

4. Sodium sulphate, anhydrous.

5. Quinol solution, 20 g/l in ether.

6. Köber reagent. Carefully mix 250 ml concentrated sulphuric acid with 136 ml water. Cool. Prepare a solution of quinol in this acid, 20 g/l.

7. Standard oestriol solutions. Prepare a stock solution in ethanol, 4 mmol/l (115 mg in 100 ml). Dilute for use with ethanol to give two standards, 100 and 400 μmol/l.

8. Bauxite chips.

Technique. Collect a 24 h specimen of urine and dilute to 2 1. Place 2 ml in each of three 150 × 25 mm glass-stoppered tubes. To each add 0.3 ml hydrochloric acid, stopper, and place in a boiling water bath for 1 h. For greater volumes of urine, make to nearest litre and use 1 ml urine and 0.15 ml acid per litre of diluted urine. Cool the tubes and to one (the internal standard) add 0.2 ml oestriol standard (400 μmol/l) and then to each add 10 ml ether. Stopper and shake vigorously for half a minute. After separation, remove the lower aqueous layer, add 0.5 ml carbonate solution and shake. Add 1 to 2 g sodium sulphate and shake again. Transfer 3 ml ether extract to clean glass stoppered tubes and prepare a blank and an external standard by adding 3 ml ether and 0.2 ml oestriol standard (100 μmol/l) and 3 ml ether to separate tubes. To each add 0.2 ml quinol solution and a bauxite chip. Evaporate to dryness at 55° C in a water bath using gentle suction at the end of the process. Add 2 ml Köber reagent, stopper and heat in a boiling water bath for 40 min. Cool under running

Feto-Placental Function Tests 161

water, add 1.7 ml water and shake gently. After 15 min read at 472, 514 and 556 nm against the blank. Calculate the corrected extinction at 514 nm using the Allen formula and take the mean of the test duplicates.

$$Ecorr_{514} = 2E_{514} - (E_{472} + E_{556})$$

Calculation. Urinary total oestrogens (μmol/24 h) =

$$\frac{\text{E corr of unknown}}{\text{E corr of internal standard} - \text{E corr of unknown}} \times \frac{0.08}{2} \times 2\,000$$

The recovery (per cent) is given by:

$$\frac{(\text{E corr of internal standard} - \text{E corr of unknown})}{\text{E corr of external standard}} \times \frac{100}{6} \times 5$$

Notes. 1. The mean recovery of E3 varies from 84 to 93 per cent.

2. Occasionally low results are attributable to incomplete hydrolysis which will not be allowed for by the internal standard. Enzymic hydrolysis may be more reliable.

3. The coefficient of variation for within-batch duplicates is 9 per cent above 35 μmol/24 h (10 mg/24 h). Between-batch precision for urine pools is 9.2 per cent at 52 μmol/24 h (15 mg/24 h) and 13.1 per cent at 40 μmol/24 h (11.5 mg/24 h).

Fluorimetric Method of Howarth and Robertshaw

The oestrogen conjugates are reacted directly with the Köber reagent by heating in a boiling water bath. Then Ittrich reagent is added and the fluorescence read. This work-simplified modification (Howarth and Robertshaw, personal communication) is based on the methods of Brombacher *et al.* (1968), and Howarth and Robertshaw (1971).

Reagents. 1. Köber reagent. Dissolve 2 g quinol, BDH, AnalaR grade, in 200 ml concentrated sulphuric acid (BDH, AnalaR or Micro AnalaR grade) by leaving for 3 to 4 h at 4°C. As the reagent tends to go brown on storage and exposure to light, prepare only small quantities.

2. Ittrich reagent, trichloracetic acid 50 g/l in chloroform. Dissolve 50 g trichloracetic acid, AnalaR grade, in 1 litre chloroform, AnalaR grade. Larger quantities can be prepared but some batches give better results if prepared immediately before use.

3. Stock standard oestriol solution, 4 mmol/l. Dissolve 115 mg oestriol in 100 ml ethanol, spectroscopic grade.

4. Working standard oestriol solution 40 μmol/l. Dilute 1 ml stock solution to 100 ml with double deionised water. Prepare freshly at least once a week.

5. Acetone.

Apparatus. Micro pipettes of 10 and 20 μl are required for test and standards. Precision is improved by using automatic pipettes to add deionised water and reagents. A centrifuge capable of taking 15 ml glass

162 *Practical Clinical Biochemistry*

stoppered centrifuge tubes is required. The tubes are stored in sulphuric acid, 100 ml/l, and used only for this purpose. Immediately before use they are removed from the acid, washed well in running tap water, followed by 6 rinses in deionised water and then dried in an oven at $95°C$. The fluorimeter used requires a primary wavelength of about 538 nm which can be obtained from a mercury arc with an interference filter; the secondary filter requires a sharp cut off at 560 nm.

Technique. Collect a 24 h sample of urine and dilute to 2 or preferably 3 litres and carry out duplicate determinations for all tests and standards. Pipette 10 μl diluted urine and 10 and 20 μl working standard into the centrifuge tubes. A further tube is required as a blank. To each add 1 ml deionised water followed by 2 ml Köber reagent and mix by flicking the tubes. Stoppering is not necessary if care is employed. Place the tubes in a briskly boiling water bath for 45 min. Then remove and cool rapidly in a sink of running cold water. Transfer to a tray containing water and ice for the next stage of the determination. The capacity of the bath and the amount of ice should be such that ice is still present at the end of the sequence.

Add 2 ml deionised water to each tube in turn, mix and cool for 3 min. From this stage onwards carry out the operations with strict attention to detail and minimum delay. The number of tubes handled together depends on the ability of the operator and the capacity of the centrifuge. With a centrifuge capacity of 8 tubes the following sequence can be employed. Starting with the blank and standard tubes, add 6 ml Ittrich reagent to the first 8 tubes, stopper in pairs and shake vigorously for 20 s, then return to the ice bath. When all 8 tubes have been shaken, remove the stoppers and transfer the tubes to the centrifuge, spin by bringing rapidly to 3 000 rpm and then switch off. During this operation add the Ittrich reagent to the next series of tubes ready for extraction. As the tubes are removed from the centrifuge, transfer to a rack at room temperature and remove the upper aqueous layer by suction. Repeat until all tubes are ready for fluorimetric reading. This operation depends upon the number of available cuvettes which need only be of good quality glass as wavelengths in the visible region are used. Several are preferable as a single tube needs drying after several readings. Transfer the acid chloroform reagent to the cuvette without forming bubbles and without spillage. Bubbles are avoided by transferring the solution with a fixed volume automatic pipette. If the outside of the cuvette is contaminated, immerse it in water and dry gently with a soft cloth. Make the readings between 20 and 25 min after shaking with the Ittrich reagent. Zero the instrument with the blank and adjust the gain so that a 20 μl standard reads 160 if the urine is diluted to 2 litres, or 240 if to 3 litres. Read the other 20 μl standard, then the 10 μl standards which should give half the scale reading. Duplicate standards should agree within 5 per cent. Read the duplicate test samples. If only one cuvette is used, moisture will gradually condense in it. Rinse with acetone and dry after each 10 readings.

Feto-Placental Function Tests

Calculation. With the fluorimeter standardised as above, the scale readings correspond directly to the urinary oestriol output in μmol/24 h. If a urine diluted to 2 litres gives the same reading as the 20 μl standard its concentration is 80 μmol/l. The daily output is thus 160 μmol, the scale reading.

Notes. 1. A suitable pool of urine can be dispensed in AutoAnalyzer cups and deep frozen for use as control solutions. Alternatively control samples can be obtained from Fermtrol and International Diagnostic Aids:—

Fermtrol Pregnancy Urine (Purce Associates Ltd., marketed by G. S. Ross Ltd, 2 Allenby Road, Biggin Hill, Westerham, Kent, U.K.),

I.D.A. Oestriol Control (International Diagnostic Aids Ltd, Ellen Street, Portslade, Brighton, BN4 1EQ, U.K.).

2. Duplicate results for test urines should agree to within 4 to 8 μmol/24 h. If not, repeat the determination in the next batch.

3. This method requires a high degree of technical ability on the part of the operator if reliability and precision are to be maintained.

Automated Methods for Urinary Oestriol

In one of the earliest automated methods (Ua Conaill and Muir, 1968) the pre-hydrolysed urine is heated with Köber reagent in an AutoAnalyzer digester unit, extracted with chloroform containing p-nitrophenol and read colorimetrically using two colorimeters in series to allow for interference. A modification (Barnard and Logan, 1970) employs fluorimetry but both methods require predilution of the sample and hydrolysis prior to reaction in the digester. Campbell and Gardner (1971) and Hainsworth and Hall (1971) introduced more fully automated methods utilising the full potential of the Ittrich procedure. The Köber reaction is performed directly on oestrogen conjugates after diluting the urine considerably. By heating at 120°C instead of 100°C, the time of reaction is shortened before extracting the Köber chromogen into the Ittrich reagent, and reading fluorimetrically. Lever *et al.* (1973) prefer to avoid the use of chloroform and hence phase separation, which has decided advantages.

Method of Hainsworth and Hall (1971). (See also Moscrop *et al.,* 1974).

The prediluted urine is sampled at 20/h, further diluted with water in a dilution circuit, mixed with Köber reagent and heated at 120°C. After cooling in a jacketed mixing coil, Ittrich reagent is added and after passing through a phase separator the fluorescence of the chloroform layer is measured.

Reagents. 1. Köber reagent. Dissolve 20 g quinol in 1 litre of sulphuric acid prepared by mixing 666 ml concentrated sulphuric acid with 333 ml water. Allow to cool. This acid can be obtained from BDH Ltd as "Sulphuric Acid Solution 66% v/v for the determination of urinary oestrogens".

164 *Practical Clinical Biochemistry*

2. Ittrich reagent, trichloracetic acid in chloroform 50 g/l. Prepare as required.

3. Stock standard oestriol solution, 4 mmol/l. Dissolve 115 mg in 100 ml ethanol. Store at 4° C.

4. Working standard oestriol solutions. Dilute 1 ml stock solution to 50 ml with water to give a solution containing 80 μmol/l and further dilute this to give solutions containing 20, 40 and 60 μmol/l. Store at room temperature but prepare freshly each month.

5. Triton X-100, 1 ml/l water.

6. Dilute Triton X-100. Add 5 ml reagent 5 to 1 litre water.

7. Quality control preparations (as Note 1, p. 163).

Equipment. All items in the manifold (Fig. 4,5) are from Technicon unless stated otherwise. Ismatec MP 13 and 25 pumps can successfully replace the AutoAnalyzer Mark II pump. A standard Technicon 40 ft (12 m) coil (internal diameter 1.6 mm) is used in the heating bath filled with Shell Nonidet P 40 and set at 120°C. A fluorimeter with flow cell is required. The Locarte Mk IV instrument is suitable. The primary beam comes from a thallium arc emitting at 535 nm (Wotan thallium lamp, A.E.G. Ltd., 27 Chancery Lane, London, W.C.2) and requires no primary filter. With a mercury arc a 538 nm interference filter is required. The secondary side requires an interference filter of 560 nm. The interface between the fluorimeter and recorder can be obtained from Locarte Co. Ltd., 24 Emperors Gate, London, S.W.7) All pump tubing is acidflex and transmission tubes are glass or Tygon as shown.

Technique. Dilute urine samples manually to at least 3 litres. Higher dilutions, although preferable (p. 168), may not be possible depending upon the sensitivity and stability of the fluorimeter. Remove any obvious sediment by centrifuging to prevent obstruction of the sampling probe.

Commence the run with phase separator and flow cell disconnected to avoid acid entering the latter. Pump the water and Köber reagent lines until a good flow pattern is established in the heating coil. Then pump the Ittrich reagent and when a good flow pattern is established connect the phase separator and flow cell. Flush the flow cell with ethanol and then air before connecting. These manipulations are done conveniently if the phase separator and flow cell are linked by acidflex tubing. When the recorder trace is steady, set the base line to zero and then sample two 40 μmol/l standards. Use the first to adjust the fluorimeter gain to give a convenient reading on the recorder, e.g. 40 divisions, and use the second to check this. Follow with a water wash, a standard curve up to 80 μmol/l and a further water wash before sampling urines. Include the 40 μmol/l standard as a drift control after every 5 specimens and add at least two quality control specimens to each batch of 40 urine samples. Allow for any drift and preferably include a standard curve at the end of the run.

When the run is finished turn the oil bath temperature to 90°C, disconnect the phase separator and pump the effluent to waste. Remove the sample tube from the Köber reagent and the water line to the dilution

Feto-Placental Function Tests

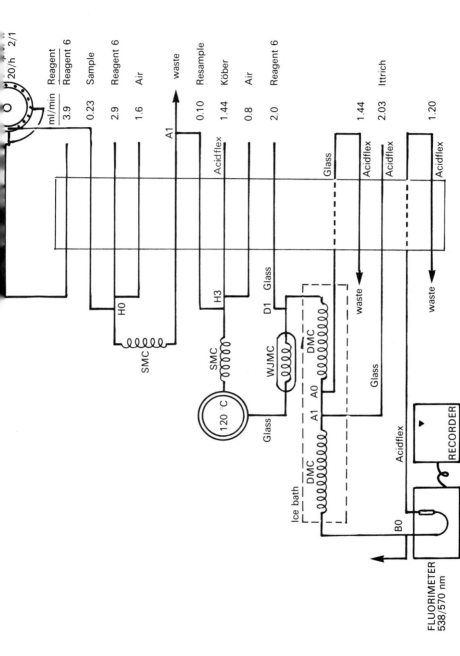

Fig. 4.5. Automated Method for the Determination of Total Oestrogens in Urine. (Modification of the method of Hainsworth and Hall, 1971.) For the Locarte fluorimeter the operating conditions are: excitation — thallium lamp without filter or mercury arc with 538 nm interference filter; emission — filter with cut-off below 560 nm or interference wedge set at 570 nm. SMC, DMC, WJMC — single, double and water-jacketed mixing coils; BO — phase separator. The heating bath mixing coil is 12 m × 1.6 mm (internal diameter).

166 *Practical Clinical Biochemistry*

circuit but continue pumping the other reagents until the system is free from acid. Pump water for a short time through the Ittrich line and draw ethanol through the phase separator and flow cell. Increase the oil bath temperature to 120° C before restarting an analytical run.

Calculation. Urinary total oestrogens, as oestriol (μmol/24 h) = Reading from recorder chart $\times$ vol diluted urine (l).

Notes. 1. The bubble pattern in the phase separator may be improved by treating it with HW Ltd's silicone DC 1107 (MS 1107). Soak in a 1 to 3 per cent solution of DC 1107 in ethyl acetate, butanone or hexane. Drain off the solvent and bond the silicone to the surface by heating for 1 to 2 h at 100° C, 15 min at 150° C or 5 min at 200 to 250° C.

2. A short length (5 to 10 cm) of narrow bore glass tubing preceding the flow cell helps to detect contamination revealed by bubbles of acid adhering to the glass. It should be watched throughout the run and if necessary the ethanol wash procedure mentioned earlier may be performed in 1 to 2 min.

3. Regular cleaning of the system with aqueous "Decon", 50 ml/l is necessary for good performance. This should not be pumped through the dilution circuit, phase separator or flow cell. The wash can be conveniently carried out before an analytical run.

4. The coefficient of variation at 49 μmol/l (14 mg/l) is 1.5 to 5 per cent within batch and 2 to 7.5 per cent between batch.

Method of Lever *et al.* (1973)

The urine is diluted, mixed with a Köber reagent containing quinol and ferrous sulphate in sulphuric acid and heated at 120° C. The resultant mixture is then diluted with a solution containing trichloracetic acid and chloral, cooled and passed directly through the flow cell of the fluorimeter. A single aqueous phase is used throughout.

Reagents. 1. Quinol-sulphuric acid reagent, 32 g/l in concentrated sulphuric acid. Dissolve an appropriate amount of quinol in cold concentrated sulphuric acid. Stand for at least 30 min to ensure complete sulphonation.

2. Ferrous sulphate solution, 24 g Fe SO_4. $7H_2O$/l in water. Prepare as required.

3. Köber reagent. Carefully add 3 volumes reagent 1 to one volume reagent 2 with cooling. The reagent is ready for immediate use and is stable for several days if protected from excessive exposure to air.

4. Stock standard oestriol solution, 500 μmol/l in sulphuric acid. Dissolve 144 mg oestriol in 10 ml cold concentrated sulphuric acid. Stand at room temperature for 20 to 60 min for sulphonation to occur and pour into ice cold water. Finally dilute to 1 litre.

5. Working oestriol standard solution. Prepare suitable dilutions to cover the range 30 to 120 μmol/l by diluting with sulphuric acid, 100 mmol/l.

Feto-Placental Function Tests

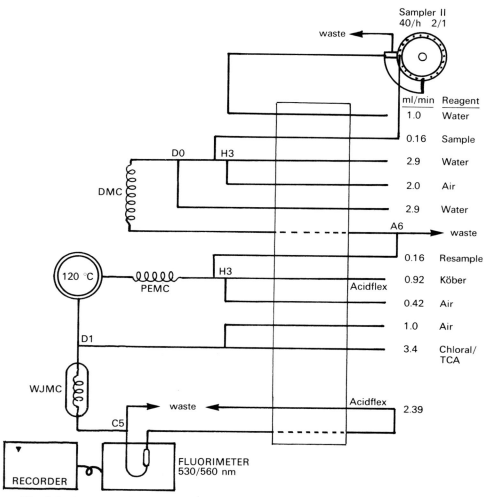

Fig. 4,6. Automated Method of the Determination of Total Oestrogens in Urine. (Method of Lever et al., 1973.) DMC, WJMC, PEMC — double, water-jacketed and polyethylene mixing coils. The heating bath coil is 6 m x 1.6 mm (internal diameter).

6. Fluorescence reagent. Dissolve 500 g trichloracetic acid and 500 g chloral hydrate in distilled water and make up to 2 l.

Equipment. The items used for the manifold (Fig. 4,6) are those employed in the previous method except that acidflex tubing is required only for the Köber reagent and the fluorimeter flow-through lines. Polyethylene transmission tubing (1.2 mm i.d.) is used in all lines containing acid.

Technique. A range of freshly prepared standards (30, 60, 90 and 120 μmol/l), controls and undiluted urine samples are sampled as previously described at 40 samples/h with a 2/1 sample to wash ratio.

168   *Practical Clinical Biochemistry*

Calculate the results from the standard curve or directly from the recorder chart once the linearity of response has been established.

Note. Modifications to the method are recommended by Little *et al.* (1975) who found unacceptable carryover at 40 samples/h. They used a 60/h 1 : 1 sampling cam with water cups placed between each sample giving an effective rate of 30/h and eliminated the air segmentation of the trichloracetic acid/chloral hydrate reagent, compensating by increasing the air segmentation of the Köber reagent to 0.06 ml/min.

Some General Problems Relating to Methods for Oestrogens in Pregnancy Urines

An important factor affecting oestriol assays using direct Köber, Ittrich fluorimetry is the presence in fresh urine of substances impairing the recovery of oestriol glucosiduronate. These substances, mostly of unknown origin, include glucose but the problem persists in its absence. In their collaborative study, Moscrop *et al.* (1974) found that the apparent oestrogen content of fresh urine increased on storage when urines were diluted to 2 litres before analysis. Higher results for fresh urine were found if the samples were diluted to 20 litres and the mean recovery of added steroid improved from 73 per cent at 2 litres to 94 per cent at 20 litres. As the specimens aged, the recovery at 2 litres dilution improved. Also the apparent daily variation for an individual was greater at 2 litres than at 20 litres dilution. During 3 weeks one patient excreted a fairly constant 120 μmol/24 h with percentage recoveries of 84 to 100 at 20 litres dilution, but at 2 litres dilution the same specimens showed an apparent daily excretion of 63 to 108 μmol/24 h with recoveries from 30 to 71 per cent. Such variations can cause diagnostic confusion. At the higher acid concentrations used by Lever *et al.* (1973) and Simkins and Worth (1975) the effect may be abolished as the latter authors and Little *et al.* (1975) using the Lever method found no such behaviour with undiluted urine. The Lever method has however a higher dilution circuit in the manifold.

The action of glucose is such that the recovery falls with increasing glucose concentration. The effect, particularly with direct fluorimetric methods applied to pregnancy urines, is well recognised and is minimised at higher dilutions of urine. Glucose in a concentration of 110 mmol/l (2 g/100 ml) reduces the apparent oestriol level by 40 per cent (Campbell and Gardner, 1971). Yeast fermentation removes glucose but may not abolish the interference and Little *et al.* (1975) found oestriol recoveries of only 57 per cent after completely removing glucose originally present at a concentration of 500 mmol/l (9 g/100 ml). Oestriol reacts with aldehydes forming derivatives which do not give the Köber reaction. With formaldehyde and acid hydrolysis, oestriol is no longer extractable into ether (Ryan and Grey, 1975). Glucose and other aldoses react like formaldehyde and the poor recovery after yeast fermentation may be due to incomplete conversion into ethanol of the acetaldehyde formed.

Feto-Placental Function Tests

Glucose is best removed by reduction to sorbitol with sodium borohydride. Worth (1973) incubated 100 mg borohydride with 5 ml undiluted urine at $37°C$ for 15 min before destroying excess borohydride with 3 drops of concentrated sulphuric acid. Ryan and Gray (1975) remove glucose by adding to 5 ml urine, 0.5 ml 100 g/l sodium borohydride in 100 mmol/l sodium hydroxide and incubating at $37°C$ for 1 h, adding a drop of octan-2-ol to prevent frothing. They then add 0.5 ml glacial acetic acid to remove borohydride and correct for the dilution. Little *et al.* (1975) found this amount of borohydride (50 mg) inadequate for glucose concentrations over 500 mmol/l (9 g/100 ml) but achieved quantitative recovery by using 0.5 ml of a 500 g/l solution. They recommend the use of this solution for all urines giving a positive Clinistix test for glucose and treat similarly all subsequent urines from the same patient whether they contain glucose or not. They do not follow the suggestion of Ryan and Gray (1975) that all urines should be treated with borohydride to avoid interference from other aldehydes which may be present in glucose-free urines.

Other interferences with urinary oestrogen methods are less common. Various drugs, particularly laxatives, which are important in urines from non-pregnant patients, give less trouble at the higher dilutions used for pregnancy oestrogens. However, Mandelamine (methenamine mandelate) interferes badly as it liberates formaldehyde during acid hydrolysis. In high doses aspirin, excreted as a glucosiduronate, interferes in methods using glucuronidase to split conjugates by competing for the enzyme (Adlercreutz, 1975). In methods using the colorimetric Köber reaction and an Allen correction, urobilin can interfere if present in excess as in the crises of congenital haemolytic anaemia (Wood, 1975).

INTERPRETATION

Methods using direct fluorimetry for total oestrogens in urine give higher results than those in which initial hydrolysis and extraction procedures are used. This may be due to several factors: oestriol may represent less than 67 per cent of total oestrogens; the recovery of oestrogens is more complete in the direct methods; other steroids of fetoplacental origin may contribute to the fluorescence. Hull *et al.* (1975) report values from 56 patients using Moscrop's modification of the method on pp. 163 to 166 (Table 4,6). At 30 weeks, Oakey *et al.* (1967) using their hydrolysis and extraction method found 31.2 to 90.3 μmol/24 h (9 to 26 mg/24 h); at 33 weeks, 31.2 to 104 μmol/24 h (9 to 30 mg/24 h); at 36 weeks, 34.7 to 139 μmol/24 h (10 to 40 mg/24 h) and at 40 weeks, 48.6 to 191 μmol/24 h (14 to 55 mg/24 h). In our experience the automated method of Hainsworth and Hall and the manual method of Howarth and Robertshaw (p. 161) give essentially similar results, although the automated method gives slightly lower results at higher levels and higher results at the lower end of the normal range. It is important therefore to interpret results in the light of

TABLE 4,6
Means and 95 per cent Probability Bounds of Urinary Oestrogen Excretion in Normal Pregnancy. (Hull et al., 1975)

| Gestation (weeks) | Urinary total oestrogen excretion | | | | | |
| | μmol/24 h | | | mg/24 h | | |
	Mean	Upper limit	Lower limit	Mean	Upper limit	Lower limit
25	64.6	117	35.8	18.6	33.7	10.3
26	69.1	125	38.2	19.9	36.1	11.0
27	74.3	134	41.0	21.4	38.7	11.8
28	79.5	144	44.1	22.9	41.5	12.7
29	85.4	155	47.2	24.6	44.5	13.6
30	91.3	165	50.3	26.3	47.6	14.5
31	97.9	177	54.2	28.2	51.1	15.6
32	105	190	58.0	30.2	54.7	16.7
33	112.5	204	62.2	32.4	58.7	17.9
34	120.5	218	66.7	34.7	62.9	19.2
35	129	234	71.5	37.2	67.4	20.6
36	139	251	76.4	39.9	72.2	22.0
37	149	269	82.1	42.8	77.4	23.6
38	159	288	87.8	45.8	82.9	25.3
39	170	309	94.1	49.1	88.9	27.1
40	183	331	101	52.6	95.3	29.1

the method used. The range of values at a given stage of pregnancy is very wide and single results for an individual are usually valueless. For correct interpretation a trend must be established by repeated estimations. Attempts have been made to shorten the urine collection period and to express the oestrogen output in relation to that of creatinine. The consensus of opinion is that the variation from day to day of such a measure is greater than that of oestrogens over a 24 h period and the practice is not recommended.

As might be expected low oestrogen excretion occurs after *fetal death* and with an *anencephalic fetus* — in both cases fetal adrenal inactivity is the cause. High excretion is a feature of a multiple pregnancy. The main use of the investigation is in the investigation of high-risk pregnancies particularly those associated with toxaemia, diabetes, retarded fetal growth or other factors likely to imperil the fetus. The topic is reviewed by Wilde and Oakey (1975).

Urinary oestrogen excretion is a useful predictor of fetal survival in that death is unusual if figures remain consistently in the normal range. The investigation is a relatively poor predictor of fetal size but for babies known to have impaired growth the mean oestrogen excretion rises only slowly after 34 weeks. There is still some overlap between the whole group of cases of *"small for dates" fetuses* and the normal range (Klopper, 1975). The investigation is useful in predicting the survival of the fetus, an

Feto-Placental Function Tests

171

increased perinatal death rate being associated with oestrogen excretion below the normal range. In *toxaemia of pregnancy*, the severity is generally correlated with low oestrogen excretion, and failure to increase, or even to decrease, with time. A successful outcome is likely when the figures remain within the normal range but a low excretion with falling levels is a warning of impending fetal death. Frequently repeated measurements with early availability of results is vital in such cases of severe toxaemia with retarded fetal growth. In *diabetic pregnancy*, the investigation is useful in that with values within the normal range, the pregnancy can usually be continued safely until fetal lung maturity is established (p. 182). Falling secretion indicates fetal distress and the need for an urgent decision on management of the case. In *Rhesus immunisation* the determination has not usually helped in predicting the outcome and determination of amniotic fluid bilirubin is preferable. The *prolongation of pregnancy* beyond 40 weeks may be accompanied by the post-maturity syndrome and a tendency for the oestrogen excretion to diminish.

Oestrogen excretion may be affected by drugs taken by the mother. Corticosteroids suppress the fetal pituitary and hence the adrenal leading to impaired oestrogen excretion. This should not be taken as an indication of fetal distress unless the daily corticosteroid intake is less than the equivalent of about 75 mg cortisol. Penicillin and its preparations also interfere with the production and excretion of oestrogens but the mechanism is not defined.

The congenital absence of placental sulphatase leads to low E3 excretion since DHA sulphate cannot be utilised in the synthetic pathway (Fig. 4,3). The progress of the pregnancy as judged by fetal growth and by function tests other than those involving E3 is normal. The condition can usually be detected in this way. After delivery, tissue enzyme studies are possible.

Determination of Progesterone and its Metabolites

Progesterone is produced by the corpus luteum of pregnancy until the placenta is established when this becomes the major source. An adequate production is necessary for the satisfactory development of the fetus, particularly in the early stages. The steroid is metabolised in the maternal liver and a minor part is excreted as pregnanediol in the maternal urine. The fetus itself plays little part in the production or metabolism of this hormone. Determination of plasma progesterone or urinary pregnanediol is technically feasible and is mainly an index of placental function after the first few weeks.

Plasma progesterone may be determined in maternal samples using the RIA or CPB techniques already discussed (p. 128).

Urinary pregnanediol determinations have already been described (p. 130). The only modification needed for the higher concentrations in pregnancy urine is to reduce the volume of urine analysed to one fifth or one tenth of that used for the non-pregnant patient and to adjust the calculation accordingly.

172 *Practical Clinical Biochemistry*

INTERPRETATION

When pregnancy occurs the luteal peak of plasma progesterone or urinary pregnanediol is not followed by the usual fall but persists or increases somewhat during the first trimester. Further increases occur in the middle trimester but a more rapid rise is seen from about the 24th week. During the first trimester, plasma progesterone values are usually below 128 nmol/l (40 μg/l) but are increased to 255 to 800 nmol/l (80 to 250 μg/l) at term. Daily urinary pregnanediol excretion averages 34 μmol (11 mg) at 12 weeks, 68 μmol (22 mg) at 24 weeks; 124 μmol (40 mg) at 30 weeks and 140 μmol (45 mg) at term. There is a wide individual variation and the 95 per cent range for the period from 30 to 40 weeks varies from 47 to 54.5 μmol/24 h (15 to 17.5 mg/24 h) at the lower end to 205 to 230 μmol/24 h (66 to 74 mg/24 h) at the upper. For an individual patient the day to day coefficient of variation is about 20 per cent.

The main use of progesterone or pregnanediol estimations has been in early abortion, threatened abortion and in toxaemia or placental insufficiency. Very *early abortion,* particularly after the induction of ovulation, has been attributed to an inadequate corpus luteum on the basis of low serum or urine results. In cases of *threatened abortion* in the first half of pregnancy, plasma progesterone measurements are unhelpful in determining the outcome, the overlap between continuing pregnancy and abortion being very marked (Nygren *et al.,* 1973). Urinary pregnanediol is a better discriminant in our experience and that of Brown *et al.* (1970). When the output is below the first percentile of the normal range, practically all cases abort and about half abort with pregnanediol between the first and tenth percentile. When the excretion is above the tenth percentile the outcome cannot be predicted with confidence as 28 per cent abort and the rest continue to term.

Where *placental insufficiency* leads to retarded fetal growth in later pregnancy, a reduced pregnanediol output is often associated with a low birth weight but the determination in an unreliable predictor of fetal death. A similar pattern exists for toxaemic states and a falling oestrogen excretion usually gives an earlier warning of fetal risk. Pregnanediol excretion is probably unsuitable for monitoring pregnancies with high fetal risk (Keller *et al.,* 1971). Increased excretion has been recorded in *Rhesus iso-immunisation* (Fairweather *et al.,* 1972).

Human Placental Lactogen in Maternal Serum

This polypeptide (HPL) is produced only in the syncytial layer of the placental trophoblastic tissue and its measurement is therefore a test of placental rather than fetal function. The control of the secretion and even the function of the product are not properly understood but it is known that near term between 1 and 3 g are secreted daily. The half-life of secreted material is only 25 min so plasma levels should respond rapidly to

Feto-Placental Function Tests

changes in production. No diurnal rhythm exists; plasma samples may be taken at any time. HPL is mainly released into the maternal circulation where the concentration is about 1 000 times that in the fetus.

Compared with many polypeptide hormones, the plasma concentration is very high leading to relatively simple and rapid methods for its determination by RIA techniques. These are exclusively used and a kit is available from the Radiochemical Centre, Amersham, Bucks, and from other manufacturers. A semi-automated procedure is described (Letchworth *et al.*, 1971).

INTERPRETATION

HPL can be detected in plasma very early in pregnancy. There is a progressive increase to a plateau at 36 to 40 weeks. Typical mean figures are 0.1 mg/l at 9 weeks, 1 mg/l at 15 weeks, 3 mg/l at 26 weeks, 5 mg/l at 32 weeks and 6 mg/l at the plateau. The figures for normal pregnancies at each period of gestation are distributed in a log normal fashion and this should be allowed for when calculating lower limits.

The usefulness of HPL determinations has been reviewed recently (Chard, 1975; Wilde and Oakey, 1975). It is useful in assessing the outcome of a *threatened abortion* particularly in the period from 9 to 19 weeks gestation when low levels are associated with abortion. By classifying results (after log transformation) into "favourable" when higher than 1.75 SD below the mean and "unfavourable" when lower than 3 SD below the mean with an "equivocal" zone in between, Gartside and Tindall (1975) correctly predicted from a single determination the immediate prognosis in 86 per cent of cases and were wrong in only 3 per cent. After 19 weeks gestation the prediction was much less reliable. HPL levels are correlated with fetal weight and tend to be low with a *"small for dates" fetus*. This presumably reflects the smaller placental mass in many such cases. In *toxaemia* the situation is somewhat confused and there is a tendency for low values to be associated with the milder forms of toxaemia and not to be clearly related to increased fetal risk. Not all workers find this and Keller *et al.* (1971) prefer HPL to urinary oestrogens in dealing with hypertensive pregnancies. In *diabetic pregnancies* which progress normally HPL results are on average higher than normal. In those with an unfavourable fetal outcome, results generally lie within the normal range or fall below it when several measurements are done. There is, however, a wide overlap. In *Rhesus iso-immunisation* the results are usually in the upper half of the normal range and are especially increased when the fetal hazard is greatest. Values more than 2 SD above the normal mean before 26 weeks suggest a severely affected baby at a stage when amniotic fluid bilirubin determinations (p. 176) are not always feasible. The increase reflects the increased placental size in these pregnancies. The level of HPL is a poor predictor of *fetal death* in Rhesus disorders as this can occur with high, normal or low

174   *Practical Clinical Biochemistry*

HPL figures. Fetal death from other causes is predictable in some cases by falling HPL results but cases are recorded where death is accompanied by continuing normal levels. These results are attributable to the lack of fetal involvement in the HPL production. The continuing presence of a normal sized placenta is reflected by continuing normal HPL results. In *prolonged pregnancy* the HPL levels fall if fetal distress supervenes and fetal distress during labour or neonatal asphyxia is predictable from HPL results less than 4 mg/l during the last 6 weeks before term. If 3 or more such figures are obtained the incidence is 71 per cent.

The Use of Human Chorionic Gonadotrophin Determinations

HCG is produced by the placenta and is excreted in the urine. It is detectable early in pregnancy and is used for its diagnosis. Peak production occurs between the 7th and 10th week with a smaller later peak at 32 to 36 weeks. Immunological methods are used for its determination, and for quantitative work, RIA techniques are preferable.

Investigations suggest that the measurement of urinary HCG is not helpful in the management of pregnancy in the second half of gestation (see Wilde and Oakey, 1975). In threatened abortion in the first half, however, measurements of urinary HCG have a useful predictive role like that of HPL. The same has been reported for plasma HCG (Nygren *et al.*, 1973).

Determination of Cystine Aminopeptidase (Oxytocinase) in Maternal Serum

The placenta produces two aminopeptidase isoenzymes capable of hydrolysing oxytocin, the posterior pituitary hormone which causes uterine contractions. They may serve to inactivate oxytocin thereby preventing the onset of labour. The enzyme activity increases during pregnancy, particularly in the last trimester.

Oxytocin is an octapeptide containing cystine and most methods have used cystine linked to an aromatic amine as substrate. Although other peptidases can attack such substrates they are present in much smaller quantities in pregnancy plasma. Tuppy and Nesvadba (1957) used L-cystine-di-β-napthylamide as substrate but later the less toxic L-cystine-di-p-nitroanilide was introduced (Tovey, 1969). Both substrates are rather insoluble but S-benzyl-L-cystine-p-nitroanilide is more soluble (Tovey *et al.*, 1973). Changes in the relative amounts of the isoenzymes of oxytocinase alters the optimal pH from 6.0 to 7.8 between the first and third trimester. At the latter pH the liberated p-nitroaniline can be determined directly by spectrophotometry making possible the use of simple kinetic methods (Peeters, 1972; Tovey *et al.*, 1973; Christensen and Hagelid, 1975).

Method of Christensen and Hagelid (1975)

The rate of hydrolysis of L-cystine-bis-p-nitroanilide is followed spectrophotometrically at pH 7.5 and room temperature by measuring the

Feto-Placental Function Tests 175

extinction of the liberated *p*-nitroaniline at 380 nm under zero-order conditions.

Reagents. 1. Substrate solution. Dissolve 38 mg L-cystine-bis-*p*-nitroanilide (Koch-Light Laboratories Ltd., Colnbrook, Bucks.) in 10 ml pure ethylene glycol monomethyl ether and store in a dark bottle at 4°C. The solution is stable for at least 14 days.

2. Tris buffer solution, pH 7.5. Prepare A: 2.42 g tris hydroxymethyl aminomethane (Merck) in 100 ml water and B: hydrochloric acid, 200 mmol/l. Mix 25 ml A with 20 ml B and dilute to 100 ml with water. Adjust to pH 7.5 if necessary and add 1 g sodium chloride and 0.3 g Triton X-100 (Koch Light Laboratories) to avoid turbidity due to limited solubility of the substrate. The solution is stable for at least 4 weeks at 4°C.

Technique. Into a spectrophotometer cuvette, path length 1 cm, place 2.0 ml buffer and 0.1 ml substrate solution. Mix, add 0.4 ml serum and mix again. Measure the extinction of the solution at 380 nm at regular intervals. There is an initial lag phase of half to 5 min. Record the rate of increase in extinction per minute ($\Delta E/min$) once the time progress curve is linear.

Calculation. As the molar extinction coefficient of *p*-nitroaniline is 1.2×10^4 and the reaction volume is 2.5 ml, the enzyme activity in IU (μmol/min) per litre of serum can be calculated.

Serum cystine-aminopeptidase (IU/l) =

$$\frac{(\Delta E/min) \times 10^6}{1.2 \times 10^4} \times \frac{2.5}{10^3} \times \frac{10^3}{0.4} = \Delta E/min \times 521$$

Notes. 1. Zero order kinetics apply even with the highest activity seen at term.

2. The reaction rate can be recorded automatically using a recording spectrophotometer or reaction rate analyser.

3. The results using this substrate correlate well with those using L-cystine-diβ-naphthylamide.

4. The coefficient of variation between batches is claimed to be 2.8 per cent.

INTERPRETATION

The median activity increases steadily from 5.0 IU/l at 30 weeks to 10.0 IU/l at 40 weeks. Over the same period the 2.5th percentile changes from 3 to 6 IU/l and the 97.5th percentile increases from 8.2 to 22 IU/l.

The usefulness of cystine aminopeptidase (CAP) activities in serum is mainly in the period from 30 weeks gestation to term. In the *"small-for-dates" fetus,* CAP activities are on average lower than in normal pregnancy and there is a considerable overlap. The rate of increase as determined by serial measurements is more helpful. In *toxaemia* there is a tendency to get low values but this is more apparent with increasing clinical severity.

176 *Practical Clinical Biochemistry*

Failure of CAP figures to rise at a normal rate is found in dysmature fetuses and a falling CAP result with time indicates the likelihood of fetal death. In *diabetic pregnancy* the situation resembles that for HPL with increased activities in those pregnancies progressing normally. As with other tests of placental rather than fetal function, fetal death which occurs without placental malfunction is not reflected by alterations in CAP. Oestriol results are more helpful in such cases.

Other Maternal Serum Enzymes

The placenta produces one or more isoenzymes of alkaline phosphatase which are relatively unaffected by heating to 65°C. Various claims have been made for this test of placental function (see Wilde and Oakey, 1975) but it is now regarded as less satisfactory than other tests. Keller *et al.* (1971) preferred HPL in a direct comparison and more recently Marshall and Parisi (1975) found it to be a poor indication of placental function or fetal status.

Diamine oxidase increases sharply in the first trimester and more slowly to term. There is however a wide normal range and day to day variation is high. The enzyme has been used as a test of placental function but is less satisfactory than others and will not be further considered here.

Determination of Bilirubin in Amniotic Fluid

As the fetal liver develops it acquires the ability to conjugate bilirubin, paralleled by a decrease in unconjugated bilirubin in the amniotic fluid. This decrease progresses until bilirubin is usually undetectable at about the 36th week (Mandelbaum *et al.,* 1967). Fetal immaturity is indicated by the persistence of bilirubin in amniotic fluid. In normal pregnancy, bilirubin concentrations are extremely low and fall from about 0.68 μmol/l (0.04 mg/100 ml) at the 32nd week to about 0.17 μmol/l (0.01 mg/100 ml) at term. The usual methods employed for the determination of serum bilirubin (Chap. 29, Vol. 1) are insufficiently sensitive and require modification. However, it is not in the prediction of fetal maturity but as an index of fetal damage by Rhesus iso-immunisation that determination of amniotic fluid bilirubin has been most used. For this purpose various methods are available: direct spectrophotometry at 450 nm, extraction into organic solution followed by spectrophotometry, or colorimetry using azo-bilirubin.

Method using Direct Spectrophotometry

Liley (1961) showed a good correlation between peak absorption at 450 nm and the severity of haemolytic disease. He allowed for background absorption by reading at 365, 450 and 550 nm. Various modifications exist for correcting for the considerable absorption of non-bilirubin substances

Feto-Placental Function Tests

which obscure the bilirubin peak at 450 nm. We have used a recording spectrophotometer to make a complete scan of the clarified fluid over the range 350-700 nm (Walker and Jennison, 1962).

Technique. Centrifuge amniotic fluid, collected in tubes covered with black paper, for 20 to 30 min. Filter successively through Whatman No. 2 and No. 42 papers until clear. Transfer to a spectrophotometer cuvette of 1 cm path and scan against a water blank from 350-700 nm. An instrument enabling a 5-fold scale expansion facilitates calculations. Draw a straight line between the readings at 365 and 550 nm and record the difference (E_{450}) between this line and the peak reading at 450 nm.

Both Liley and Walker and Jennison prepared action charts relating E_{450} with the duration of pregnancy in an attempt to predict the outcome in Rhesus incompatibility.

Notes. 1. Burnett (1972), investigating the instrumental and procedural sources of error found the error in E_{450} due to instrumental factors to be considerably larger than commonly appreciated. Whereas Liley plotted the logarithm of the extinction against wavelength to obtain a reasonably straight line in the absence of bilirubin, the use of a linear interpolation on the direct scan relating extinction itself to wavelength can introduce errors as can the failure to establish that the instrument gives a straight base line with a blank. Burnett recommended that the spectrophotometer employed should have high photometric precision, readable to 0.001 extinction units. The calculation should be carried out by computation to avoid errors introduced in a manual graphical procedure. The spectrophotometer should be properly zeroed using water in a matched cuvette.

2. In some fluids the absorption at lower wavelengths increases sufficiently rapidly to make fitting of the straight line as a tangent to the curve at 350 nm very difficult.

3. The presence of methaem pigments (methaemoglobin, methaemalhumin) markedly decreases E_{450} sometimes to negative values (Kapitulnik *et al.*, 1970). These substances occur in amniotic fluid contaminated with blood during a previous amniocentesis or intrauterine transfusion as well as in cases of imminent or actual fetal death.

4. A complete scan detects the presence of haemoglobin with the Soret band between 412 and 415 nm. A peak in this region may also indicate interfering methaem derivatives.

Method using Extraction into Organic Solvents and Spectrophotometry

Unconjugated bilirubin is soluble in chloroform but multiple extraction is required for full recovery. The reconcentration of the solvent before assay may result in loss of bilirubin. Mallikarjuneswara *et al.* (1970) overcame this problem by using the basic substance, aniline, soluble only in the non-aqueous phase, to liberate bilirubin from protein thus enabling quantitative transfer to the organic phase. Using aniline in chloroform more

178   *Practical Clinical Biochemistry*

than 99 per cent of the bilirubin can be removed from four volumes of amniotic fluid in one extraction.

Reagents. 1. Extracting solvent, chloroform-aniline. Dissolve 1 ml aniline in chloroform and dilute to 100 ml with chloroform.

2. Buffer. Dissolve 5.4 g dipotassium hydrogen phosphate (K_2HPO_4), 6 g ascorbic acid and 40 mg sodium salicylate in about 80 ml water. Adjust to pH 8.5 with 10 mol/l sodium hydroxide and dilute to 100 ml with water. Store under a layer of xylene in darkness in a refrigerator to prevent oxidation of ascorbic acid. Storage in an automatic dispenser avoids contamination with xylene.

Technique. Thoroughly mix the amniotic fluid to form a uniform suspension and transfer 20 ml to a glass stoppered centrifuge tube. Add 10 ml buffer and 5 ml solvent and shake for 2 min before centrifuging at 2 500 to 3 000 rpm for 20 min. Carefully transfer 3 ml of the solvent layer to a stoppered 10 mm cuvette. Read extinction at 453 nm against a solvent blank.

Calculation. According to the Committee on Bilirubin Standards (see Chap. 29, Vol. 1 for a discussion on the standardisation of bilirubin) a solution of bilirubin in chloroform of 1 μmol/l has an extinction of 0.0607 at 453 nm using a 10 mm cuvette. Allowing for the concentration factor of 4 in the method an amniotic fluid containing 1 μmol/l should read 0.243.

Therefore, amniotic fluid bilirubin (μmol/l)

$$= E_{453} \times \frac{1}{0.243} = E_{453} \times 4.10$$

or $\times$ 0.24 as mg/100 ml

Notes. 1. Wash all glassware before use with dilute ammonia, dilute acetic acid, distilled water and finally ethanol before air drying.

2. Bilirubin is stable in chloroform containing aniline and is unaffected by light conditions in the laboratory. Bilirubin in the sample may be unstable before extraction. It should be kept chilled and in the dark but after extraction, centrifugation can be carried out at room temperature.

3. Addition of 1 g aniline to 100 ml chloroform does not increase the extraction of conjugated bilirubin.

4. Comparison of centrifuged and uncentrifuged samples of amniotic fluid shows 25 (8 to 47) per cent more bilirubin in the latter.

5. Blood in amniotic fluid does not interfere in this method but gross contamination with meconium does. This can be detected from the absorption curve, the extinction at 400 nm being more than 70 per cent and that at 550 nm more than 10 per cent of that at 453 nm respectively.

Colorimetric Determination using Azo-bilirubin (Watson *et al.,* 1965)

The usual methods for serum lack sensitivity but Watson *et al.* modified the Lathe and Ruthven method by avoiding dilution of the sample, while

Feto-Placental Function Tests 179

Kapitulnik *et al.* (1970) used a modification of the method of Malloy and Evelyn using a 1 in 3 instead of a 1 in 10 dilution.

Reagents. 1. Solution A. Dissolve 1 g sulphanilic acid in 2 ml concentrated hydrochloric acid and dilute to 100 ml with water.

2. Solution B. Dissolve 0.5 g sodium nitrite in water and dilute to 100 ml with water.

3. Diazo reagent. Mix 10 volumes of solution A with 0.3 volumes of solution B immediately before use.

4. Methanol.

5. Diluting fluid for bilirubin standard, buffer saline pH 7.4 containing albumin. Dissolve 9.6 g $Na_2HPO_4,2H_2O$, 1.8 g KH_2PO_4 and 0.9 g sodium chloride in water, add 1 g purified albumin and make up to 1 litre.

6. Stock standard bilirubin solution, 35 μmol/l. Dissolve 2.04 mg pure crystalline bilirubin in buffer saline pH 7.4 and make up to 100 ml.

7. Dilute bilirubin solution for standard curve. Prepare solutions containing 1.75 to 35 μmol/l (0.1 to 2.0 mg/100 ml) by diluting 0.1, 0.2, 0.3 etc ml to 2 ml with buffer saline pH 7.4.

Technique. Pipette 2 ml centrifuged and filtered aliquots of amniotic fluid into each of two acid-washed cuvettes of 2 cm light path. To one, the test, add 0.5 ml diazo reagent and to the other, the blank, add 0.5 ml solution A. Pipette 2 ml of each standard and 0.5 ml diazo reagent into separate cuvettes. Mix and add 2.5 ml methanol to each, mix again and after 5 min read the extinction of test, blank and standards against water at 535 nm.

Calculation. Amniotic fluid bilirubin (μmol/l) =

$$\frac{\text{Reading of unknown} - \text{reading of blank}}{\text{Reading of standard}} \times 35 \text{ or} \times 2.04 \text{ as mg/100 ml}$$

if the undiluted standard is used. The reading is taken from the standard curve if this has been prepared.

INTERPRETATION

This depends on the method employed and local usage. Various action charts have been prepared relating the degree of risk to the bilirubin level at varying periods of gestation. Liley (1961) used the E_{450} readings for centrifuged and filtered amniotic fluid and a local variant of this chart devised by Walker and Jennison (1962) is shown in Fig. 4,7. Mallikarjuneswara *et al.* (1970) recalculated the Liley chart for their method. On this chart (Fig. 4,8) the action line of Whitfield *et al.* (1968) is superimposed. For both action lines the pregnancy is allowed to continue with bilirubin results to the left of the line but early delivery is recommended if the result is to the right. Watson *et al.* (1965) found that values greater than 14 μmol/l (0.8 mg/100 ml) at 32 to 33 weeks gestation were incompatible with a live birth. A concentration of 1.8 μmol/l (0.1 mg/100 ml) was associated in 97 per cent of babies with haemolytic disease requiring at least one replacement transfusion.

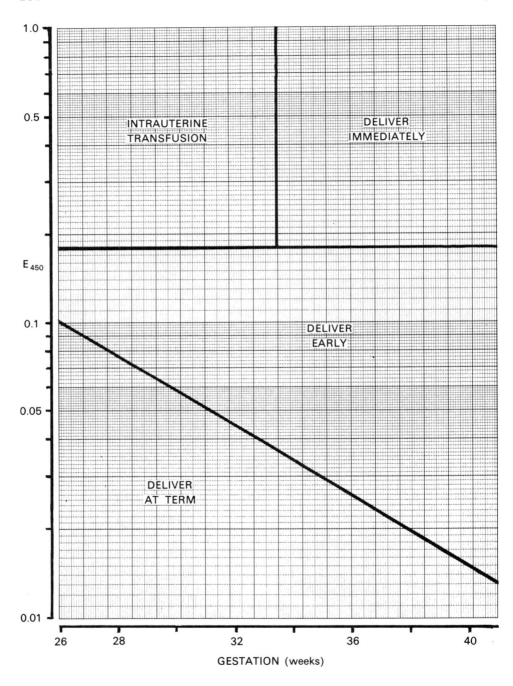

Fig. 4,7. Action Chart for Amniotic Fluid Bilirubin Results. E_{450} is defined in the text. (After Walker and Jennison, 1962.)

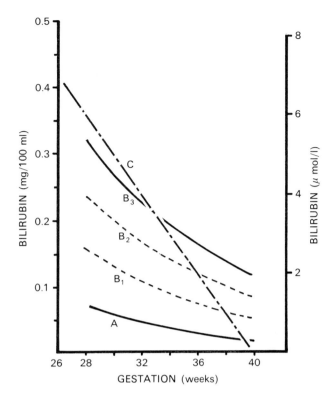

Fig. 4,8. Action Chart for Amniotic Fluid Bilirubin Results. The vertical axes indicate the concentration of unconjugated bilirubin in uncentrifuged amniotic fluid. The curves define five zones corresponding to different degrees of fetal involvement: A — normal or mildly affected; B1, B2, B3 — moderately affected to varying degrees; C — severely affected with possibility of early fetal death. The straight line $(-\cdot - \cdot - \cdot -)$ is the action line of Whitfield et al. (1968); the pregnancy is allowed to continue with results falling to its left. (After Mallikarjuneswara et al., 1970).

Although recording spectrophotometers with scale expansion facilities give better precision for direct methods, the presence of methaem derivatives makes direct quantitation of bilirubin difficult or impossible. Kapitulnik et al. (1970) found good correlation between direct spectrophotometric and diazo coupling methods for 72 clear or yellow fluids and the regression line passed through the origin. For 10 brown-tinted fluids, spectrophotometric values were much lower than expected from the chemical determinations which correlated with the clinical state. In 7 fluids the E_{450} value was negative although chemical determination indicated fetal danger. These observations emphasise the need to scan over the range 350 to 700 nm as a peak at 410 nm and little or no inflection at 540 and 580 nm usually indicate the presence of methaemalbumin. A curve showing a similar or less pronounced peak at 410 nm with definite minor peaks at

182   *Practical Clinical Biochemistry*

540 and 580 nm indicates haemoglobin. Watson *et al.* (1965) consider that caseous material, calcium hyaluronate and blood pigments which in varying degree absorb at 450 nm make direct photometry an inaccurate measure of bilirubin. The diazo method, however, has disadvantages including the necessity for a blank correction which often presents a serious problem. Amniotic fluid is colloidal and sample blanks cannot always correct adequately for turbidity.

It seems likely that for clear, yellow fluids all methods give similar results which correlate with the fetal state but for brown-tinted fluids the diazo methods agree more closely with fetal outcome.

Interpretation can be difficult if the time of gestation is uncertain or if the amniotic fluid volume is abnormal. Cherry *et al.* (1965) suggested the use of the bilirubin/protein ratio as a better index. Total protein can be estimated by the biuret reaction or by turbidimetric methods using salicylsulphonic acid and Watson *et al.* found values of 0.70 to 3.85 g/l at 32 to 33 weeks of pregnancy. A standard of dilute serum should be used not purified albumin. Mallikarjuneswara *et al.* (1970) quote the following ratios for μmol/g protein (mg/g protein): normal or mildly affected, less than 4.25 (0.25); moderately to severely affected, 4.25 to 6.8 (0.25 to 0.4); severaly affected, greater than 6.5 (0.4).

Phospholipids in Amniotic Fluid

A common problem in immature neonates is the development of the respiratory distress syndrome (hyaline membrane disease). This feature of fetal lung immaturity has to be borne in mind when early induction of labour for other reasons is contemplated and a balance has to be struck between the respiratory hazards and the risk of prolonging the pregnancy. The adequate expansion of the alveoli of the normal lung at birth depends in part, on the presence of surfactant at that site. The material accumulates as the lung matures and passes into the amniotic fluid.

Dipalmitoyl lecithin is an important phospholipid component of surfactant and appears in the amniotic fluid in increasing amounts from about 35 weeks gestation. The absolute concentration, the total amount in the fluid or the ratio of lecithin to sphingomyelin, assumed to be produced at a constant rate by extra-pulmonary sources, have all been used as an index of fetal lung maturity.

The extraction of lipids into a methanol-chloroform mixture (Folch *et al.*, 1957) is used in most methods for amniotic fluid lipids (Williams *et al.*, 1969; Hodge, 1973; Blass *et al.*, 1974; Warren *et al.*, 1974). Chromatographic separation on silica gel is usual but the developing solvents vary. Wagstaff *et al.* (1974) used chloroform-methanol-water; Williams *et al.* (1969) and Hodge (1973) used chloroform-methanol-acetic acid-water whereas Blass *et al.* (1974) used dichloromethane-ethanol-water for extremely rapid separation.

Feto-Placental Function Tests 183

The separated phospholipids can be detected by charring with sulphuric acid, exposure to iodine vapour, or by spraying with Rhodamine B dye with or without the presence of dichlorofluorescein, with bromothymol blue or with molybdic acid-stannous chloride reagent. Quantitation can be made directly by area measurement, by multiplying the length of each spot by its mid-point width, by reflectance or transmittance densitometry, or chemically by removal of the silica gel spot and digestion of the phospholipid with or without extraction from the gel. For a discussion of problems involved see Wagstaff *et al.* (1974) who preferred densitometry after staining with molybdic acid-stannous chloride. Williams *et al.* (1969) extracted from the silica gel, digested and determined the phosphorus colorimetrically. Hodge (1973) digested in the presence of the silica gel but added phosphorus standard to a similar amount of silica gel scraped from the plate.

Other methods have used GLC to measure palmitic acid in hydrolysates of amniotic fluid. It is mainly derived from the active substance, dipalmitoyl lecithin. Simplified tests have relied on the stability of the foam layer produced by shaking amniotic fluid, a property due to surfactant. For a review of these tests see Wilde and Oakey (1975).

The Determination of Amniotic Fluid Lecithin using Thin Layer Chromatography. Method of Hodge, 1973

The extracted phospholipids are chromatographed on silica gel plates. After location, appropriate areas are scraped from the plate and digested with sulphuric acid in the presence of hydrogen peroxide. The liberated phosphorus is determined by a micro-modification of the Fiske and Subbarow procedure.

Reagents. 1. Methanol.

2. Chloroform.

3. Prespread thin layer (250 μm) chromatography plates supplied by Anachem Ltd., Silica Gel G, 20 × 10 cm.

4. Developing solvent. Chloroform-methanol-glacial acetic acid-water in the ratio 50 : 25 : 7 : 3 v/v. Make up fresh each time.

5. Lecithin standard. Prepare a solution containing 1 mg/ml in chloroform. Store at 4°C.

6. Location reagent. Dissolve 17 mg 2',7'-dichlorofluorescein and 50 mg Rhodamine B in 35 ml aqueous ethanol, 950 ml/l. Add 75 ml diethyl ether, 8 ml water and mix thoroughly.

7. Sulphuric acid, 5 mol/l. Slowly add 280 ml concentrated acid to approximately 500 ml water and make up to 1 litre.

8. Hydrogen peroxide solution, "100 volumes" (BDH Aristar)

9., Ammonium molybdate solution, 4 g/l. Dissolve 0.4 g ammonium molybdate tetrahydrate in water and make up to 100 ml.

10. Reducing agent. Add 0.5 g 1-amino-2-naphthol-4-sulphonic acid to

184 *Practical Clinical Biochemistry*

195 ml sodium bisulphite solution (150 g/l). To this mixture add 5 ml sodium sulphite solution (200 g/l) and mix until dissolved.

11. Standard inorganic phosphorus solution, 2 mmol/l, 0.262 g KH_2PO_4 per litre.

12. Sodium sulphate, anhydrous.

Technique. Into a stoppered tube take 1.6 ml uncentrifuged amniotic fluid, submitted to the laboratory within 2 h of collection, and add 4 ml methanol and 2 ml chloroform. If the assay is not to be carried out immediately, mix thoroughly and store in a refrigerator. To continue the extraction shake mechanically for 10 min. Add 2 ml chloroform and 2 ml water shaking vigorously between each addition and centrifuge to separate the phases. Remove the lower chloroform layer and filter through about 1 g anhydrous sodium sulphate into a conical centrifuge tube. Re-extract the aqueous layer twice with 2 ml portions of chloroform, shaking mechanically for 5 min, and centrifuging as before. Filter each chloroform extract through the anhydrous sodium sulphate into the previous extract. Finally wash the sodium sulphate with a further 2 ml chloroform. Evaporate the combined extracts to dryness at 40°C under a stream of nitrogen. When almost dry, rinse the sides of the tube with 0.5 to 1.0 ml chloroform and re-evaporate. Redissolve in 40 μl chloroform rinsing down the sides of the tube.

Chromatography. Take a thin layer plate 10 cm long and of suitable width and draw a fine pencil line across the width about 1 cm from the end. Apply the extracted phospholipids as a 8 mm line using a 10μl syringe. Re-wash the tube with two further 20 μl portions of chloroform and apply these washings to the plate. Apply approximately 40 μl lecithin standard to the plate as marker. Prepare the solvent and use a little to rinse the tank before placing some in the bottom and allowing it to saturate the atmosphere for about 5 min. Develop the chromatogram for about 8 to 9 cm (until the solvent front reaches the end of the plate) and dry in a stream of air. Spray the plate with fluorescent indicator and dry under a stream of warm air until the spots become visible. Examine the plate under UV light (350 nm) and mark the outlines of the spots with a needle. Mark out two blank areas of equal size.

Phosphorus estimation. Scrape the spots into Pyrex tubes. The first tube containing the lipid-free silica gel serves as blank. To the second such tube add 100 μl phosphorus standard (0.2 μmol). To all tubes add 300 μl sulphuric acid and 100 μl hydrogen peroxide. Mix carefully and heat at 180°C for 30 min. Remove from the oven, cool a little, and add a further 100 μl hydrogen peroxide. Heat at 180°C for a further 30 min. Remove from the oven and cool to room temperature. Add 1 ml water, mix thoroughly and centrifuge hard. Into separate capped plastic tubes pipette 500 μl supernatant from each digest and add 500 μl ammonium molybdate and 50 μl reducing agent. Heat at 95°C for 10 min, cool and read at 700 nm using a 1 cm path length. A micro cuvette is desirable.

Feto-Placental Function Tests   185

Calculation. Amniotic fluid lecithin (μmol/l)

$$= \frac{\text{Reading of unknown}}{\text{Reading of standard}} \times 0.2 \times \frac{1\ 000}{1.6}$$

$$= \frac{\text{Reading of unknown}}{\text{Reading of standard}} \times 125 \text{ or } \times 9.38 \text{ as mg}/100 \text{ ml dipalmitoyl lecithin.}$$

Notes. 1. The greater sensitivity of the malachite green method (Chap. 25, Vol. 1) for inorganic phosphorus avoids heating and gives a more convenient final volume. To $200\ \mu$l of digest add 3 ml malachite green reagent and read at 630 nm. The calculation is unchanged.

2. The specimen must not be centrifuged and must be extracted as soon as possible after collection. The lecithin content decreases on storage at room temperature or when frozen (Bhagwanani *et al.*, 1972), or after centrifugation (Nelson, 1969).

3. The phospholipid composition of serum is quite different from that of amniotic fluid and specimens must not be contaminated with blood or meconium.

4. The method is time consuming but it does quantitatively estimate the lecithin and is not subject to the problems discussed by Wagstaff *et al.* (1974) in relation to direct densitometry.

5. Hodge found low sphingomyelin concentrations in late pregnancy which are difficult to quantitate and can introduce large errors in the lecithin/sphingomyelin ratio.

INTERPRETATION

Values above 47 μmol/l (3.5 mg/100 ml) are considered to indicate lung maturity although the spread of results at any stage in pregnancy is very wide (Hodge, 1973; Warren *et al.*, 1974). With levels less than 40 μmol/l (3.0 mg/100 ml) the respiratory distress syndrome is probable and above 55 μmol/l (4.0 mg/100 ml) it is unlikely. For low or intermediate results delay in induction is advisable if possible. The concentration may be misleading if the amniotic fluid volume is abnormal as in some diabetic pregnancies. For this reason Falconer *et al.* (1973) prefer to measure the volume simultaneously and to calculate the total lecithin content. The mean figures μmol (mg) are: 17.5 (13) at 28 to 32 weeks; 25.5 (19) at 32 to 34 weeks; 69 (52) at 34 to 36 weeks; 60 (45) at 36 to 38 weeks and 77.5 (58) at 38 to 40 weeks. They consider a figure of less than 27 μmol (20 mg) to indicate a risk of the respiratory distress syndrome.

Determination of Amniotic Fluid Volume

The amniotic fluid volume increases up to 30 to 35 weeks of gestation and then becomes less, particularly if pregnancy is prolonged beyond 40

186   *Practical Clinical Biochemistry*

weeks. Variations in volume are considerable even in normal pregnancy but pathological conditions can alter the volume more markedly. It may be useful to measure the volume of fluid as such but it also allows the total quantity of substances in the amniotic sac to be calculated (see previous section).

The usual method involves a dilution principle. A known volume of a substance of known concentration is injected into the liquor and after equilibration, its concentration in a sample of the amniotic fluid is measured. Equilibration is complete by 20 min.

Method of Falconer *et al.* (1973)

The degree of dilution of a solution of *p*-aminohippurate (PAH) injected into the amniotic fluid is determined by diazotisation and coupling with N-1-naphthyl-ethylenediamine.

Reagents. 1. Sterile solution of sodium PAH, 2 g in 10 ml, "for injection".

2. Hydrochloric acid, 1.2 mol/l. Dilute 24 ml concentrated acid to 200 ml with water.

3. Sodium nitrite solution, 1 g/l. Dissolve 100 mg $NaNO_2$ in 100 ml water. Prepare freshly every few days and store at $4°C$.

4. Ammonium sulphamate solution, 5 g/l. Dissolve 0.5 g in 100 ml water and prepare freshly every two weeks.

5. Coupling reagent. Dissolve 100 mg N-1-naphthyl-ethylenediamine hydrochloride in 100 ml water. Keep in the dark.

Technique. The amniocentesis is performed using a needle fitted with a tap using full precautions. A sample of fluid is collected (zero time sample). An accurately calibrated syringe is filled with 2.0 ml PAH injection, connected to the needle and injected into the amniotic fluid. Using a clean syringe the contents of the needle are transferred to the amniotic fluid by re-aspirating into the syringe and re-injecting several times before sealing the needle. Further samples of amniotic fluid are taken into a clean syringe at 10, 15 and 20 min after the injection. All samples and the injection fluid are analysed together.

Dilute all amniotic fluids 101-fold by adding 0.1 ml to 10 ml water in clean tubes. Dilute 0.5 ml of the PAH injection to 200 ml with water. Mix thoroughly and dilute 1 ml of the solution to 100 ml with water to give a final dilution of 1 in 40 000. Into clean tubes pipette 2 ml diluted amniotic fluid and 3 ml water or 5 ml diluted PAH solution for the standard or 5 ml water for the reagent blank. To each add 1 ml hydrochloric acid and 0.5 ml nitrite solution. Mix and leave for 5 min. Add 0.5 ml ammonium sulphamate solution to destroy excess nitrous acid. Mix, leave for 3 min and then add 0.5 ml coupling reagent. After 10 to 15 min read all solutions against the reagent blank in the colorimeter at 540 nm.

Calculation. As the final dilution of the amniotic fluid before adding the

Feto-Placental Function Tests 187

acid and nitrite is $101 \times 5/2$ times and that of PAH is 40 000 times, the dilution of the PAH injected is given by

$$\frac{S}{T-Z} \times \frac{40\ 000 \times 2}{505} \quad \text{or} \quad \frac{S}{T-Z} \times 158.4$$

Where S = extinction of the standard PAH solution
T = extinction of amniotic fluid sample at 10, 15 or 20 min
Z = extinction of zero time amniotic fluid sample
Hence

$$\text{Amniotic fluid volume (ml)} = \frac{S}{T-Z} \times 158.4 \times \text{volume PAH injected (ml)}$$

The apparent volume is calculated for each time of sampling. The 15 and 20 min samples usually agree to within 6 per cent.

INTERPRETATION

The normal ranges for amniotic fluid volume vary with the period of gestation. The following are typical: 20 weeks, 200 to 400 ml; 25 weeks, 250 to 750 ml; 30 and 35 weeks, 500 to 1 050 ml; 40 weeks, 250 to 950 ml; 43 weeks, less than 100 to 750 ml.

An increase in volume to more than 2 litres is referred to as hydramnios. The causes include general disorders in the mother, placental abnormalities and fetal abnormalities. Thus it may be a feature of any oedematous state in the mother, of toxaemia of pregnancy and of diabetic pregnancy. Placental factors include a large placenta, multiple pregnancy, placental infarction or venous stasis, and occlusion of the umbilical vein. Fetal factors include Rhesus immunisation, fetal liver disease and, in about a quarter of cases, fetal congenital abnormalities such as anencephaly, spina bifida, lung hypoplasia, heart disease, and obstructions in the oesophagus, stomach or upper small intestine. The latter group may impair the normal swallowing of the fluid by the fetus.

The opposite condition, oligohydramnios, is very rare and is characterized by an abnormally small fluid volume and early onset of labour. Some cases involve fetal renal agenesis which would abolish the normal fetal urine flow into the amniotic fluid.

Other Determinations on Amniotic Fluid

As the fetus matures its contributions to the amniotic fluid composition alter. These changes, reflected in the concentration of electrolytes, urea and creatinine or in the osmolality, have been used to assess fetal maturity (see review by Wilde and Oakey, 1975). They are probably less satisfactory than radiological or ultrasound methods.

The other main use has been in the diagnosis of congenital abnormalities of the fetus — see reviews by Nyhan (1971) and Wilde and Oakey (1975).

188   *Practical Clinical Biochemistry*

Examples include analysis of the fluid itself for pregnanetriol in congenital adrenal hyperplasia (Chap. 3) and for α-fetoprotein in varying degrees of neural tube defects. The cells present in the fluid may be cultured and examined for chromosomal abnormalities or for specific enzymes characteristic of specific genetic disorders.

REFERENCES

Abraham, G. E. (1974). *J. clin. Endocr. Metab.*, 39, 340.
Abraham, G. E., Maroulis, G. B. and Marshall, J. R. (1974). *Obstet. Gynec.*, 44, 522.
Abraham, G. E., Odell, W. D., Edwards, R. and Purdy, J. M. (1970). *Acta Endocrinol.*, Suppl. 147, 332.
Abraham, G. E., Odell, W. D., Swerdloff, R. S. and Hopper, K. (1972). *J. clin. Endocr. Metab.*, 34, 312.
Abraham, G. E., Swerdloff, R., Tulchinsky, D. and Odell, W. D. (1971). *J. clin. Endocr. Metab.*, 32, 619.
Adlercreutz, H. (1975). *Lancet*, 1, 1386.
Ahmed, J. and Mester, J. (1973). *Clin. chim. Acta*, 48, 37.
Akande, E. O. (1975). *Br. J. Obstet. Gynaec.*, 82, 552.
Andre, C. M. and James, V. H. T. (1964). *Steroids*, 24, 295.
August, G. F., Tkachuk, M. and Grumbach, M. M. (1969). *J. clin. Endocr. Metab.*, 29, 891.
Bardin, C. W., Ross, G. T. and Lipsett, M. B. (1967). *J. clin. Endocr. Metab.*, 27, 1558.
Barnard, W. P. and Logan, R. W. (1970). *Clin chim. Acta*, 29, 401.
Bauld, W. S. (1954). *Biochem. J.*, 56, 426.
Beazley, J. M. (1972). *Brit. J. hosp. Med.*, 7, 573.
Besser, G. M., McNeilly, A. S., Anderson, D. C., Marshall, J. C., Harsoulis, P., Hall, R., Ormston, B. J., Alexander, L. and Collins, W. P. (1972). *Brit. med. J.*, 3, 267.
Bhagwanani, S. G., Fahmy, D. and Turnbull, A. C. (1972). *Lancet*, 1, 159.
Bierich, J. R. (1975). *Clinics Endocr. Metab.*, 4, 1.
Bishop, P. M. F. and Sommerville, I. F. in *Biochemical Disorders in Human Disease*. 3rd Edn. Ed. by R. H. S. Thompson and I. D. P. Wootton, Churchill, London, 1970, p. 797.
Blass, K. G., Thibert, R. J. and Draisey, T. F. (1974). *J. Chromatog.*, 89, 197.
Boyer, R. M., Perlow, M., Hellman, L., Kapen, S. and Weitzman, E. (1972). *J. clin. Endocr. Metab.*, 35, 73.
Boyer, R. M., Perlow, M., Kapen, S., Lefkowitz, G., Weitzmann, E. and Hellman, L. (1973). *J. clin. Endocr. Metab.*, 36, 561.
Brombacher, P. J., Gijzen, A. H. J. and Verbessen, P. E. (1968). *Clin. chim. Acta*, 20, 360.
Brown, J. B. (1952). *J. Endocr.*, 8, 196.
Brown, J. B. (1955a). *Biochem. J.*, 60, 185.
Brown, J. B. (1955b). *Mem. Soc. Endocr.*, 3, 1.
Brown, J. B. (1955c). *Lancet*, 1, 320.
Brown, J. B., Evans, J. H., Beischer, N. A., Campbell, D. G. and Fortune, D. W. (1970). *J. Obstet. Gynaec. Brit. Cwlth.*, 77, 690.
Brown, J. B., MacLeod, S. C., Macnaughtan, C., Smith, M. A. and Smyth, B. (1968a). *J. Endocr.*, 42, 5.
Brown, J. B., Macnaughtan, C., Smith, M. A. and Smyth, B. (1968b). *J. Endocr.*, 40, 175.
Brown, J. B. and Matthew, J. (1962). *Rec. Progr. Horm. Res.*, 18, 337.
Burnett, R. W. (1972). *Clin. Chem.*, 18, 150.

References 189

Campbell, D. G. and Gardner, G. (1971). *Clin. chim. Acta*, 32, 153.

Chard, T. (1975). *Postgrad. med. J.*, 51, 221.

Chen, J. C., Zorn, E. M., Hollberg, M. C. and Wieland, R. C. (1971). *Clin. Chem.*, 17, 581.

Cherry, S. H., Kochwa, S. and Rosenfield, R. E. (1965). *Obstet. Gynec.*, 26, 826.

Chevins, R., Launay, J. M., Julien, R. and Dreux, C. (1974). *Clin. chim. Acta*, 55, 333.

Christensen, A. and Hagelid, P. E. (1975). *Acta Endocr.*, 78, 364.

Christner, J. E. and Fetter, M. C. (1974). *Steroids*, 24, 327.

Cleary, R. E. and Young, P. C. M. (1974). *Am. J. Obstet. Gynec.*, 118, 18.

Cohen, M. and Cohen, H. (1974). *Am. J. Obstet. Gynec.*, 118, 200.

Comhaire, F. and Vermeulen, A. (1975). *J. clin. Endocr. Metab.*, 40, 824.

Corker, C. S., Exley, D. and Naftolin, F. (1970). *Acta Endocr.*, Suppl. 147, 305.

Corker, C. S. and Naftolin, F. (1971). *J. Obstet. Gynaec. Brit. Cwlth.*, 78, 330.

Crosignani, P. G., Reschini, E., D'Alberton, A., Trojsi, L., Cantalamessa, L. and Guistina, G. (1974). *Am. J. Obstet. Gynec.*, 120, 376.

Demetriou, J. A. and Austin, F. G. (1971). *Clin. chim. Acta*, 33, 21.

DeVane, G. W., Czekala, N. M., Judd, H. L. and Yen, S. S. C. (1975). *Am. J. Obstet. Gynec.*, 121, 496.

Dignam, N. J., Parlow, A. F. and Daane, T. A. (1969). *Am. J. Obstet. Gynec.*, 105, 679.

Doering, C. H., Kraemer, H. C., Brodie, H. K. H. and Hambing, D. A. (1975). *J. clin. Endocr. Metab.*, 40, 492.

Doerr, P., Goebel, R. and Kuss, E. (1973). *Acta Endocr.*, 73, 314.

Doring, G. H. (1969). *J. Reprod. Fertil.*, Suppl. 6, 77.

Dubin, N. H., Crystle, C. D., Grannis, G. F. and Townsley, J. D. (1973). *Am. J. Obstet. Gynec.*, 115, 835.

Dufau, M. L., Catt, K. J., Isuruhara, T. and Ryan, D. (1972). *Clin. chim. Acta*, 37, 109.

Easterling, W. E. Jr., Talbert, L. M. and Potter, H. D. (1974). *Am. J. Obstet. Gynec.*, 120, 385.

England, B. G., Niswender, G. D. and Midgley, A. R. Jr. (1974). *J. clin. Endocr. Metab.*, 38, 42.

Exley, D. and Moore, B. (1973). *J. Steroid Biochem.*, 4, 257.

Fairweather, D. V. I., Billewicz, W., Loraine, J. A. and Bell, E. T. (1972). *J. Obstet. Gynaec. Brit. Cwlth.*, 79, 97.

Falconer, G. F., Hodge, J. S. and Gadd, R. L. (1973). *Brit. med. J.*, 2, 689.

Fisher, R. A., Anderson, D. C. and Burke, C. W. (1974). *Steroids*, 24, 809.

Folch, J., Lees, M. and Sloane-Stanley, G. H. (1957). *J. biol. Chem.*, 226, 497.

Foreman, C. and Ryan, R. J. (1967). *J. clin. Endocr. Metab.*, 27, 444.

Fraser, I. S. and Baird, D. T. (1974). *J. clin. Endocr. Metab.*, 39, 564.

Furr, B. J. A. (1973). *Acta Endocr.*, 72, 89.

Furuyama, S., Mayes, D. M. and Nugent, C. A. (1970). *Steroids*, 16, 415.

Furuyama, S. and Nugent, C. A. (1971). *Steroids*, 17, 663.

Gartside, M. W. and Tindall, V. R. (1975). *Brit. J. Obstet. Gynaec.*, 82, 303.

Ginsburg, J., Isaacs, A. J., Gore, M. B. R. and Howard, C. W. H. (1975). *Brit. med. J.*, 3, 130.

Goebel, R. and Kuss, E. (1974). *J. clin. Endocr. Metab.*, 39, 969.

Hagerman, D. D. amd Williams, K. L. (1969). *Am. J. Obstet. Gynec.*, 104, 114.

Hainsworth, I. R. and Hall, P. E. (1971). *Clin. chim. Acta*, 35, 201.

Hobkirk, R. and Metcalf-Gibson, A. (1963). *Standard Methods of Clinical Chemistry*, 4, 65.

Hodge, J. S. (1973). *Ann. clin. Biochem.*, 10, 167.

Hollberg, M. C., Zorn, E. M. and Wieland, R. G. (1968). *Steroids*, 12, 241.

Holub, W. R. (1971). *Clin. Chem.*, 17, 1083.

Horton, R., Kato, T. and Sherins, R. (1967). *Steroids*, 10, 245.

Howarth, A. T. and Robertshaw, D. A. (1971). *Clin. Chem.*, 17, 316.

190   *Practical Clinical Biochemistry*

Hull, M. G. R., Braunsberg, H. and Irving, D. (1975). *Clin. chim. Acta*, **58**, 71.

Ismail, A. A. A., Niswender, G. D. and Midgley, A. R. Jr. (1972). *J. clin. Endocr. Metab.*, **34**, 177.

Ittrich, G. (1958). *Z. physiol. Chem.*, **312**, 1.

Jacobs, H. S. (1975). *Postgrad. med. J.*, **51**, 209.

Jacobsen, A., Marshall, J. R., Ross, G. T. and Cargille, G. M. (1968). *Am. J. Obstet. Gynec.*, **102**, 284.

Jaing, N. S. and Ryan, R. J. (1969). *Proc. Mayo Clinic*, **44**, 461.

Johansson, E. D. B. (1969). *Acta Endocr.*, **61**, 592.

Johansson, E. D. B., Neill, J. D. and Knobil, E. (1968). *J. clin. Endocr. Metab.*, **82**, 143.

Jones, G. S., Maffezzoli, R. D., Strott, C. A., Ross, G. T. and Kaplan, G. (1970). *Am. J. Obstet. Gynec.*, **108**, 847.

Judd, H. L., Judd, G. E., Lucas, W. E. and Yen, S. S. C. (1974). *J. clin. Endocr. Metab.*, **39**, 1020.

Kapitulnik, J., Kaufmann, N. A. and Blondheim, S. H. (1970). *Clin. Chem.*, **16**, 756.

Katagiri, H., Stanczyk, F. Z. and Goebelsmann, U. (1974). *Steroids*, **24**, 225.

Kato, H. and Horton, R. (1968). *Steroids*, **12**, 681.

Katz, M. and Carr, P. J. (1974). *J. Obstet. Gynaec. Brit. Cwlth.*, **81**, 791.

Keller, P. J., Baertschi, U., Bader, P., Gerber, C., Schmid, J., Soltermann, R. and Kopper, E. (1971). *Lancet*, **2**, 729.

Kellie, A. E., *The Scientific Basis of Medicine. Annual Reviews*, Athlone Press, London, 1973, p. 203.

Kim, M. H., Hosseinian, A. H. and Dupon, C. (1974). *J. clin. Endocr. Metab.*, **39**, 706.

Kletzky, O. A., Nakamura, R. M., Thorneycroft, I. H. and Mishell, D. R., Jr. (1975). *Am. J. Obstet. Gynec.*, **121**, 668.

Klopper, A. I. (1971). *Clin. chim. Acta*, **34**, 215.

Klopper, A. (1975). *Postgrad. med. J.*, **51**, 227.

Klopper, A. I. and Billewicz, W. (1963). *J. Obstet. Gynaec. Brit Cwlth.*, **70**, 1024.

Klopper, A., Michie, E. A. and Brown, J. B. (1955). *J. Endocr.*, **12**, 209.

Klopper, A., Wilson, G. R. and Cooke, I. (1969). *J. Endocr.*, **43**, 295.

Köber, S. (1931). *Biochem. Z.*, **239**, 209.

Korenman, S. G., Tulchinsky, D. and Eaton, L. W. (1970). *Acta Endocr.*, Suppl. **147**, 291.

Kuss, E. and Goebel, R. (1972). *Steroids*, **19**, 509.

Lee, P. A., Jaffe, R. B. and Midgley, A. R. Jr. (1974). *J. clin. Endocr. Metab.*, **39**, 664.

Leigh, R. J., Fleetwood, J. A., Hall, R. and Latner, A. L. (1974). *Proc. Roy. Soc. Med.*, **67**, 1223.

Letchworth, A. T., Boardman, R., Bristow, C., Landon, J. and Chard, T. (1971). *J. Obstet. Gynaec. Brit. Cwlth.*, **78**, 542.

Lever, M., Powell, J. C. and Peace, S. M. (1973). *Biochem. Med.*, **8**, 188.

Liley, A. W. (1961). *Am. J. Obstet. Gynec.*, **82**, 1359.

Lind, T. (1975). *Brit. J. hosp. Med.*, **14**, 631.

Lindberg, P. and Edqvist, L. E. (1974). *Clin. chim. Acta*, **53**, 169.

Little, A. J., Aulton, K. and Payne, R. B. (1975). *Clin. chim. Acta*, **65**, 167.

Loraine, J. A. and Bell, E. T. *Hormone Assays and their Clinical Application*, 3rd Edn., Livingstone, Edinburgh & London, 1971.

Loriaux, D. L., Guy, R. and Lipsett, M. B. (1973). *J. clin. Endocr. Metab.*, **36**, 788.

Lurie, A. O. and Patterson, R. J. (1970). *Clin. Chem.*, **16**, 856.

Mallikarjuneswara, V. R., Clemetson, C. A. E. and Carr, J. J. (1970). *Clin. Chem.*, **16**, 180.

Mandelbaum, R., La Croix, G. C. and Robinson, A. R. (1967). *Obstet. Gynec.*, **29**, 471.

Marshall, J. C. (1975). *Clinics Endocr. Metab.*, **4**, 545.

Marshall, B. R. and Parisi, F. (1975). *Obstet. Gynec.*, **45**, 136.

Martin, B. T., Cooke, B. A. and Black, W. P. (1970). *J. Endocr.*, **46**, 369.

Masson, G. M. (1973). *J. Obstet. Gynaec. Brit. Cwlth.*, **80**, 201, 206.

References 191

Mayes, D. and Nugent, C. A. (1968). *J. clin. Endocr. Metab.*, 28, 1169.
Midgley, A. R., Jr. (1966). *Endocrinology*, 79, 10.
Midgley, A. R., Jr. (1967). *J. clin. Endocr. Metab.*, 27, 295.
Midgley, A. R., Jr. and Niswender, G. D. (1970). *Acta Endocr.*, Suppl. 147, 320.
Mikhail, G., Wu, C-H., Ferin, M. and van der Wiele, R. L. (1970). *Steroids*, 15, 333.
Moore, J. W. and Cooper, W. (1974). *Clin. chim. Acta*, 56, 215.
Mortimer, C. H., Besser, G. M., McNeilly, A. S., Marshall, J. C., Harsoulis, P., Tunbridge, W. M. G., Gomez-Pan, A. and Hall, R. (1973). *Brit. med. J.*, 4, 73.
Moscrop, K. H., Antcliff, A. C., Braunsberg, H., James, V. H. T., Goudie, J. H. and Burnett, D. (1974). *Clin. chim. Acta*, 56, 265.
Murphy, B. E. P. (1968). *Canad. J. Biochem.*, 46, 299.
Murphy, B. E. P. (1969). *Rec. Progr. Horm. Res.*, 25, 563.
Nelson, G. H. (1969). *Am. J. Obstet. Gynec.*, 105, 1072.
Nygren, K-G., Johansson, E. D. B. and Wide, L. (1973). *Am. J. Obstet. Gynec.*, 116, 916.
Nyhan, W. L. *Biochemistry of Development*, ed. Benson, P. F., Heinemann, London, 1971, p. 14.
Oake, R. J., Davies, S. J., MacLachlan, M. S. F. and Thomas, J. P. (1974). *Quart. J. Med.*, 43, 603.
Oakey, R. E., Bradshaw, L. R. A., Eccles, S. S., Stitch, S. R. and Heys, R. F. (1967). *Clin. chim. Acta*, 15, 35.
Onikki, S. and Adlercreutz, H. (1973). *J. Steroid Biochem.*, 4, 633.
Outch, K. H., Dennis, P. M. and Larsen, A. (1972). *Clin. chim. Acta*, 40, 377.
Patten, P. T., Anderson, A. B. M. and Turnbull, A. C. (1973). *J. Obstet. Gynaec. Brit. Cwlth.*, 80, 952.
Peeters, J. A. B. M. (1972). *Clin. Chem.*, 18, 563.
Pirke, K. M. and Doerr, P. (1975). *Acta Endocr.*, 79, 357.
Podoba, V., Rizkallah, T. H. and Kelly, W. G. (1973). *Am. J. Obstet. Gynec.*, 117, 321.
Pohlman, C., Chen, J. C., Zorn, E. M. and Wieland, R. C. (1971). *Clin. Chem.*, 17, 585.
Pratt, J. J., van der Linden, G., Doorenbos, H. and Woldring, M. G. (1974). *Clin. chim. Acta*, 50, 137.
Rosenfield, R. L., Eberlein, W. R. and Bongiovanni, A. M. (1969). *J. clin. Endocr. Metab.*, 29, 854.
Roth, J. C., Kelch, R. P., Kaplan, S. L. and Grumbach, M. M. (1972). *J. clin. Endocr. Metab.*, 35, 926.
Ryan, M. and Gray, B. C. (1975). *Clin. chim. Acta*, 60, 197.
Sanghvi, A., Wight, C., Serenko, A. and Balachandran, R. (1974). *Clin. Chim. Acta*, 56, 49.
Schiller, H. S. and Brammall, M. A. (1974). *Steroids*, 24, 665.
Schwarzstein, L., de Laborde, H. P., Aparicio, N. J., Turner, D., Markin, A., Rodriguez, A. F., Hullier, L. and Rosner, J. M. (1975). *J. clin. Endocr. Metab.*, 40, 313.
Shaaban, M. M. and Klopper, A. (1973). *J. Obstet. Gynaec. Brit. Cwlth.*, 80, 776.
Shahmanesh, M., Ellwood, M., Nelson, E. and Hartog, M. (1975). *Postgrad. med. J.*, 51, 59.
Shaw, R. W., Butt, W. R., London, D. R. and Marshall, J. C. (1975). *Clin. Endocr.*, 4, 267.
Shutt, D. A. (1969). *Steroids*, 13, 69.
Simkins, A. and Worth, H. G. J. (1975). *Ann. clin. Biochem.*, 12, 233.
Slob, A. and Winkel, P. (1973). *Clin. chim. Acta*, 44, 307.
Smals, A. G. H., Kloppenborg, P. W. C. and Benraad, T. J. (1975). *Acta Endocr.*, 78, 604.
Sommerville, I. F., Gough, N. and Marrian, G. F. (1948). *J. Endocr.*, 5, 247.
Swain, M. C. (1972). *Clin. chim. Acta*, 39, 455.
Swapp, G. H., Masson, G. M. and Klopper, A. I. (1975). *Brit. J. Obstet. Gynaec.*, 82, 132.
Swerdloff, R. S. and Odell, W. D. (1975). *Postgrad. med. J.*, 51, 200.

Thorneycroft, I. H., Ribiero, W. O., Stone, S. C. and Tillson, S. A. (1973). *Steroids*, **21**, 111.

Thorneycroft, I. H., Sribyatta, B., Tom, W. K., Nakamura, R. M. and Mishell, D. R. Jr. (1974). *J. clin. Endocr. Metab.*, **39**, 754.

Tovey, J. E. (1969). *Clin. Biochem.*, **2**, 289.

Tovey, J. E., Dawson, P. J. G. and Fellowes, K. P. (1973). *Clin. Chem.*, **19**, 756.

Townsley, J. D., Gartman, L. J. and Crystle, C. D. (1973). *Am. J. Obstet. Gynec.*, **115**, 830.

Tredway, D. R., Goebelsmann, U., Thorneycroft, I. H. and Mishell, D. R. Jr., (1974). *Am. J. Obstet. Gynec.*, **120**, 1035.

Tulchinsky, D., Hobel, C. J. and Korenman, S. G. (1971). *Am. J. Obstet. Gynec.*, **111**, 311.

Tulchinsky, D., Hobel, C. J., Yeager, E. and Marshall, J. R. (1972). *Am. J. Obstet. Gynec.*, **112**, 1095.

Tuppy, H. and Nesvadba, H. (1957). *Mschr. Chem.*, **88**, 977.

Ua Conaill, D. and Muir, G. G. (1968). *Clin. Chem.*, **14**, 1010.

Wagstaff, T. I., Whyley, G. A. and Freedman, G. (1974). *Ann. clin. Biochem.*, **11**, 74.

Walker, A. H. C. and Jennison, R. F. (1962). *Brit. med. J.*, **1**, 152.

Warren, C., Holton, J. B. and Allen, J. T. (1974). *Ann. clin. Biochem.*, **11**, 31; *Brit. med. J.*, **1**, 94.

Watson, D., Mackay, E. V. and Trevella, W. (1965). *Clin. chim. Acta*, **12**, 500.

Whitfield, C. R., Neely, R. A. and Telford, M. E. (1968). *J. Obstet. Gynaec. Brit. Cwlth.*, **75**, 121.

Wilde, C. E. and Oakey, R. E. (1975). *Ann. clin. Biochem.*, **12**, 83.

Williams, J. H., Kuchmak, M. and Witter, R. F. (1969). *Clin. chim. Acta*, **25**, 447.

Wilson, G. R. (1973). *Clin. chim. Acta*, **46**, 297.

Wood, G. P. (1975). *Obstet. Gynec.*, **45**, 133.

Worth, H. G. J. (1973). *Clin. chim. Acta*, **49**, 53.

Wu, C-H., Lundy, L. E. and Lee, S. G. (1973). *Am. J. Obstet. Gynec.*, **115**, 169.

Yen, S. S. C., Vanden Berg, G., Rebar, R. and Ehara, Y. (1972). *J. clin. Endocr. Metab.*, **35**, 931.

Yoshimi, T. and Lipsett, M. B. (1968). *Steroids*, **11**, 527.

Youssefnejadian, E. and Sommerville, I. F. (1973). *J. Steroid Biochem.*, **4**, 659.

CHAPTER 5

ADRENALINE, NORADRENALINE AND RELATED COMPOUNDS

THE secretion of adrenaline by the adrenal medulla has been known since the end of the last century. From its formula it will be seen that it has the two phenolic groups of catechol and is an amine, hence the term catecholamine. Other catecholamines related to adrenaline are noradrenaline and 3-hydroxytyramine (dopamine), both intermediates in the formation of adrenaline from tyrosine (see Fig. 5,1). Tyrosine is first hydroxylated at the 3-position to give 3,4-dihydroxyphenylalanine (dopa) which is decarboxylated to form dopamine. Hydroxylation on the side chain produces noradrenaline, into the amino group of which a methyl group is finally introduced to give adrenaline. Both adrenaline and noradrenaline are physiologically active pressor amines. Catecholamines are found in the urine partly free and partly conjugated as glucuronides and sulphates.

The adrenal medulla is not the only tissue capable of producing catecholamines. The endings of adrenergic nerve fibres of the autonomic nervous system secrete noradrenaline and localised collections of neurones within the brain secrete noradrenaline or dopamine. Adrenaline secretion appears to be entirely from the adrenal medulla.

Several tumours share a common ancestry being derived embryologically from the neural crest. Of these the phaeochromocytoma has long been known to produce catecholamines. Its site of occurrence is most commonly in the adrenal medulla but it may arise anywhere along the sympathetic chain, a property which sometimes makes location very difficult. Actively secreting carotid body and glomus jugulare tumours in the neck have been described. All these tumours are usually benign but can cause severe, sometimes fatal, disturbances. They are associated with hypertension, often paroxysmal in type, and other manifestations of sympathetic overactivity. Their diagnosis is important since surgical removal usually relieves the hypertension and avoids the serious consequences of sudden excessive release of catecholamines. Tumours arising in adults from sympathetic ganglia, called ganglioneuromas also secrete catecholamines in some cases and are benign. A highly malignant tumour in children is the neuroblastoma which usually secretes very large amounts of catecholamine metabolites. These are present in the urine although the excretion of the biologically active free amines is not greatly increased. Dopamine excretion may be much increased in certain cases of neuroblastoma and malignant phaeochromocytoma. See Gjessing (1968) for a discussion of the origin of the various neural crest tumours.

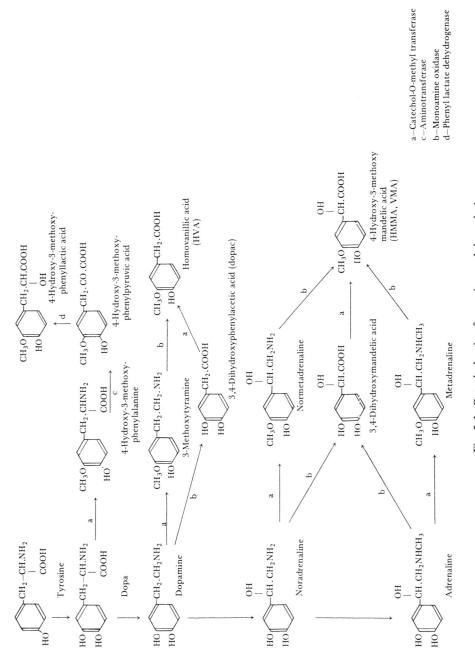

Fig. 5,1. Catecholamine formation and degradation.

The Determination of Catecholamines

Both biological and chemical methods have been used for determining these substances. The former usually estimate only the free, i.e. non-conjugated, physiologically active substances. Chemical methods have been reviewed by Goldenberg *et al.* (1954) and Persky (1955). Some of these determine only adrenaline and noradrenaline, others include 3-hydroxytyramine. Oxidation converts adrenaline into adrenochrome and in alkaline solution this changes into adrenolutine (Fig. 5,2), the trihydroxyindole reaction. Adrenolutine has a yellowish green fluorescence which however disappears rapidly in presence of oxygen. Noradrenaline is converted into similar compounds, noradrenochrome and noradrenolutine.

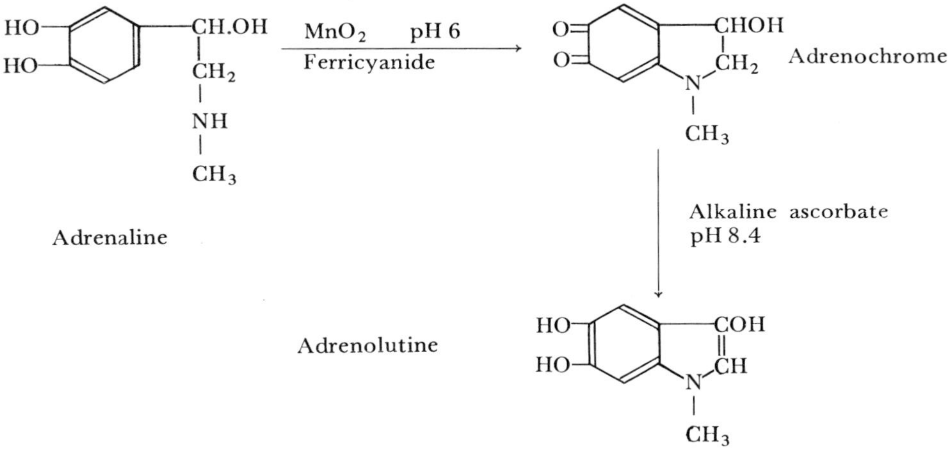

Fig. 5,2. Oxidation of Adrenaline.

Several different oxidising agents have been employed, including manganese dioxide (Lund, 1949), and ferricyanide (von Euler and Floding, 1955; Sobel and Henry, 1957). With iodine (von Euler and Hamberg, 1949) used for colorimetric determination of catecholamines in tissues, coloured 2-iodo derivatives of the adrenochromes are obtained. Crout (1961) used the trihydroxyindole reaction for the fluorimetric determination of catecholamines as did Griffiths *et al.* (1970) for determining plasma adrenaline and noradrenaline. All the agents oxidise both adrenaline and noradrenaline at a pH above 5 but only adrenaline is oxidised below pH 4, a property used for their differential estimation.

The pink coloured quinones produced by this oxidation can be transformed to highly fluorescent derivatives by the addition of alkali and the exclusion of oxygen. Lund (1949) first used ascorbic acid for this purpose but this may not be the most suitable reagent since high blanks and instability can result if meticulous care is not taken. Haggendal (1963) found that dimercaprol with sodium sulphite gave increased stability and reduced blank readings. Merrils (1963) used alkaline thioglycollate which

196 *Practical Clinical Biochemistry*

stabilises noradrenolutine, whereas adrenolutine fades rapidly giving another method for differential determination of adrenaline and nor-adrenaline. This method was adapted for the AutoAnalyzer by Merrils (1963) and further investigated by Robinson and Watts (1965). Addition of acetic acid to the stabilised solution increases the sensitivity of the method which has been used by Renzini *et al.* (1970) and Griffiths *et al.* (1970) to determine plasma adrenaline and noradrenaline.

A third method for the differential estimation of adrenaline and noradrenaline uses differential spectrofluorimetry, reading at different activating and emission wavelengths (Vendsalu, 1960).

An alternative to the trihydroxyindole reaction is the condensation of the two *o*-quinone groups of adrenochrome with ethylenediamine in alkaline solution (Weil-Malherbe and Bone, 1952) in which adrenaline readily undergoes auto-oxidation. Dopamine gives a strongly fluorescent product in this reaction as do catechol and some of its derivatives which may be present in urine.

Separation of Catecholamines from Biological Fluids

Either the catechol or the amine group can be used to separate catecholamines from contaminating substances. Reactions for either or both have been used. On stirring the solution containing catecholamines with alumina at pH 8.4, the catechol group is adsorbed (Lund, 1949; Weil-Malherbe and Bone, 1952). The alumina must be activated and the catecholamine protected from auto-oxidation by EDTA. The alumina is then separated by decantation, washed, and the catechols eluted with dilute acid. Adsorption of the amine group on weak cation exchange resins such as Amberlite IRC 50 was originally used by Bergstrom and Hanssen (1951). Strong acid resins, for example Dowex 50 (Bertler *et al.*, 1958; Vendsalu, 1960) are now more commonly employed since they can separate the amines from the O-methyl metabolites and dopamine with good recovery (Haggendal, 1963). Weil-Malherbe and Bone (1957) first used alumina to take up the catechols and Zeocarb to adsorb the amines; Renzini *et al.* (1970) used alumina and Amberlite CG 50.

The trihydroxyindole reaction (p. 195) can be applied to extracts obtained by any of these methods of separation. The ethylenediamine method is suitable only with the ion exchange resins as little is to be gained by adsorbing the total catechols and then applying a method which is dependent upon the catechol group.

For further information concerning the separation and determination of catecholamines see Callingham (1963, 1967).

Determination of Total Catecholamines in Urine

This is a modified version of the method of Bell, Horrocks and Varley given in the second edition of this book. The catecholamines are adsorbed

Adrenaline, Noradrenaline and Related Compounds 197

from untreated urine on to a column of Amberlite IRC 50, eluted and condensed in alkaline solution with ethylenediamine and the resulting fluorescence read.

Reagents. 1. Sulphuric acid, 500 mmol/l.

2. Sodium hydroxide, 1 mol/l.

3. Amberlite IRC 50 (British Drug Houses, Analytical reagent), acid form.

4. Phosphate buffer, pH 6.5, 500 mmol/l. Mix 31.8 ml of a solution of $Na_2 HPO_4, 2H_2 O$ (89.07 g/l) and 68.2 ml of $KH_2 PO_4$ solution (69.085 g/l).

5. Ethylenediamine dihydrochloride, 2 mol/l. Dissolve 26.6 g in water and make up to 100 ml. Ethylenediamine dihydrochloride can be prepared from freshly distilled ethylenediamine. Dissolve 50 ml in 200 ml ethanol and mix with 1 500 ml ethanolic hydrochloric acid containing 150 ml concentrated acid. Filter the crystals with suction, wash with ethanol and dry in an incubator (Weil-Malherbe and Bone, 1954). Ethylenediamine dihydrochloride as bought can be recrystallised from ethanol (700 ml/l with water).

6. Ammonia, sp. gr. 0.88.

7. Solid sodium chloride.

8. Isobutanol.

9. Hydrochloric acid, 6 mol/l.

10. Sodium hydroxide, 10 mol/l.

11. Orthophosphoric acid, sp. gr. 1.75.

12. Stock standard solutions. (*a*) Adrenaline 600 μmol/l. Dissolve 11.0 mg adrenaline in 10 ml of 1 mol/l hydrochloric acid and make to 100 ml with water. (*b*) Mixed standard. Dissolve 11.0 mg adrenaline, 19.1 mg noradrenaline bitartrate and 11.4 mg dopamine hydrochloride in separate 100 ml volumes of 10 mmol/l hydrochloric acid and mix in the ratio of 1 : 2.2 : 8.5 adrenaline, noradrenaline and dopamine. These are the mean proportions found by Weil-Malherbe in the urine of normal persons. The mixed standard contains 600 μmol/l.

13. Standard solutions for use. Dilute the stock standards 1 to 100 with water. The solutions then contain 6 μmol/l.

Technique. Collect a 24 h specimen of urine into a bottle containing 50 ml of 500 mmol/l sulphuric acid and measure the volume. Take one hundredth of this, making to about 15 ml for smaller volumes, and adjust to pH 6.5 with 1 mol/l sodium hydroxide.

Prepare a 5 × 1 cm column of the resin and wash in turn using a flow rate of about 5 ml/min with (1) 50 ml sulphuric acid; (2) 50 ml water; (3) 50 ml 1 mol/l sodium hydroxide; (4) 50 ml water; (5) 50 ml phosphate buffer; (6) 50 ml water.

Alternatively the resin can be prepared in bulk as follows: Wash with water, stand, and decant. Stir with 5 volumes of hydrochloric acid for 30 min, remove excess acid and wash several times with water, decanting each time. Add 3 volumes of water followed by 2 volumes 10 mol/l sodium hydroxide added over 15 min while stirring mechanically. Wash again

198   *Practical Clinical Biochemistry*

several times with distilled water. Then suspend the resin in an equal volume of water and add phosphoric acid until the pH remains at 6.5 while stirring continuously for 30 min. For use place the required amount of the resin into the column, drain, and wash with 25 ml of water.

Run the urine, adjusted to pH 6.5, through the column at a rate of 2 to 3 ml/min. Follow with 50 ml water. Then elute the adsorbed catecholamines with sulphuric acid. Discard the first 5 ml and collect the next 20 ml.

Fluorimetry. Measure 5 ml (= 1/400th of the total urine volume) of the eluate into a glass-stoppered tube and 0.5 ml of the diluted adrenaline standard plus 4.5 ml water into a similar tube (or 1.5 ml of mixed standard plus 3.5 ml water). To each add 0.5 ml ethylenediamine dihydrochloride and 1 ml ammonia. Place in a water bath at 50°C for 20 min, cool, add solid sodium chloride (2 to 3 g) and 6 ml isobutanol, stopper, shake thoroughly for 3 min and then centrifuge to separate the layers. Remove the isobutanol layer for fluorimetry. For the blanks take a further 5 ml eluate (test blank), 0.5 ml standard plus 4.5 ml water (standard blank) and 5 ml water (reagent blank) and to each add 1 ml ammonia. Heat in the water bath at 50°C for 20 min, cool, and add 0.5 ml ethylenediamine dihydrochloride and proceed as described for the test and standard. Read against the reagent blank in the fluorimeter activating at 436 nm and reading fluorescence at about 530 nm.

Blanks are only required if an abnormally high result is obtained. Then it is particularly important to carry through a test blank since urines occasionally contain substances which fluoresce on addition of ammonia. The catecholamines are destroyed when heated with ammonia before adding the ethylenediamine thus allowing the fluorescence from other substances to be measured.

Calculation. Urinary total catecholamines (μmol(24 h) as adrenaline

$$= \frac{\text{Reading of unknown}}{\text{Reading of standard}} \times 0.5 \times \frac{6}{1\,000} \times 400, \text{ i.e. } \times 1.2$$

$$\text{or} = \frac{\text{Reading of unknown}}{\text{Reading of standard}} \times 3.6 \text{ (for mixed standard):}$$

Subtract any urine blank from the total test reading.

To convert to μg/24 h multiply μmol/24 h by 183.

Notes. 1. In the above technique only the free catecholamines are determined. Most earlier workers used a period of heating at pH 1 to 2 to hydrolyse conjugated catecholamines. To do this adjust the urine to pH 1.5 with more 500 mmol/l sulphuric acid, transfer to a small bottle, stopper firmly, heat in a boiling water bath for 20 min, cool, and adjust to pH 6.5 with 1 mol/l sodium hydroxide. Proceed as described above. The result then gives free and conjugated amines. Some later workers, however, have determined only the free compounds (see for example, MacMillan, 1957). The reason for preferring not to hydrolyse the conjugated amines is discussed on the opposite page.

Adrenaline, Noradrenaline and Related Compounds

2. *Use as a screening test.* The above technique can be used as a visual screening test with a simple u.v. lamp should a suitable fluorimeter not be available. For this the mixed standard (1.5 ml) is more suitable. A very high proportion of patients with hypertension not due to phaeochromocytoma have an excretion of free total catecholamines less than this. Accordingly if the fluorescence of test and standard are compared using a BTH Mercra Lamp, Type MBW/V 125 W, urine from most patients with phaeochromocytoma should show a markedly stronger fluorescence than the standard, whereas others will fluoresce less, usually much less, than the standard.

3. It should be noted that adrenaline gives a greater amount of fluorescence than noradrenaline and dopamine. The difference varies with the instrument used but is about three times as great.

INTERPRETATION

In a series of 422 hypertensive patients without phaeochromocytoma Bell (1960) found daily excretion of total unconjugated catecholamines in urine to range from 0 to 1.3 μmol (0 to 240 μg expressed as adrenaline), with a mean of 0.46 μmol (84 μg). The distribution was skew at the upper end, 5 per cent having values over 0.87 μmol (160 μg) and 1.5 per cent over 1.12 μmol (205 μg). In 11 patients with phaeochromocytoma the two lowest results were 1.09 and 1.75 μmol (200 and 320 μg), the remainder varying from 3.3 to 22 μmol (600 to 4 000 μg).

In phaeochromocytoma if the hypertension is paroxysmal considerable variations in catecholamine excretion occur and amounts near to and possibly within the normal range can be obtained when the blood pressure is at its lowest. The excretion in one patient varied between 3.3 and 13.6 μmol (600 and 2 500 μg) while a patient who excreted 1.1 μmol (200 μg) between attacks put out 11 μmol (2 000 μg/24 h) during a severe hypertensive phase. On the other hand, a patient whose hypertension did not vary much excreted between 5.2 and 6.0 μmol (950 and 1 100 μg).

Since the fluorescence given by adrenaline is approximately three times that of the other catecholamines, results expressed in terms of the mixed standard are numerically about three times greater than those given above. So almost all patients with hypertension not due to phaeochromocytoma will have values below 3.3 μmol/24 h (600 μg/24 h).

If hydrolysed urine is used Bell (1960) reported that over 70 per cent of the total catecholamines were unconjugated and the distribution was similar in normal, hypertensive and phaeochromocytoma patients. However, he found a few cases in which the unconjugated catecholamine excretion was normal yet the proportion was only 8 to 45 per cent of the total. The high values for the total was due to the presence of large amounts of dopamine. Crout and Sjoerdsma (1959) showed that ingestion of bananas produced increased excretion in the urine of conjugated noradrenaline and dopamine (also of 5-hydroxyindole acetic acid) which could reach several μmol. Because of this occasional finding it is considered preferable to determine only the free catecholamines.

200 *Practical Clinical Biochemistry*

Increased catecholamine excretion occurs after exercise and as a response to pain or stress including anaesthesia particularly after ether. Various drugs have been shown to alter catecholamine metabolism and hence their excretion. Increases occur when patients are given phenothiazines, monoamine oxidase inhibitors, theophylline or aminophylline. Decreased excretion occurs after reserpine.

Direct interference during the fluorimetric procedure is seen with other substances. Tetracyclines, erythromycin and ampicillin are interfering antibiotics, and chloral and formaldehyde may sometimes cause trouble. More important, however, are various drugs used in the treatment of hypertension which may cause false positives when hypertensive patients are investigated. The drugs involved are guanethidine and especially α-methyldopa. It is desirable that all drugs be withdrawn before the test is carried out. In particular, interference from α-methyldopa may persist for several days.

Determination of Urinary Adrenaline and Noradrenaline by Ferricyanide Oxidation (von Euler and Floding, 1955; Weil-Malherbe and Bone, 1957)

Ferricyanide oxidation can also be applied to the eluate from the Amberlite IRC 50 column obtained as described in the previous method.

Reagents. 1. Acetate buffer, pH 6.0, approximately 1 mol/l. Dissolve 136 g sodium acetate (CH_3COONa, $3H_2O$) in about 900 ml water, adjust to pH 6.0 with glacial acetic acid and make to 1 litre with water.

2. Sodium hydroxide, 2.5 mol/l.

3. Zinc sulphate solution, 5 g $ZnSO_4,7H_2O/l$.

4. Potassium ferricyanide solution, 2.5 g/l. Prepare freshly at frequent intervals.

5. Sodium hydroxide, 5 mol/l.

6. Ascorbic acid, 20 g/l. Prepare freshly by dissolving 100 mg in 5 ml water.

7. Alkaline ascorbate solution. Mix 9 volumes sodium hydroxide (reagent 5) with 1 volume ascorbic acid immediately before use.

8. Standard solution of noradrenaline 600 μmol/l. Prepare a stock standard of 19.1 mg noradrenaline bitartrate in 100 ml 10 mmol/l hydrochloric acid and dilute 1 to 100 with water to give a standard for use containing 6 μmol/l.

Technique. Adjust the 20 ml of eluate obtained as described for total catecholamines to pH 6.0 with 2.5 mol/l sodium hydroxide and make to 25 ml. Transfer 5 ml of this (= 1/500th of the original 24 h specimen) to a suitable glass-stoppered centrifuge tube. To a similar tube add 0.4 ml standard and make to 5 ml with water; for the reagent blank take 5 ml water. To each add 1 ml acetate buffer, followed by 0.1 ml zinc sulphate and 0.1 ml potassium ferricyanide. Mix and then stand for 3 min. Add 1 ml alkaline ascorbate and read in the fluorimeter as in the previous method after 2 to 3 min. For the blanks take 5 ml eluate (test blank) and 0.4 ml

Adrenaline, Noradrenaline and Related Compounds

standard made to 5 ml (standard blank) and treat as the test except that 1 ml sodium hydroxide (reagent 5) is added instead of the alkaline ascorbate. The standard blank can be omitted and in most cases the test blank as well. However, whilst the true fluorescence is a greenish-yellow, occasionally turbidity occurs giving a blue fluorescence. If the tube is then centrifuged the correct fluorescence is seen in the liquid and the blue fluorescence in the deposit.

Calculation. Urinary adrenaline + noradrenaline (μmol/24 h).

$$= \frac{\text{Reading of unknown} - \text{reading of unknown blank}}{\text{Reading of standard} - \text{reading of standard blank}} \times \frac{0.4}{1\ 000} \times 6 \times 500$$

$$= \frac{\text{Reading of unknown}}{\text{Reading of standard}} \times 1.2$$

To convert to μg/24 h (expressed as noradrenaline) multiply μmol/24 h by 169.

INTERPRETATION

In a series of 100 cases of hypertension not due to phaeochromocytoma a daily excretion of more than 1.2 μmol (200 μg) was only once slightly exceeded (Bell, 1960). The lowest result from a patient with confirmed phaeochromocytoma was 2.4 μmol (400 μg). Later a value of 1.2 μmol (200 μg) was obtained at one time in a patient with fluctuating hypertension due to a tumour. The method can thus be used as a screening test using this standard and the Mercra lamp referred to above should a fluorimeter not be available.

Note. In normal urine there is very little adrenaline. In patients with phaeochromocytoma, although noradrenaline is the catecholamine usually present in the greatest proportion, considerable amounts of adrenaline may be present occasionally. In such cases the adrenaline only can be determined by carrying out the oxidation at pH 3.5 instead of at pH 6.0. For this use an acetate buffer pH 3.5. Dissolve 136 g sodium acetate (CH_3COONa, $3H_2O$) in approximately 900 ml water, adjust to pH 3.5 with glacial acetic acid and make to 1 litre with water. Substitute 1.0 ml of this for the pH 6.0 buffer at the appropriate place in the above technique.

Noradrenaline is thus obtained by difference, and dopamine can be obtained from the value for total catecholamines by the previous technique.

Determination of Adrenaline and Noradrenaline in Urine by the Combined Alumina-Trihydroxyindole Method. (Quek *et al.*, 1975).

The method given above is adequate for detecting relatively large increases of adrenaline and noradrenaline when a sensitive fluorimeter is not available. A more suitable technique uses much smaller urine samples to avoid quenching effects and employs separation on alumina columns. The urine sample, adjusted to pH 8.2 to 8.5 in the presence of EDTA, is

202 *Practical Clinical Biochemistry*

adsorbed on a column of alumina, which is then washed with sodium acetate and water before eluting with dilute acetic acid. The pH of the eluate is adjusted for the oxidation by adding borate. The trihydroxyindole reaction is then applied.

Reagents. 1. Aluminium oxide (BDH), washed several times with deionised water to remove fine particles and dried at 100 to 120°C. Store in a tightly stoppered bottle. The removal of fines is essential if adequate flow through the chromatographic columns is to be achieved.

2. EDTA (disodium salt), 100 g/l.

3. Sodium hydroxide, 1 mol/l and 5 mol/l.

4. Sodium acetate, 0.2 mol/l. Dissolve 27.2 g of the trihydrate in water and make to a litre. Store in the refrigerator.

5. Acetic acid, 0.4 mol/l. Dilute 23 ml glacial acetic acid to 1 litre with water.

6. Disodium tetraborate ($Na_2 B_4 O_7, 10 H_2 O$), 30 g/l.

7. Potassium ferricyanide, 5 g/l. Prepare freshly every month.

8. Alkaline ascorbate reagent. Prepare just before use. Weigh 100 mg ascorbic acid and dissolve in 5 ml deionised water. Mix one part of this with nine parts 5 mol/l sodium hydroxide.

9. Noradrenaline stock standard, 6 mmol/l (1.01 g/l), 19 mg noradrenaline bitartrate made up to 100 ml in 100 mmol/l hydrochloric acid. Store in the refrigerator and renew after 6 months.

10. Dilute stock standard, 12 μmol/l (2 mg/l). Dilute 100 μl of the stock standard to 50 ml with 100 mmol/l hydrochloric acid. Store in the refrigerator and renew monthly.

11. Noradrenaline working standard, 0.12 μmol/l (20 μg/l). Prepare freshly by diluting 100 μl dilute stock standard to 10 ml with 0.4 mol/l acetic acid.

Technique. Collect 24 h urine specimens in bottles containing 15 ml hydrochloric acid (500 ml concentrated acid/l with water) and keep refrigerated.

To 25 ml of the mixed specimen in a beaker, add 5 drops EDTA and rapidly adjust to pH 8.2 to 8.5 with 5 mol/l and 1 mol/l sodium hydroxide using indicator paper or a pH meter. Rapidly centrifuge about 10 ml of this and use within an hour.

Just before or during the centrifugation of the sample depending on the rate of flow through the columns prepare the column of alumina. These columns are the same as those used for the chromatography of pregnanediol (p. 133), being 1 cm internal diameter glass tubes with a sintered glass disc porosity No. 1 at the lower end. A column of length about 20 cm is suitable. Seal the lower end of the column with a finger and add a few ml deionised water, pour in 1.5 g alumina and tap the tube until air bubbles are released and the alumina settles. Add a further 5 ml water and when this has passed through, prime with 5 ml sodium acetate. Allow to drain and carefully pipette 1 ml of the treated urine onto the surface of the alumina and when this has percolated through, wash the column with

Adrenaline, Noradrenaline and Related Compounds 203

10 ml sodium acetate and 10 ml deionised water allowing the column to drain completely between additions and taking care not to disturb the alumina. Discard all effluents up to this stage. To elute the catecholamines add 10 ml acetic acid and collect the eluate which can be assayed immediately or within the next 24 h if kept at 4° C.

For developing the fluorescence four tubes are required. Disposable plastic tubes are satisfactory. Put these up as follows:

	Standard (S)	Standard blank (SB)	Test (T)	Test blank (TB)
Column eluate (ml)	—	—	1.0	1.0
Working standard (ml)	1.0	1.0	—	—
Disodium tetraborate (ml)	2.5	2.5	2.5	2.6
Potassium ferricyanide (ml)	0.1	0.1	0.1	—
Stopper or seal with Parafilm, mix by inversion and stand 3 to 5 min. Then add				
Alkaline ascorbate (ml)	1.0	1.0	1.0	1.0

Mix again by inversion and read the fluorescence within 20 min. Each test is followed by its corresponding blank at an activating wavelength of 405 nm and emission at 495 nm.

Calculation. Urinary catecholamines, adrenaline + noradrenaline (μmol/24 h)

$$= \frac{T-TB}{S-SB} \times \frac{0.12}{1\,000} \times \frac{24 \text{ h urine volume (ml)}}{0.1}$$

By this method the urinary excretion of adrenaline + noradrenaline is less than 0.6 μmol/24 h (100 μg/24 h).

Determination of Adrenaline and Noradrenaline in Tissue Extracts Using Iodine Oxidation (von Euler and Hamberg, 1949; von Euler *et al.*, 1954)

This simple colorimetric method can be applied to trichloracetic acid extracts of tissues to determine the proportion of adrenaline and noradrenaline present in surgically removed adrenal glands. It is based on the differential oxidation of the two catecholamines at different pH values producing the pink-coloured iodo derivatives (p. 195).

Reagents. 1. Silver sand.

2. Trichloracetic acid, 100 g/l.

3. Sodium hydroxide, 2.5 mol/l.

4. Acetate buffer, pH 3.5, approximately 1 mol/l. Dissolve 136 g sodium acetate ($CH_3COONa.3H_2O$) in approximately 900 ml water, adjust to pH 3.5 with glacial acetic acid and make up to 1 litre with water.

5. Acetate buffer, pH 6.0, approximately 1 mol/l. Prepare as above and adjust to pH 6.0 with glacial acetic acid.

6. Iodine, 12.7 g/l in potassium iodide 20 g/l.

204 Practical Clinical Biochemistry

7. Sodium thiosulphate, 100 mmol/l, 24.8 g/l.

8. Stock standard solutions of adrenaline and noradrenaline containing 100 mg/l of each amine in 10 mmol/l hydrochloric acid. Adjust an appropriate amount of standard to pH 4.0 with 100 mmol/l sodium hydroxide then dilute to give a solution containing 50 mg/l.

Technique. Weigh 3 to 4 g freshly removed tissue and transfer to a mortar. Add sufficient silver sand and then cold trichloracetic acid to cover the tissue, and grind with a pestle. Allow to settle and decant the supernatant through a filter paper into a stoppered measuring cylinder. Add further acid to the residue and repeat the extraction three more times combining the extracts. When the filtration has finished make the extract up to 10 ml for each gram of tissue. Take 10 ml of the extract, adjust to pH 4.0 with sodium hydroxide, stirring continuously to avoid loss of catecholamines by oxidation in alkaline solution. Make the volume of extract up to 20 ml. Each ml is now equal to 0.05 g of the original tissue.

Determine the volume of extract to take by trial and error. It is useful to start with 1 ml, oxidise at pH 6.0, and decide from the resultant colour how much extract to use next. Pipette duplicate amounts of each standard (2 ml) and unknown into separate tubes and make up to 4 ml with water. To one set of tubes add 1 ml acetate buffer, pH 3.5, and 0.2 ml iodine solution. Shake, stand for exactly 1.5 min and add 0.2 ml sodium thiosulphate solution to discharge the excess iodine. To the other set of tubes add 1.0 ml acetate buffer, pH 6.0, and 0.2 ml iodine solution. Mix and stand for 3 min then add 0.2 ml sodium thiosulphate solution. Read at 530 nm against a water blank or a blank containing all reagents. The choice of wavelength is that at which the absorption curves for the products obtained from the oxidation of adrenaline at pH 3.5 and pH 6.0 cross, the isosbestic point. This depends on the conditions employed and the instrument used but subsequent calculations are simplified if this wavelength is employed.

Calculation.

$$\text{Tissue noradrenaline, mg/g} = \frac{d(b-a)}{1-e} \times 0.1 \times \frac{20}{\text{volume of extract used (ml)}}$$

$$\text{Tissue adrenaline, mg/g} = c \left(a - \frac{e(b-a)}{1-e} \right) \times \frac{0.1 \times 20}{\text{volume of extract used (ml)}}$$

where
  (a) Reading at pH 3.5 (1.5 min iodine treatment).
  (b) Reading at pH 6.0 (3 min iodine treatment).
  (c) Calibration factor for adrenaline. 100/reading for 100 μg.
  (d) Calibration factor for noradrenaline. 100/reading for 100 μg at pH 6.0.
  (e) Relative amount of noradrenaline oxidised at pH 3.5 in 1.5 min, i.e. Reading for standard at pH 3.5/Reading for standard at pH 6.0.

Adrenaline, Noradrenaline and Related Compounds 205

If 1 ml of diluted extract is used with a noradrenaline standard of 100 μg, this is equivalent to 20 × 100 μg/g, i.e. 2 mg/g.

INTERPRETATION

Normal adrenal tissue contains up to 1.0 mg catecholamines/g of which 90 per cent is adrenaline. Phaeochromocytomas contain greatly increased amounts of catecholamines with noradrenaline predominating. Thus for 31 tumours investigated, 25 contained more noradrenaline with a range of 1.1 to 22.5 mg/g tissue. Adrenaline was barely detectable in 18 of these but was the predominant material in 6 with a range from 1.1 to 11.0 mg/g tissue. In only one of these 31 tumours was noradrenaline not detected. In contrast ganglioneuromas and neuroblastomas (see p. 193) possess no storage capacity and values of the order of 100 to 200 μg/g tissue are usually found.

Determination of Catecholamine Metabolites

Methods are also available for determining certain metabolites of adrenaline and noradrenaline. The pathways by which these are formed are shown in Fig. 5,1, p. 194. Noradrenaline and adrenaline are converted by catechol-O-methyl transferase into normetadrenaline and metadrenaline (also termed normetanephrine and metanephrine), then by the action of monoamine oxidase into 4-hydroxy-3-methoxy-mandelic acid (HMMA), often incorrectly termed vanillylmandelic or vanilmandelic acid (VMA). Alternatively, though quantitatively less so, oxidation to 3,4-dihydroxy-mandelic acid may occur first followed by conversion to 4-hydroxy-3-methoxy-mandelic acid.

Dopamine is metabolised along similar lines through 3-methoxytyramine to homovanillic acid (4-hydroxy-3-methoxy-phenylacetic acid). In certain patients with malignant phaeochromocytoma or neuroblastoma, atypical or deranged metabolism can occur whereby large amounts of dopa enter the circulation. Dopa can be decarboxylated in the kidney so that large amounts of dopamine are excreted in the urine, or it can be methylated and then undergo transamination to the corresponding keto acid, 4-hydroxy-3-methoxy-phenyl pyruvic acid, which is unstable and is converted to the corresponding hydroxy acid, 4-hydroxy-3-methoxy-phenyllactic acid. This may be detected in small amounts in the urine of many patients suffering from neuroblastoma but it is found in characteristically large amounts in the group 2 patients (see later, p. 213).

Determination of Metadrenaline and Normetadrenaline in Urine (Pisano, 1960; Crout *et al.,* 1961)

Pisano (1960) developed a relatively simple method for determining normetadrenaline and metadrenaline in urine. These compounds are

206 *Practical Clinical Biochemistry*

adsorbed on to Amberlite CG 50, eluted with ammonia and converted to vanillin by oxidation with periodate, the vanillin formed being read at 350 and 360 nm.

$$CH_3O-\underset{HO}{\bigcirc}-CH-CH_2NH_2 \quad \underset{NaIO_4}{\longrightarrow} \quad CH_3O-\underset{HO}{\bigcirc}-CHO + H.CHO+NH_3+NaIO_3$$

Vanillin

Reagents. 1. Hydrochloric acid, 6 mol/l.
2. Sodium hydroxide, 2.5 mol/l.
3. Sodium hydroxide, 10 mol/l.
4. Amberlite CG 50, 100 to 200 mesh, Rohm and Hass (supplied by British Drug Houses). This is a chromatographic grade of the IRC 50 resin used for total catecholamine determination. Obtain the acid form and purify as follows. Suspend in about 3 volumes of water, stir for 10 min, then allow to stand for 30 min and discard the supernatant. Repeat the process several times until the supernatant is clear after standing 10 to 15 min. Add 3 volumes of water followed by 2 volumes of 10 mol/l sodium hydroxide over a period of 15 min while stirring mechanically. Continue stirring for a further 2 h. Remove excess hydroxide by decanting and wash the resin well with several changes of water. To clear further add 5 volumes of hydrochloric acid, stir for about 30 min, remove excess acid and wash several times with distilled water with decanting. Reconvert to the alkaline form by repeating the stirring with the sodium hydroxide for 30 min. Wash several times with distilled water. Then suspend the resin in an equal volume of water and add glacial acetic acid stirring continuously until the pH remains at 6.0 to 6.5 for 30 min. When the acetic acid is added the pH drops sharply but on stirring rises slowly until equilibrium is reached. This last stage is critical so sufficient time must elapse to ensure the pH remains at the correct level. Once prepared the resin keeps well.

After use the resin can be regenerated by first converting to the acid form, then to the sodium form.
5. Ammonia, 4 mol/l. Mix 100 ml ammonia (sp. gr. 0.88) with 360 ml water.
6. Sodium metaperiodate solution. Dissolve 100 mg $NaIO_4$ in 5 ml water as required.
7. Sodium metabisulphite, 100 g/l water. Kept stoppered this is stable at $3°$ C for at least one month.
8. Standard solution of normetadrenaline, 1 mmol/l. Prepare a solution containing 220 μg/ml normetadrenaline hydrochloride (Normetanephine, Sigma) in 10 mmol/l hydrochloric acid. This contains the equivalent of 183 mg/l of free base.

Technique. Collect a 24 h specimen in acid as for total catecholamines, filtering if necessary. Transfer one 200th of this into a capped test tube,

Adrenaline, Noradrenaline and Related Compounds 207

add 1/10th its volume of hydrochloric acid and place in a boiling water bath for 20 min. Cool, adjust to pH 6.0 to 6.5 with 2.5 mol/l sodium hydroxide and dilute to approximately 20 ml with water.

Prepare a column of resin about 5 × 1 cm and wash with 15 ml water to remove the buffer solution. Apply the hydrolysed urine at a flow rate not exceeding 1 ml/min. Then wash the column with 15 to 20 ml water and elute with ammonia until 10 ml of eluate is obtained. Take two 4 ml aliquots. To one (the test) add 100 μl metaperiodate, mix and allow oxidation to proceed for 1 min. Then add 100 μl metabisulphite to remove excess periodate. To the other (the blank) add 100 μl metabisulphite, then 100 μl periodate. For the standard add 100 μl normetadrenaline standard ($\equiv$ 0.1 μmol) to 10 ml ammonia and treat as the test solution. Read each test against it own blank and the standard against an ammonia blank at 350 and 360 nm. Pisano uses the reading at 360 nm for the calculation (see note below).

Calculation.   Urinary   normetadrenaline + metadrenaline   (μmol/24 h) (expressed as normetadrenaline)

$$= \frac{\text{Reading of unknown}}{\text{Reading of standard}} \times 0.1 \times 200$$

$$= \frac{\text{Reading of unknown}}{\text{Reading of standard}} \times 20$$

To convert to mg/24 h multiply μmol/24 h by 0.183.

Notes. 1.   The reading at 360 nm should be approximately 75 per cent of that at 350 nm. Interfering substances, for example p-octopamine, which oxidizes to p-hydroxybenzaldehyde with a peak at 330 nm, if present can reduce the reading at 360 nm to about 50 per cent that at 350 nm. Such readings should be regarded with suspicion.

2. *Drug interference.* Altered excretion of metadrenalines occurs following administration of drugs which alter catecholamine metabolism. Monoamine oxidase inhibitors reduce HMMA formation and increase metadrenaline excretion. Increased output also occurs with the phenothiazine, prochlorperazine, which reduces the uptake of noradrenaline by tissues. Laevodopa reduces the excretion.

Other drugs appear to interfere with the method itself. Phenothiazines and the tricyclic antidepressant, imipramine, have caused trouble. It is desirable to withdraw the drug before the investigation, if possible. A different, potentially serious source of interference (Johnson *et al.,* 1972) is methyl glucamine (meglumine) which occurs in at least 15 radiographic contrast media in combination with the iodinated substances, iodipamide, iothalamate or diatriazoate. Meglumine salts are replaced by sodium salts of the same iodinated compounds in other contrast media which do not interfere. Meglumine is adsorbed onto the resin, is eluted with the metadrenaline fraction and then competes for metaperiodate preventing

208 *Practical Clinical Biochemistry*

vanillin formation and so giving falsely low results. If this interference is suspected, read also at 330 and 300 nm. If the reading at 330 nm exceeds that at 350 nm and is similar at 300 nm, meglumine interference is likely and the result is unreliable. Further specimens are best obtained after a lapse of at least three days but internal standards can be employed if necessary.

INTERPRETATION

The daily excretion in normal persons is less than 5.5 μmol (1.0 mg). In patients with phaeochromocytoma Pisano reported a daily excretion of 16.5 to 620 μmol (3 to 113 mg), Bell 15 to 165 μmol (2.8 to 30 mg).

Determination of Urinary 4-Hydroxy-3-Methoxy-Mandelic Acid

Sandler and Ruthven (1959, 1961) adsorbed HMMA on to Dowex IX 2 ion exchange resin as acetate and after eluting oxidised to vanillin which was then assayed spectrophotometrically. Gitlow *et al.* (1960a) and Robinson *et al.* (1959) used two-dimensional chromatography. A useful simple colorimetric screening test based on the coupling of this substance with diazotised *p*-nitroaniline was devised by Gitlow *et al.* (1960b). Finally, Pisano *et al.* (1962) developed a method for extracting the HMMA and oxidising it to vanillin which is then read spectrophotometrically.

Simple Colorimetric Screening Test (Gitlow *et al.,* 1960b)

The HMMA is extracted from acidified urine by ethyl acetate, coupled with diazotised *p*-nitroaniline, the coloured compound extracted into amyl alcohol and read at 450 and 550 nm. As the amount of HMMA excreted rises the ratio of these two readings falls, approximately to that given when pure HMMA is similarly treated.

Reagents. 1. Hydrochloric acid, 5 mol/l.

2. Ethyl acetate.

3. Potassium carbonate solution, 50 g/l.

4. *p*-Nitroaniline solution, 500 mg dissolved in 10 ml concentrated hydrochloric acid and 490 ml water.

5. Sodium nitrite solution, 2 g/l.

6. Diazotised *p*-nitroaniline. Mix reagents 4, 5 and water in the proportions 1 : 1 : 2.

7. Ethanolamine—amyl alcohol. Wash amyl alcohol in turn with hydrochloric acid, water, potassium carbonate and water. Add 1 volume of ethanolamine to 100 volumes of amyl alcohol.

Technique. Collect a fasting morning specimen of urine in acid as for catecholamines after the patient has had no medicines, coffee, fruits and substances containing vanillin for 48 h. Bring the urine immediately to between pH 2 and 4 with hydrochloric acid and keep at 10° C. Determine

Adrenaline, Noradrenaline and Related Compounds

the creatinine content and measure a volume of urine which contains 5 μmol (0.5 mg) creatinine into a 15 ml centrifuge tube. Bring the volume to 2 ml with water and add 0.1 ml hydrochloric acid. Extract once with 4 ml, then twice with 2 ml ethyl acetate. Carefully remove the ethyl acetate each time with a capillary pipette, avoiding water droplets. Pool in a small beaker (30 ml) and evaporate under a warm stream of air using a suitable dryer. Dissolve the dry material in 2 ml water and shake with 1 ml potassium carbonate. Then add rapidly with constant shaking 1 ml diazotised p-nitroaniline and follow with 5 ml amyl alcohol-ethanolamine. Shake, centrifuge and read against a water blank at 450 and 550 nm. Calculate the ratio E_{450}/E_{550}.

INTERPRETATION

The mean value for this ratio in normal subjects was given by Gitlow *et al.* as 2.09 (range 1.58 to 2.26); in patients with primary hypertension 1.82 (range 1.42 to 2.25); in patients with phaeochromocytoma 0.74 (range 0.41 to 1.16). The corresponding figures for HMMA excretion in mg/g creatinine in these groups were 1.6 (0.7 to 2.25), 1.5 (0.5 to 4.0) and 16 (7.5 to 30). The figures in the units mmol/mol creatinine are 0.9 (0.4 to 1.25), 0.8 (0.3 to 2.25) and 8.6 (4.2 to 16.8).

It is emphasised that this is a screening test and that should a positive result be obtained, i.e. a value for the ratio of less than 1.30, further investigations should be carried out. Thus Gitlow *et al.* obtained low values in two patients who excreted excess of 5-HIAA.

The method is sensitive to interference by such foodstuffs as bananas, coffee, tea, chocolate and vanilla flavouring. Certain drugs also interfere directly with the diazo-reaction. These include aspirin, p-aminosalicylic acid, bromsulphthalein, α-methyl dopa and tetracycline.

Quantitative Determination (Pisano, Crout and Abraham, 1962; see also Sandler and Ruthven, 1963)

HMMA is extracted from acidified urine into ethyl acetate, then back extracted with alkali and oxidised to vanillin with metaperiodate. After purification by further extraction the vanillin is read spectrophotometrically. An internal standard is used as HMMA recovery varies from one urine to another.

Reagents. 1. Hydrochloric acid, 6 mol/l.

2. Sodium chloride.

3. Ethyl acetate.

4. Potassium carbonate, 1 mol/l.

5. Sodium metaperiodate, $NaIO_4$, 20 g/l. Dissolve 1 g in 50 ml water. Prepare freshly each week.

6. Sodium metabisulphite solution, 100 g/l in water. Keep refrigerated and prepare freshly each week.

210   *Practical Clinical Biochemistry*

7. Acetic acid, 5 mol/l. Dilute 30 ml glacial acetic acid to 100 ml with water.

8. Phosphate buffer, 1 mol/l, pH 7.5. Add approximately 45 ml 1 mol/l potassium hydroxide (56 g/l) to 50 ml 1 mol/l potassium dihydrogen phosphate (36 g KH_2PO_4/l) until the pH is 7.5.

9. Cresol red indicator, 400 mg/l in water.

10. Toluene.

11. HMMA standard, 3 mmol/l (594 mg/l) in water.

Technique. Collect a 24 h specimen of urine into a bottle containing 10 ml hydrochloric acid. Keep cool. The volume of urine taken depends on the volume of specimen and the result expected. For a suspected normal value use 5 ml urine and transfer this amount to three 50 ml glass stoppered tubes. These are test, test + standard, and urine blank tubes. To the test + standard tube add 50 μl ($\equiv$ 0.15 μmol) of standard solution and to each tube 500 μl hydrochloric acid, sufficient solid sodium chloride (about 3 g) to saturate the solution and 25 ml ethyl acetate. Stopper and shake mechanically for 5 min to extract the phenolic acids. Centrifuge and transfer 20 ml of the ethyl acetate layer to a second glass stoppered tube and extract the phenolic acids into 1.5 ml potassium carbonate by shaking for 3 min. Centrifuge again and carefully transfer 1 ml of the carbonate layer to a third tube. To the test and internal standard tubes add 100 μl periodate solution and place all 3 tubes in a water bath at 50° C for 30 min to convert the HMMA into vanillin. Cool and to all tubes add 100 μl metabisulphite solution followed by 100 μl metaperiodate to the blank tube. Neutralise with 300 μl acetic acid and 600 μl phosphate buffer. The pH should be checked to be below 8.8, i.e. should be yellow to a drop of cresol red. Shake for 3 min with 25 ml toluene to extract the vanillin. Centrifuge and transfer 20 ml of the toluene layer to a further 50 ml glass stoppered tube and extract the vanillin into 4 ml potassium carbonate. Centrifuge and read against a carbonate blank at 360 nm.

Calculation. Urinary 4-hydroxy-3-methoxy-mandelic acid (μmol/l).

$$\frac{\text{Reading of test} - \text{Reading of blank}}{\text{Reading of test} + \text{standard} - \text{Reading of test}} \times \frac{0.15 \times 1\,000}{\text{volume of urine used (ml)}}$$

For a normal urine using 5 ml this becomes

$$\frac{\text{Reading of test} - \text{Reading of blank}}{\text{Reading of test} + \text{standard} - \text{Reading of test}} \times 30$$

To convert to mg/l multiply μmol/l by 0.198.

INTERPRETATION

Pisano *et al.* (1962) gave the normal range for daily excretion as 9.0 to 35.5 μmol (1.8 to 7.1 mg). Much increased values up to 2 650 μmol (530 mg) were found in patients with phaeochromocytoma.

The recovery of added HMMA varies from about 50 to 90 per cent

Adrenaline, Noradrenaline and Related Compounds

depending on other urinary constituents. Drugs such as clofibrate excreted as glucuronides compete for the metaperiodate so that incomplete oxidation occurs. The blank is usually of little significance but random urine samples from children with a neuroblastoma occasionally contain large amounts of vanillin-like material. Green and Walker (1970) showed that dietary vanillin contributes little to the blank and that a vanillin-free diet is not necessary. Restriction of bananas and chocolate is desirable. Certain drugs, for example, nalidixic acid (Negram) increase values by direct interference which can be corrected for by the blank procedure (Elder, 1968).

Drugs which alter catecholamine metabolism may alter the excretion of HMMA. Decreases are seen after the administration of monoamine oxidase inhibitors, guanethidine, laevodopa and imipramine. Variable effects occur after reserpine and phenothiazines.

Summary. *Phaeochromocytoma.* Now that determinations of three classes-catecholamines, normetadrenalines and HMMA—can be carried out comparatively simply, we can compare the results in patients with a phaeochromocytoma. Although HMMA is present in largest amounts, a better indication of relative value is to express each daily excretion in relation to the upper limit of the normal range. Thus Crout *et al.* (1961) found in 15 of 23 patients that free catecholamines show the greatest relative increase above normal, and HMMA the least. We have found that during hypertensive phases the free amines are most increased though all three determinations show diagnostic increases, while during quiescent periods the determination of the metadrenalines is the most sensitive.

Kelleher *et al.* (1964) also found determination of metadrenalines easier and more helpful than that of HMMA. On the other hand Sandler (1964) while accepting that the metadrenalines undergo the largest proportional increase thought their estimation (Pisano, 1960) to be more tedious than that of HMMA. Georges and Whitby (1964) considered the estimation of metadrenaline unsatisfactory on the grounds of much greater relative interference by substances absorbing at wavelengths of 330 to 340 nm.

Additional information has become available during the last ten years on which to base a decision. Although gross increases in catecholamine excretion usually associated with phaeochromocytoma can be detected by the methods described, 14 of 49 urine specimens from our series of patients with raised metadrenaline output had a catecholamine (adrenaline + noradrenaline) excretion of less than 1.2 μmol/24 h (200 μg/24 h). Sheps *et al.* (1966) also reported normal urinary catecholamines in 7 of 28 cases. The method is subject to interference by methyl dopa currently widely used for treating hypertension which further reduces its value in the routine screening for phaeochromocytoma.

Determination of metadrenaline excretion on 89 urines from 23 of our patients with proven phaeochromocytoma gave a mean figure of 38 μmol/24 h (7.0 mg/24 h) 5.4 times the upper limit of 7.0 μmol/24 h (1.3 mg/24 h) for non-phaeochromocytoma hypertensive patients. Only 3

212   *Practical Clinical Biochemistry*

results were less than 14 μmol/24 h, twice the non-phaeochromocytoma upper limit. The mean excretion of HMMA in 78 urines from 19 of these patients was 81.5 μmol/24 h (16.3 mg/24 h) 2.04 times the upper limit of the non-phaeochromocytoma range of 40 μmol/24 h (8 mg/24 h). Fifty-one results (65 per cent) were less than 80 μmol/24 h (16 mg/24 h) and 11 (14 per cent) less than 50 μmol/24 h (10 mg/24 h) a value exceeded on several occasions by non-phaeochromocytoma patients on first admission to hospital.

This confirms that metadrenaline excretion is relatively more increased in phaeochromocytoma. In our opinion it is less subject to interference than the HMMA estimation and is the preferred screening test for phaeochromocytoma. This was also the view of Sheps *et al.* (1966) after reviewing the results from 28 patients with phaeochromocytoma. The statement by Crout *et al.* (1961) that an excretion of less than 5.5 μmol/24 h (1.0 mg/24 h) of metadrenalines in a patient with sustained hypertension can be taken to exclude phaeochromocytoma, and values of over 13.7 μmol/24 h (2.5 mg/24 h) to be diagnostic for this, would appear to be valid. For intermediate values they recommend determination of the free amines. If the hypertension is paroxysmal and normal values are found for the metadrenalines, urine should be collected over a timed period during the paroxysm for determination of free catecholamines.

If the hypertension is paroxysmal but metadrenaline excretion is normal it is unlikely that the results of methods described here would justify surgical intervention. The determination of plasma catecholamines on blood obtained by catheterisation of the vena cava at various levels has been described and might give some indication of the site of the tumour. In our experience a tumour as small as 5 g is detectable by a combination of clinical examination, biochemical findings and aortography so such an approach would rarely seem to be necessary. Absence of symptoms is less important. One of our patients was symptom-free until a pregnancy compressed the tumour and resulted in the excretion of 85 μmol/24 h (17 mg/24 h) of HMMA and 71 μmol/24 h (13 mg/24 h) of metadrenalines. A normal excretion of HMMA but increased output of metadrenalines, 27.5 μmol/24 h (5 mg/24 h), was found postpartum before removal of the tumour which weighed 110 g and contained 5 mg noradrenaline/g tissue.

Neuroblastoma. The excretion of these substances has also been studied in children with neuroblastoma (see Voorhess and Gardner, 1960, who give several earlier references). Several workers report a marked increase in the excretion of HMMA, but in a smaller proportion of cases dopamine appears to be excreted in the largest amount. Bell (1968) from a study of 34 cases recognised three types of excretion pattern as regards catecholamines, metadrenalines and HMMA. One showed an increase in all three, the second a marked increase in catecholamines with not more than a small increase in the others, while the third had a normal or only slightly increased excretion of catecholamines with a variable increase in the other two (Table 5,1).

Adrenaline, Noradrenaline and Related Compounds

TABLE 5,1
Excretion Patterns in Neuroblastoma (Bell, 1966, 1968)

	Number of cases	Total catecholamines (as dopamine) mmol/mol creatinine (mg/g creatinine)	4 Hydroxy-3-methoxy-mandelic acid	
			Gitlow test	Pisano (p. 209) mmol/mol creatinine (mg/g creatinine)
Group 1	21	2.5−47 (3.4−64)	0.49−1.0	27−325 (48−580)
Group 2	7	7.3−170 (10−232)	1.3−2.1	3.7−14.4 (5.6−25.5; 3 below 10)
Group 3	6	0.92−1.34 (1.25−1.8)	0.53−0.87	10.2−35.5 (18−63)
Non-neuroblastoma	64	0.17−1.1 (0.23−1.5)	1.2−2.15	Less than 5.6 (Less than 10)

Either the Gitlow test (p. 208) or the screening test for catecholamines (p. 199) were positive in all cases.

	Number of cases	Positive Gitlow test	Positive screening test for catecholamines
Group 1	21	21	21
Group 2	7	0	7
Group 3	6	6	0

In no case in which a neuroblastoma was shown to be present were both tests negative. The simpler of the tests, the Gitlow, was positive in over 70 per cent of cases. Bell takes as the criteria for a positive test a ratio of 1.0 or less coupled with an extinction of 0.5 or more.

For several articles concerned with various aspects of the above monoamines see the Symposium edited by Varley and Gowenlock (1963) and Bohun (1966).

REFERENCES

Bell, M. (1960), "Thesis for the Degree of M.Sc.", Manchester University.
Bell, M. (1966), in "Recent Results in Cancer Research", Volume 2, *Neuroblastomas—Biochemical Studies,* edited C. Bohun, Springer-Verlag, Berlin, p. 42.
Bell, M. (1968), in "Recent Results in Cancer Research", Volume 13, *Tumours in Children,* edited H. B. Marsden and J. K. Steward, Springer-Verlag, Berlin, p. 138.

214 *Practical Clinical Biochemistry*

Bergstrom, S. and Hansson, G. (1951), *Acta physiol. Scand.*, 22, 87.

Bertler, J., Carlson, A. and Rosengren, E. (1958), *Acta physiol. Scand.*, 44, 273.

Bohun, C. (1966), editor, "Recent Results in Cancer Research", Volume 2, *Neuroblastomas–Biochemical Studies*, Springer-Verlag, Berlin.

Callingham, B. A. (1963), in *"The Clinical Chemistry of Monoamines"*, edited by H. Varley and A. H. Gowenlock, Elsevier, Amsterdam.

Callingham, B. A. (1967), in *"Hormones in Blood"*, edited C. H. Gray and A. L. Bacharach, 2nd edition, Academic Press, p. 519.

Crout, J. R. (1961), "Standard Methods in Clinical Chemistry", edited David Seligson, Academic Press, 3, 62.

Crout, J. R., Pisano, J. J. and Sjoerdsma, A. (1961), *Amer. Heart J.*, 61, 375.

Crout, J. R. and Sjoerdsma, A. (1959), *New Eng. J. Med.*, 261, 23.

Elder, G. H. (1968), *Clin. chim. Acta*, 19, 507.

Euler, U. S. von and Floding, I. (1955), *Acta physiol. Scand.*, 33, Suppl. 118, p. 45.

Euler, U. S. von, Franksson, C. and Hellstrom, J. (1954), *Acta physiol. Scand.*, 31, 6.

Euler, U. S. von and Hamberg, U. (1949), *Science*, 110, 561.

Georges, R. J. and Whitby, L. G. (1964), *J. clin. Path.*, 17, 64.

Gitlow, S. E., Mendlowitz, M., Khasis, Sarah, Cohen, G. and Sha, Joanne (1960a), *J. clin. Invest.*, 39, 221.

Gitlow, S. E., Ornstein, L., Mendlowitz, M., Khasis, Sarah, and Kruk, E. (1960b), *Amer. J. Med.*, 28, 921.

Gjessing, L. R. (1968), in "Advances in Clinical Chemistry", edited O. Bodansky and A. L. Latner, Academic Press, 11, p. 82.

Goldenberg, M., Serlin, I. Edwards, T. and Rapport, M. M. (1954), *Amer. J. Med.*, 16, 310.

Green, M. and Walker, G. (1970), *Clin. chim. Acta*, 29, 189.

Griffiths, J. C., Laing, F. Y. T. and McDonald, T. J. (1970), *Clin. chim. Acta*, 30, 395.

Haggendal, J. (1963), *Acta physiol. Scand.*, 44, 273.

Johnson, L. R., Reese, M. and Nelson, D. H. (1972), *Clin. Chem.*, 18, 209.

Kelleher, J., Walter, G., Robinson, R. and Smith, P. (1964), *J. clin. Path.*, 17, 399.

Lund, A. (1949), *Acta Pharmacol.*, 5, 75, 121, 231.

Macmillan, M. (1957), *Lancet*, 1, 715.

Merrils, R. J. (1963), *Anal. Biochem.*, 6, 272.

Persky, H. (1955), in "Methods of Biochemical Analysis", edited D. Glick, Interscience, New York, 2, 57.

Pisano, J. J. (1960), *Clin. chim. Acta*, 5, 406.

Pisano, J. J., Crout, J. R. and Abraham, D. (1962), 7, 285.

Quek, E. S. C., Buttery, J. E. and de Witt, G. F. (1975), *Clin. chim. Acta.*, 58, 137.

Renzini, V., Brunori, C. A. and Valori, C. (1970), *Clin. chim. Acta*, 30, 587.

Robinson, R., Ratcliffe, J. and Smith, P. (1959), *J. clin. Path.*, 12, 541.

Robinson, R. L. and Watts, D. T. (1965), *Clin. Chem.*, 11, 986.

Sandler, M. (1964), *J. med. Lab. Technol.*, 21, 306.

Sandler, M. and Ruthven, C. R. J. (1959), *Lancet*, 2, 113, 1034.

Sandler, M. and Ruthven, C. R. J. (1961), *Biochem. J.*, 80, 78.

Sandler, M. Ruthven, C. R. J. (1963), Broadsheet, No. 44 (NS), Association of Clinical Pathologists, BMA House, Tavistock Square, London, W.C.1.

Sheps, S. G., Tyce, G. M., Flock, E. V. and Maher, F. T. (1966), *Circulation*, 34, 473.

Sobel, C. and Henry, R. J. (1957), *Amer. J. clin. Path.*, 27, 240.

Varley, H. and Gowenlock, A. H. (editors) (1963), *"The Clinical Chemistry of Monoamines"*, Elsevier, Amsterdam.

Vendsalu, A. (1960), *Acta physiol. Scand.*, 49, Suppl. 173.

Voorhess, M. L. and Gardner, L. I. (1960), *Lancet*, 2, 651.

Weil-Malherbe, H. and Bone, A. D. (1952), *Biochem. J.*, 51, 311.

Weil-Malherbe, H. and Bone, A. D. (1954), *Biochem. J.*, 58, 132.

Weil-Malherbe, H. and Bone, A. D. (1957), *J. clin. Path.*, 10, 138.

CHAPTER 6

VITAMINS

LABORATORY methods for investigating vitamin deficiencies have used the determination of the vitamin in blood or urine, either under ordinary conditions or after test doses; the determination in serum or urine of metabolic products derived from the vitamin, or of some substance in serum or urine the concentration of which is influenced by the amount of the vitamin in the body. For surveys of techniques showing the presence of vitamin deficiencies see Györgi and Pearson (1967) and of our present knowledge of the vitamins Sebrell and Harris (1967).

The original division into fat soluble and water soluble substances made when it was found that growth promoting factors were present in both the fat of milk and in the whey is still useful. There are important differences between the two groups. Thus the former being insoluble in water are carried in the plasma attached to protein and so are not excreted in the urine. They are also stored in substantial amounts in some tissues particularly the liver so that a deficiency arises much less quickly than with water soluble vitamins which are less often stored to any appreciable extent (however, B_{12} is a notable exception, see p. 243) so that any excess uptake is usually rapidly excreted in the urine. Whereas a deficiency of fat soluble vitamins can arise in conditions in which there is impaired absorption of fat alone, more general malabsorption can affect both classes.

When the existence of vitamins was first recognised their chemical structure was unknown and they were distinguished alphabetically sometimes differently in different countries. Now that names are available based on their chemical nature or occasionally on their physiological behaviour these should be used wherever possible.

We shall first consider the fat soluble vitamins: retinol (vitamin A), cholecalciferol (D), and the tocopherols (E), then the water soluble B group and ascorbic acid (C). We have used mass concentration rather than molar concentration for the results of vitamin determinations as vitamins are prescribed therapeutically in mass units.

RETINOL (VITAMIN A) AND CAROTENES

The name retinol is derived from its role in the retina in the rods of which it is present as the aldehyde retinal, combined with the protein opsin in rhodopsin, visual purple, required for vision in a dim light.

Retinol is obtained from foods either as the vitamin itself or from the plant pigments, carotenes, which can be converted into it in the wall of the

216   *Practical Clinical Biochemistry*

small intestine, Carotenes which can be used in this way are α, β, γ, carotenes and cryptoxanthine. The formula for vitamin A is

$$
\begin{array}{c}
CH_3 \quad CH_3 \\
\diagdown C \diagup \\
\diagup \diagdown \\
CH_2 \qquad C-CH=CH-C=CH-CH=CH-C \;=\; CH-CH_2OH \\
| \qquad\quad \| \qquad\qquad\; | \qquad\qquad\qquad\; | \\
CH_2 \qquad C-CH_3 \qquad CH_3 \qquad\qquad CH_3 \\
\diagdown \diagup \\
CH_2
\end{array}
$$

Retinol

If we write this as $X_1 - CH_2OH$ where X_1 represents the whole of the formula to the left of the dotted line, then the carotenes can be represented by the formula $X_1 - CH = CH - X_2$. In the case of β-carotene X_2 is the same as X_1 but not in the other three carotenes though the differences in X_2 are small and occur only in the ring. Theoretically it should thus be possible to obtain two molecules of retinol from one molecule of β-carotene but not from the other carotenes. However, it appears that only one molecule is obtained from one molecule of each of the carotenes.

It is evident that both retinol and carotenes in the food are important in ensuring an adequate supply of this vitamin. While the vitamin is stored in the liver and to a lesser extent in the kidneys, carotenes are stored in adipose tissue.

Determination of Retinol and Carotenes in Serum using the Carr-Price Reaction (Kimble, 1938-39; Kaser and Stekol, 1943)

Proteins are precipitated with ethanol and the retinol and carotenes extracted into light petroleum. After reading the intensity of the yellow colour due to the carotenes the light petroleum is evaporated off and the residue dissolved in chloroform. Carr-Price reagent is added and the amount of blue colour produced read. Since carotenes also give some colour, a correction for this is made in order to obtain that due to the retinol present.

Reagents. 1. Absolute ethanol.

2. Light petroleum, b.p. 40° to 60°C.

3. A cylinder of carbon dioxide.

4. Chloroform.

5. Acetic anhydride. Use good quality analytical reagent.

6. Carr-Price reagent. Antimony trichloride, 250 g/l in chloroform. Keep at room temperature in a tightly-stoppered brown bottle, filtering before use if necessary.

7. Stock standard, 500 mg β-carotene/l in light petroleum.

Vitamins 217

8. Working standard, 10 mg/l. Dilute the stock standard 1 in 50 with light petroleum.

Technique. Pipette 3 ml serum into a stoppered centrifuge tube and add 3 ml absolute ethanol, slowly drop by drop with shaking, in order to obtain a finely divided precipitate of protein. Add 6 ml light petroleum and shake vigorously for 10 min, then centrifuge at a low speed for about 1 min. Pipette off as much as possible of the light petroleum layer, taking care not to remove any of the watery layer with it.

Determination of the Carotenes

Place the light petroleum extract in the colorimeter cuvette and read at 440 nm or with a violet filter using light petroleum as blank. Prepare a standard curve from the working standard as follows:

Serum carotenes (mg/l)	0	0.50	1.00	2.00	4.00	6.00
Standard solution (ml)	0	0.25	0.50	1.00	2.00	3.00
Light petroleum (ml)	10	9.75	9.50	9.00	8.00	7.00

Serum carotene concentration is read directly from this curve. The fact that 2 ml of light petroleum contain the carotenes from 1 ml serum has been taken into account.

Note. Carotenes do not keep well since they easily oxidise. They then give a less yellow coloured solution in the light petroleum. Even freshly bought specimens are not always satisfactory. We have found carotenes supplied by Roche Products Ltd. to be reliable.

INTERPRETATION

The normal range may be taken as 0.5 to 2.0 mg/l, though upper limits a little higher have been given and Campbell and Tonks (1949) gave a lower limit of 0.2 mg/l (see Krebs and Hume, 1949). Serum carotene concentration is greatly influenced by dietary carotenes and becomes very low in a few weeks if absent from the diet. On the other hand an increase in serum carotenes is found if large amounts of carotene-rich vegetables are consumed. This usually means large quantities of carrots, the richest source of carotenes. Other foods rich in carotenes include spinach, parsley, watercress, lettuce, and tomatoes. In general, the greener the vegetable the higher the carotene content. Serum carotenes may then reach and exceed 5 mg/l. This condition, *carotenaemia,* is accompanied by a yellow skin pigmentation which may simulate jaundice (see Chapter 28, Vol. I). Increased values for serum carotenes have been reported in myxoedema, diabetes mellitus, and chronic nephritis. Low values have been found in a high proportion of patients with the malabsorption syndrome (Wenger *et al.,* 1957).

218   *Practical Clinical Biochemistry*

Determination of Retinol

Measure 4 ml of the light petroleum solution, prepared as above, into one of the colorimeter tubes and evaporate off the solvent by placing in a water bath at 40° to 50°C preferably passing a stream of dry carbon dioxide over the solvent surface. Dissolve the residue in 0.5 ml of chloroform and add a drop of acetic anhydride to remove traces of water which might cause cloudiness when the Carr-Price reagent is added. Zero the colorimeter with chloroform, using an orange filter or transmission at 620 nm, and with the tube in position, add quickly 3 ml of Carr-Price reagent from a pipette with a wide tip. The colour develops rapidly reaching a clearly defined maximum in 5 to 15 sec, and then fades quickly. Note this maximum reading of the colorimeter. A rather more stable colour is obtained if the Carr-Price reagent is cooled to 0 to 5°C before use.

It is important that the glassware used should be perfectly dry. This also applies to the chloroform and the Carr-Price reagent. When small amounts of water are present it may be impossible to read the colour. If any cloudiness develops repeat the test.

A correction is made for the colour given by the carotenes present. Prepare two standard curves for the colorimeter, one for retinol allowed to react with Carr-Price reagent, the other for carotenes similarly treated. Then, when the serum carotene level has been determined, read the amount of colour due to this from the carotene curve and subtract from the actual colorimeter reading. The colorimeter reading due to retinol is thus obtained and the serum retinol is read from the retinol standard curve. This applies so long as 4 ml of the light petroleum extract is taken for the determination. If a smaller volume has to be used, multiply the colorimeter reading by 4 divided by the volume of extract used.

(*a*) Retinol standard curve. Prepare a solution containing 4.0 mg retinol/l in chloroform and set up a series of tubes:

Serum retinol (mg/l)	0	0.10	0.20	0.40	0.60	0.80	1.00
Retinol solution (ml)	0	0.05	0.1	0.2	0.3	0.4	0.5
Chloroform (ml)	0.5	0.45	0.4	0.3	0.2	0.1	0

Add 3 ml Carr-Price reagent and read as described.

(*b*) Correction curve for the carotenes present. Dilute 1 ml of the stock β-carotene standard solution (p. 216) to 25 ml with chloroform, thus obtaining a solution containing 20 mg/l. Set up a series of tubes:

Serum carotenes (mg/l)	0	1.0	2.0	3.0	4.0	5.0
Carotene solution (ml)	0	0.1	0.2	0.3	0.4	0.5
Chloroform (ml)	0.5	0.4	0.3	0.2	0.1	0

Add 3 ml Carr-Price reagent and read as described.

Vitamins 219

Other methods. Sobel and Snow (1947) used the colour given with activated glycerol dichlorhydrin. This colour is more stable than that given by the Carr-Price reagent and traces of water present do not interfere, but the colour is less intense. More recently Dugan *et al.* (1964) used trifluoroacetic acid instead of Carr-Price reagent. This also is less susceptible to interference from traces of water present.

Determination of Retinol by a Spectrophotometric Method using the Ultraviolet Spectrophotometer (Bessey *et al.,* 1946; Karmaker and Rajagopal, 1952; Paterson and Wiggins, 1954)

Retinol has an absorption peak at 327 nm and can be determined by reading the extinction at this wavelength before and after irradiating with ultraviolet light to destroy the retinol present. The method given is that of Paterson and Wiggins.

Reagents. 1. Absolute ethanol.
2. Normal heptane (free from aromatic hydrocarbons).
3. Standard solution of retinol. Prepare a solution containing 1.0 mg/l in normal heptane.

Technique. Shake 4 ml serum or heparinised plasma with 8 ml absolute ethanol and 8 ml normal heptane for 15 min in a mechanical shaker. Allow the layers to separate. Remove the heptane layer and divide it into two approximately equal parts. Irradiate one part in a glass-stoppered soda glass tube for 3 h with ultraviolet light. The time required to give complete destruction of retinol varies with different lamps and should be studied. Read the extinction of the non-irradiated part at 327 nm using the irradiated part as a blank and the retinol concentration from a standard curve by plotting the extinction of standards irradiated in the same way. Suitable quantities are:

Serum retinol (mg/l)	0	0.20	0.40	0.60	0.80	1.00
Standard solution (ml)	0	1.0	2.0	3.0	4.0	5.0
Heptane (ml)	10	9.0	8.0	7.0	6.0	5.0

Alternatively, read the extinction of the same heptane extract before and after irradiation, against a heptane blank. A smaller volume of serum can then be used. Smaller volumes may also need to be used in bloods taken in retinol absorption tests (see below). Plasma and heptane extracts both before and after irradiation can be kept in the refrigerator at 4° C up to 48 h without appreciable change occurring.

220 *Practical Clinical Biochemistry*

INTERPRETATION

Several workers in England have found the normal range between about 0.20 and 0.50 mg/l (Yudkin, 1941; Sinclair, 1947; Campbell and Tonks, 1949; Krebs and Hume, 1949; Krebs, 1950). Higher figures have been given elsewhere, 0.33 to 0.63 mg/l (Haig and Patek, 1942, in the U.S.A.); 0.30 to 0.90 mg/l (Lindquist, 1938, in Scandinavia).

It may be assumed that there is no deficiency when the serum level is above 0.20 mg/l. When the concentration falls below about 0.10 mg/l dark adaptation begins to be impaired. The absorption of both retinol and carotenes from the intestine is defective when there is diminished fat absorption, and there is also increased loss in the faeces when liquid paraffin is being taken. The capacity to store retinol may also be affected in liver disease and conversion of carotenes to retinol is impaired in myxoedema.

Retinol absorption tests have been used to study absorption in steatorrhoea. A large dose of the vitamin is given orally and the rise in the serum level studied. Thus Sinclair (1947) determined serum retinol fasting and 4 and 7 h after giving 3 mg retinol/kg body weight. Barnes *et al.* (1950), gave 18 mg daily for 4 days before the test, and then for the test 2.25 mg/kg, and determined the serum level at 0, 2, 4, 6, 9, and 24 h. In normal patients a maximum of 6 to 9 mg/l serum is reached in about 4 h, after which it falls steadily Absorption is impaired in steatorrhoea so that a much smaller rise is found. Paterson and Wiggins (1954) who discussed a number of factors of importance in this test, also gave 2.25 mg/kg with a maximum of 105 mg in the form of retinol or the palmitate in arachis oil to avoid the nausea produced in some people by fish oils. They did not withhold meals. They concluded that although a rise in serum retinol to about 1.5 mg/l some 4 to 5 h after the dose almost certainly excludes steatorrhoea, flat absorption curves with maxima lower than this, do not confirm a diagnosis of steatorrhoea. Sammons *et al.* (1961), however, found that 17 of 18 normal individuals exceeded 1.5 mg/l, whereas none of 11 patients with steatorrhoea did so. Kagan *et al.* (1950) in studies on children with nephrosis used 4.0 mg/kg body weight and determined serum retinol at 0, 3, 6, and 24 h.

Note. Previously values were given in International Units (I.U.). One I.U. of retinol is defined as having the activity of 0.344 μg of the acetate. This is equal to 0.300 μg retinol and to 0.6 μg of pure β-carotene.

CHOLECALCIFEROL (VITAMIN D_3)

Cholecalciferol is the naturally occurring member in man of a group of substances which are able to cure rickets. It is known as D_3, the only other

Vitamins
221

of importance being ergocalciferol, D_2. The structure of cholecalciferol is shown.

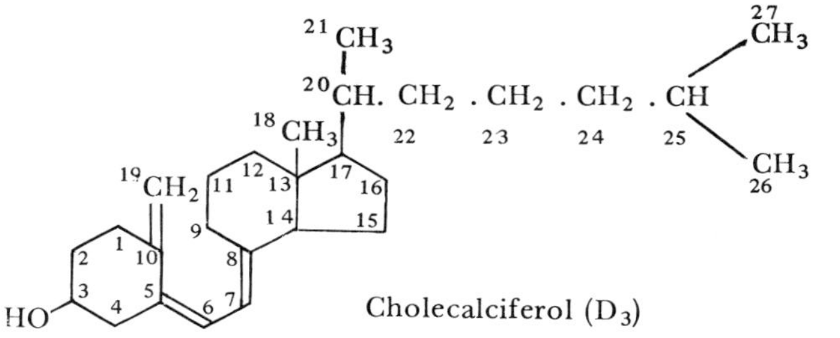

Cholecalciferol (D_3)

However, recent work has shown that this is not the active substance, the 1,25-dihydroxy derivative, into which it is converted in two stages. Cholecalciferol absorbed in the small intestine is hydroxylated on C-25 in the liver, then circulates to the kidney where hydroxylation on C-1 takes place. The 1,25-dihydroxycholecalciferol then passes to the target organ.

Cholecalciferol is present in appreciable amounts in only a few foods. Egg yolk, artifically-reinforced margarine and oily fish are the main sources in normal diets, the concentration in fish liver oils being much higher. Many diets in the United Kingdom are quite deficient in it. However, a variable but significant amount is produced in the skin by the action of ultraviolet light on 7-dehydrocholesterol an action which opens up the ring between C atoms 9 and 10. This variable contribution makes it difficult to assess the

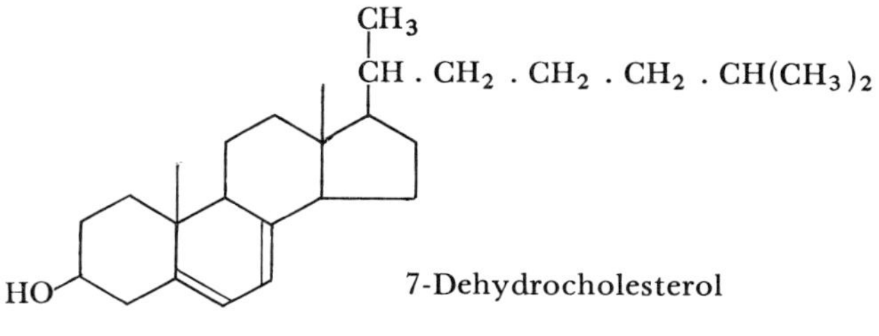

7-Dehydrocholesterol

dietary requirements of the vitamin. A generally accepted figure is in the region of $10 \mu g/day$ or 400 IU (1 IU = 25 ng). The dietary contribution is important and any defect of absorption from the intestine is likely to lead to clinical deficiency. Because the daily intake is so low the concentration in the plasma is too low for satisfactory chemical assay so that its determination has been by biological or immunological methods. In the clinical chemistry laboratory the only tests used to study conditions of deficiency or excess intake have been serum and urine calcium and phosphate and serum alkaline phosphatase. These are described in Chapter 25, Vol. I.

Ergocalciferol (D_2) has been used therapeutically. It is formed by the action of ultraviolet light on ergosterol which is present in some low forms

222   *Practical Clinical Biochemistry*

of plant life, for example yeasts. It differs in chemical structure from cholecalciferol only in having a double bond between C atoms 22 and 23 and an additional methyl group on C-24.

THE TOCOPHEROLS (VITAMIN E)

Vitamin E activity is shown by four naturally occurring tocopherols, α, β, γ, and δ, with the general formula below, of which α-tocopherol is the most potent,

The Tocopherols

	α	β	γ	δ
R_1	Me	Me	H	H
R_2	Me	H	Me	H
R_3	Me	Me	Me	M

and also four tocotrienols with three double bonds in the side chain at C-3' 7' and 11'. These were first found to be necessary for normal reproduction in the rat. Nothing definite is known about its specific action in man. For a short assessment of the present situation see the *Lancet* (1974) in which it is suggested that an important function is to maintain cellular and intra-cellular membrane integrity possibly by interaction with poly-unsaturated fatty acids. A simple method for determining plasma tocopherol is available using the Emmerie-Engel reaction which is based on the reduction by tocopherols of ferric to ferrous ions which then form a red complex with α,α'-dipyridyl. Tocopherols and carotenes are first extracted into xylene and the extinction read at 460 nm to measure the carotenes. A correction is made for these after adding ferric chloride and reading at 520 nm.

Determination of Serum Tocopherol (Quaife *et al.*, 1949; Baker and Frank, 1968).

    Reagents. 1. Absolute ethanol, aldehyde-free.
    2. Xylene.
    3. α,α'-Dipyridyl, 1.20 g/l in *n*-propanol.
    4. Ferric chloride solution, 1.20 g $FeCl_3,6H_2O$/l in ethanol. Keep in a brown bottle.
    5. Standard solution of D-Lα-tocopherol, 10 mg/l in ethanol.
    Technique. Into three stoppered centrifuge tubes measure 1.5 ml serum, 1.5 ml standard, and 1.5 ml water (blank) respectively. To test and blank add 1.5 ml ethanol and to the standard 1.5 ml water. Then add 1.5 ml xylene to all the tubes, stopper, mix well, and centrifuge. Transfer 1 ml of the xylene layers into other stoppered tubes taking care not to include any ethanol or protein. Add 1 ml α,α'-dipyridyl reagent to each tube, stopper

Vitamins 223

and mix. Pipette 1.5 ml of the mixture into colorimeter cuvettes and read the extinction of test and standard against the blank at 460 nm. Then in turn beginning with the blank add 0.33 ml ferric chloride solution, mix, and after exactly 1.5 min read test and standard against the blank at 520 nm.

Calculation

Serum tocopherols (mg/l) =

$$\frac{(\text{Reading of unknown at } 520\,\text{nm} - \text{Reading at } 460\,\text{nm} \times 0.29)}{\text{Reading of standard at } 520\,\text{nm}} \times 10$$

since the standard contains 10 mg/l.

INTERPRETATION

Healthy adults have a value in the region 10 to 12 mg/l, infants 2 to 4 mg/l rising to adult values in later childhood. In absorption defects low values are obtained ranging from 1 to 8 mg/l while it may be increased in cardiovascular disease (10 to 34) and in diseases associated with hyper-cholesterolaemia (15 to 38). Plasma tocopherol may be raised in pregnancy though in newborn infants it is appreciably lower than in the mother. Some premature infants have been born with inadequate reserves and develop an anaemia which requires treatment with α-tocopherol as well as with iron and folic acid.

A deficiency may be shown by a low plasma tocopherol, by increased urinary creatine, by diminished red cell survival, and increased *in vitro* haemolysis of red cells exposed to oxidising agents. These are all found in many conditions associated with malabsorption and malnutrition and are reversed on giving tocopherol.

Tocopherols have been claimed to be useful in the treatment of intermittent claudication but apart from this and the anaemia of premature infants referred to above, trials in a variety of conditions such as habitual abortion, sterility, and muscular dystrophies, do not appear to have shown any benefit from giving tocopherol. Whether it should be given when the signs of a deficiency described above are present is open to argument (see *Lancet*, 1974).

THIAMINE (VITAMIN B$_1$)

Thiamine, the first of the B group of water soluble vitamins to be recognised, is present in cocarboxylase as the pyrophosphate. Cocarboxylase

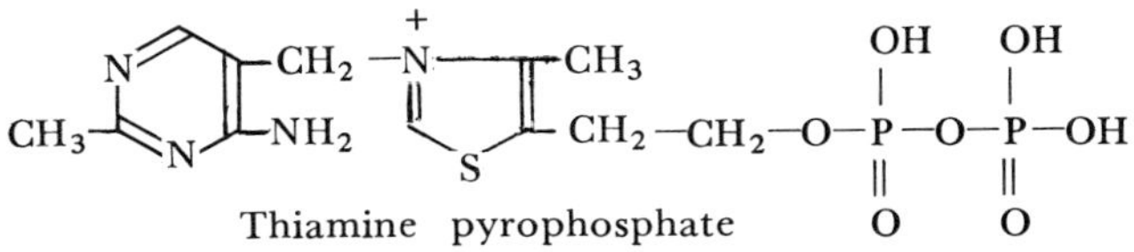

Thiamine pyrophosphate

224   *Practical Clinical Biochemistry*

is the coenzyme of several enzymes involved in α-keto acid metabolism including carboxylase which catalyses the decarboxylation of pyruvate to active acetate which is incorporated into acetyl coenzyme A. This is the end stage of the glycolytic pathway but transketolase and transaldolase occur in the metabolism of pentoses by the hexose monophosphate shunt. They respectively transfer glycol aldehyde (a 2 C fragment) and dihydroxyacetone radicles (a 3 C fragment) as shown below (p. 228).

As regards biochemical laboratory methods two main approaches have been made to the problem of detecting a deficiency of thiamine, the estimation of blood pyruvate and of the vitamin itself in urine. There is only a small amount of thiamine in blood and a simple method for its estimation in routine work is not yet available. Friedemann and Kmieciak (1943) used a thiochrome method. Microbiological methods have been employed, using the fungus *Phycomyces blakesleeanus,* which requires thiamine for its growth (see Meiklejohn, 1937; and Sinclair, 1938, 1939), and *Lactobacillus fermenti* (Sarett and Cheldelin, 1944; Cheldelin *et al.,* 1946). See also Baker and Sobotka (1962). More recently the thiamine status has been evaluated by determining the red cell transketolase activity with and without added thiamine pyrophosphate (see p. 228).

Determination of Thiamine in Urine by the Thiochrome Reaction (Johnson *et al.,* 1945)

Thiamine has been determined in urine by oxidising it to thiochrome by alkaline ferricyanide. This tricyclic derivative is then extracted into isobutanol and measured fluorimetrically.

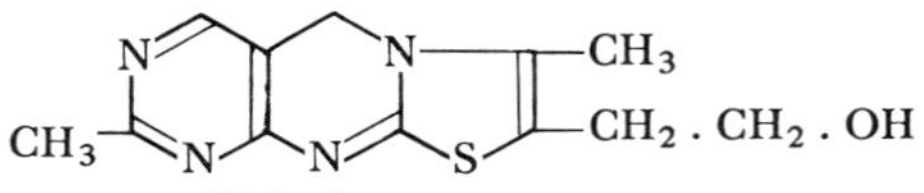

Thiochrome

Reagents. 1. Activated Decalso or Permutit. There is considerable variation between different samples. A product is required which will adsorb thiamine well and settle out rapidly. When about 200 mg are shaken with water in a 10 ml measuring cylinder all the particles should settle rapidly to the bottom in not more than 2 min. To obtain a suitable product, suspend material which will pass a 100-mesh sieve in acetic acid (10 ml/l water) in large cylinders. Separate the granules which settle down to the bottom in 2 min from the lighter particles, by decanting. Boil these three times with the dilute acetic acid with settling and decanting between fresh additions of acetic acid. Wash the product with distilled water and dry at 110° C. If addition of potassium ferricyanide results in the formation of Prussian blue, wash the product in a warm, fairly strong, solution of hydrochloric acid. Carry out test runs with synthetic thiamine. Unsatisfactory products can be reactivated by the method of Najjar and Wood

Vitamins 225

(1940). The activity of a satisfactory product remains constant for months if it is kept dry.

2. Potassium chloride solution, approximately 250 g/l.

3. Sodium hydroxide solution, 150 g/l.

4. Potassium ferricyanide solution, 2.5 g/l, prepared fresh daily.

5. Isobutanol or *n*-butanol. This should give almost no blank. Test each new batch before use. If desired collect after use and recover by redistillation.

6. Acetic acid, approximately 10 ml/l in water.

7. Stock standard thiamine hydrochloride solution, 40 mg/l in water.

8. Working standard, 2 mg/l. Dilute 5 ml stock standard to 100 ml with water and add 400 mg oxalic acid.

Technique. Collect urine in glass vessels and store in amber bottles, adding 100 mg of oxalic acid for every 25 ml of urine. Measure 2 ml urine (0.5 ml if the result is likely to be high), 2 ml working standard and 2 ml water (as blank) into glass-stoppered test tubes and to each add about 200 mg of the activated Decalso or Permutit and mix with 10 rapid shakes. The adsorption is optimal at pH 3 to 6, which is assured by use of the oxalic acid. Now add about 8 ml acetic acid, and mix by inversion 10 times. Stand for a short time and remove the supernatant fluid. Repeat this washing process which is important since if ineffective the final fluorescence has a silvery-blue admixture to the true thiochrome mauve, thus giving unsatisfactory readings. If any trouble is experienced in this connection, further washings are made. The thiamine is firmly adsorbed so that repeated washings only remove interfering substances.

Add 0.5 ml potassium chloride solution and shake gently, taking care to avoid splashing the solid far up the side. Elution is complete within thirty seconds. Add 0.1 ml potassium ferricyanide and 0.25 ml sodium hydroxide, shaking gently after each addition. Add 2 ml isobutanol, stopper and shake vigorously for about a minute (25 shakes up and down). Stand to allow separation of the two phases, or centrifuge for a short time. Transfer the supernatant fluid to a cuvette and read in the fluorimeter at 435 nm using excitation at 365 nm and zeroing with the blank extract.

INTERPRETATION

The excretion of thiamine is greatly affected by variations in the dietary intake. Further variations result from different methods used in its estimation. Daily excretion ranges from 50 to 500 μg, but while some workers have reported even lower figures, an excretion of under 90 μg/24 h has been regarded as evidence of a deficient intake (Melnick, 1942). The Oxford Nutrition survey considered less than 50 μg/l as abnormal and below 20 μg/l as showing extreme abnormality.

More reliable results are obtained by studying the amount excreted after a test dose. Several variants have been used. Melnick and Field (1942) injected intramuscularly a dose of 0.35 mg/m^2 of surface area, and collected urine for the next 4 h period. At least 50 μg (about 8 per cent of

226   *Practical Clinical Biochemistry*

the test dose) should be excreted in that time. Najjar and Holt (1940) injected 1 mg of thiamine intravenously and obtained at least 110 μg in the following 4 h in adults. Mason and Williams (1942) gave 1 mg by mouth and found over 100 μg in the urine in 24 h.

These tests are more sensitive than the estimation of blood pyruvate. Diminished excretion of thiamine following a test dose gives the earliest indication of a deficiency. Simple estimation of pyruvate is the least sensitive, the increase in pyruvate after administration of glucose being intermediate between these.

Determination of Blood Pyruvate

So far this has been much the most used biochemical procedure for showing the presence of thiamine deficiency, either as a single test or as part of a pyruvate tolerance test. Thiamine deficiency is accompanied by deficiency of cocarboxylase impairing the decarboxylation of pyruvate so that its concentration in blood rises. For many years the technique most used was based on the formation of its 2,4-dinitrophenylhydrazone which gives a red compound with alkali. Acetone, acetoacetate, and some of the other aldehydes and ketones which might be present also form hydrazones but these and excess dinitrophenylhydrazine are not extracted into sodium carbonate as is the hydrazone from pyruvate. However, some additional colour is produced from other ketoacids. The simplified technique of Friedemann and Haugen (1943) was given in earlier editions of this book.

Later an enzymic method was introduced using lactate dehydrogenase which is specific for pyruvate. Though the method of choice its general use was somewhat delayed because of the need to use an ultraviolet spectrophotometer, but now these instruments are generally available as are the necessary reagents the enzymic method should be used.

Enzymic Method (Gloster and Harris, 1962; Boehringer leaflet)

The conversion of pyruvate to lactate

$$CH_3.CO.COO^- + NADH_2 \rightarrow CH_3.CHOH.COO^- + NAD$$

is catalysed by lactate dehydrogenase. The reaction proceeds almost to completion at pH 6.9 and its course can be followed by reading the change in extinction at 340 nm at which $NADH_2$ absorbs while NAD does not. The method given is a modification of that published by Boehringer.

Reagents. 1. Trichloracetic acid, 100 g/l in hydrochloric acid, 500 mmol/l.

2. Phosphate buffer, 1.1 mol/l. Dissolve 19.14 g dipotassium hydrogen phosphate in 100 ml glass-distilled water.

3. Reduced nicotinamide adenine dinucleotide. Dissolve 5 mg in 1 ml glass-distilled water. This is best made freshly but can be kept for a few days at 4°C.

Vitamins 227

4. Lactate dehydrogenase, 0.75 mg enzyme protein in 1 ml ammonium sulphate solution. This and the previous reagent can be obtained from the Boehringer Corporation (London) Ltd.

5. Pyruvate standard, 20 mg/l. Dissolve 2.13 mg lithium pyruvate in 100 ml water.

Technique. Take about 5 ml blood into a syringe. Avoid venous stasis and, especially, activity of forearm muscles (Braybrook *et al.*, 1975). At once inject into 5 ml trichloracetic acid contained in a weighed centrifuge tube. Shake the tube well and reweigh to obtain the weight of blood added. From this the volume can be obtained by dividing by 1.060, the specific gravity. Alternatively it may be thought that the volume of blood can be measured with sufficient accuracy in the syringe. Centrifuge at 2000 r.p.m. for 10 min. Add 0.7 ml of phosphate buffer to 2 ml of the supernatant fluid and to 2 ml water (as blank) and transfer 2 ml to 10 mm quartz cuvettes. Add a further 1 ml of phosphate buffer and then 50 μl NADH$_2$. Mix well by stirring. After 2 min read the extinction at 340 nm against the blank. Repeat the reading 1 min later to ensure a steady state. This reading should be between 0.500 and 0.800. Then add 50 μl lactate dehydrogenase and mix well with a glass rod. Read the extinction after 2 min and at minute intervals for a further 3 min until no further change occurs. For normal bloods taken from resting persons a difference in extinction between 0.050 and 0.100 is usually obtained. Check at intervals by putting the pyruvate standard through the procedure.

Calculation. If v ml of blood is taken then $2v/(5 + v)$ ml of blood is present in 2 ml of the supernatant fluid; 0.7 ml of phosphate is added to this and 2 ml taken; the final volume is 3.1 ml. At 340 nm in a 10 mm cuvette a change of extinction (ΔE) of 0.100 is equivalent to 16.1 nmol pyruvate per ml of reaction mixture. Hence:

$$\text{Blood pyruvate } (\mu\text{mol/l}) = \frac{5 + v}{2v} \times \frac{2.7}{2.0} \times \frac{\Delta E}{0.100} \times 3.1 \times 16.1$$

$$= 337 \times \frac{(5 + v)}{v} \times \Delta E$$

$$\text{Or} = 337 \times \frac{(5 + v)}{v} \times \Delta E \times 8.8 \ \mu\text{g/100 ml.}$$

Note. Sets of reagents for this enzymic determination can be obtained from Boehringer. In this case the blood is taken into an equal volume of perchloric acid (5 ml of the 70 per cent acid diluted to 100 ml with redistilled water) instead of trichloracetic acid.

INTERPRETATION

The normal range for blood pyruvate by this enzymic method is 34 to 80 μmol/l (300 to 700 μg/100 ml). This is lower than that from the dinitrophenylhydrazone method which was about 56 to 114 μmol/l (500 to

228 *Practical Clinical Biochemistry*

1 000 μg/100 ml). In marked thiamine deficiency values up to 220 to 330 μmol/l (2 to 3 mg/100 ml) are found. Increases in pyruvate have also been reported in diabetes mellitus (see Chapter 16, Vol. I) in congestive heart failure (Kleeberg and Gitelson, 1954) in diarrhoea and other digestive disturbances, in severe liver damage and in some acute infections.

Bueding *et al.* (1941) suggested using the increase in blood pyruvate which results from taking glucose. Such an increase is found in normal persons, but reaches a maximum in an hour and returns to normal limits within 3 h. In thiamine deficiency a greater increase occurs and a longer time is required for the return to normal. This test is said to show abnormal results before the fasting blood pyruvate is increased. Williams *et* al. (1943) gave glucose in a dose of 0.4 g/kg body weight, intravenously as a 50 per cent solution. Blood for determination of pyruvate is taken fasting, and half, one, and two hours after giving glucose. Alternatively, the glucose can be given as in the glucose tolerance test, (Chapter 14, Vol. I), that is, 50 g in a cupful of water with the patient fasting. The rise in pyruvate should not produce a blood level of more than about 100 μmol/l (1.1 mg/100 ml); a greater rise is evidence in favour of thiamine deficiency.

Technique Using Red Cell Transketolase Activity (Brin *et al.*, 1960; Brin, 1962-7)

Brin was largely responsible for developing the use of the activity of this enzyme which is concerned with transaldolase in pentose metabolism. The sequence of changes can be summarised:

2 ribose phosphate + xylulose phosphate $\xrightarrow{\text{Transketolase}}$
(C_5) (C_5)

sedoheptulose phosphate + glyceraldehyde phosphate $\xrightarrow{\text{Transaldolase}}$
(C_7) (C_3)

erythrose phosphate + fructose phosphate
(C_4) (C_6)

Then erythrose phosphate + ribose phosphate $\xrightarrow{\text{Transketolase}}$
(C_4) (C_5)

fructose phosphate + glyceraldehyde phosphate
(C_6) (C_5)

And 2 glyceraldehyde phosphate $\xrightarrow{\text{Transaldolase}}$ fructose phosphate
(C_3) (C_6)

So overall we have 6 $C_5 \rightarrow$ 5 C_6 since in order to get two molecules of glyceraldehyde phosphate the first three reactions have to be doubled.

In the technique used (Brin, 1967; Pearson, 1967) haemolysed red cells are incubated with ribose-5-phosphate with and without the addition of thiamine pyrophosphate. When there is a deficiency of the latter, pentose

Vitamins 229

disappears and hexose is formed at a lower rate. The results obtained suggest that a difference of 0-15 per cent is normal, between 15 and 25 per cent shows a marginal deficiency, and more than 25 per cent a severe deficiency with clinical signs. Either pentose or hexose can be determined, the former using the orcinol reaction and the latter the anthrone.

RIBOFLAVIN (VITAMIN B_2)

Riboflavin, or Vitamin B_2 as it was first known, is present as the monophosphate in flavin mononucleotide (FMN) and, linked with adenosine phosphate, in flavin adenine dinucleotide (FAD); both are coenzymes in a number of enzyme systems. Thus the former is present in cytochrome-*c*-reductase and L-amino acid oxidase, the latter in D-amino acid oxidase, xanthine oxidase and succinate dehydrogenase. Chemically it contains a ribitol molecule attached to a flavin (isoalloxazine).

$$CH_2-CHOH . CHOH . CHOH . CH_2OH$$

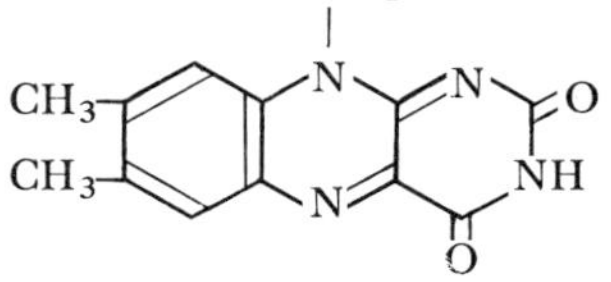

Riboflavin

It is more heat resistant than thiamine and in solution gives an intense yellow-green fluorescence, properties which led to its discovery.

No well-defined deficiency disease characterises riboflavin deficiency but there is present a variety of lesions of the skin, mouth and tongue, and bilateral vascularisation of the cornea.

Determination of Riboflavin in Urine (Najjar, 1941; Johnson *et al.*, 1945; see also, Slater and Morrell, 1946)

The riboflavin is extracted with an acetic acid-pyridine-butanol mixture after interfering urinary pigments have been oxidised with permanganate. The concentration of riboflavin is then measured fluorimetrically.

Reagents. 1. Dry powdered oxalic acid.

2. A mixture of equal volumes of pyridine and glacial acetic acid.

3. Potassium permanganate solution, 40 g/l.

4. Hydrogen peroxide, 10 volumes per cent.

5. Isobutanol or *n*-butanol. Examine each batch before use in ultraviolet light. Redistil if there is perceptible fluorescence.

6. Anhydrous sodium sulphate.

7. Stock standard riboflavin solution, 40 mg/l.

8. Working standard, 1 mg/l. Dilute 2.5 ml stock standard to 100 ml with water and add 400 mg oxalic acid.

230   *Practical Clinical Biochemistry*

Technique. Collect a 24 h specimen as described under thiamine, using oxalic acid and keeping in an amber bottle. Carry out all operations in a diffuse light, avoiding direct sunlight. Measure 0.5 ml urine, working standard and water (as blank) into separate 10 ml glass-stoppered test tubes and add 0.5 ml pyridine-acetic acid mixture. Add a drop of potassium permanganate solution and shake gently for about a minute. Then add 2 drops of hydrogen peroxide and again shake gently. The permanganate should be destroyed within a few seconds, if not, add a further drop of hydrogen peroxide and warm slightly to $21°C$. Add 1.5 ml isobutanol, stopper, and shake vigorously up and down 25 times, that is, for about a minute. Stand to allow the layers to separate, add a small amount of anhydrous sodium sulphate, rotate between the hands to clear the alcohol layer, and stand a minute or two for the layers to separate. Transfer 1 ml of the clear upper alcohol layer to a glass cuvette and read at 535 nm in the fluorimeter using excitation at 450 nm, zeroing against the blank. The alcohol solutions remain stable for at least 2 h. To get a true riboflavin reading, after the initial reading has been made, expose the urine extract to strong ultraviolet light for exactly an hour to destroy the riboflavin and read again. The amount of fluorescence not destroyed by ultraviolet light is, however, remarkably constant, being about half the initial reading in most urines, and much less, about one-fifth, in urines collected after a test dose of riboflavin has been taken.

Calculation.

$$\text{Urinary riboflavin (mg/l)} = \frac{\text{Reading of unknown}}{\text{Reading of standard}}$$

INTERPRETATION

The daily excretion is greatly influenced by the amount taken in the diet. On a satisfactory intake it is between 0.5 and 0.8 mg. Tests using a standard dose are more satisfactory than an estimation made on a 24 h specimen. If 16 μg/kg body weight is given intravenously at least 25 per cent of the amount given should be excreted during the following 4 h (see Najjar and Holt, 1941; Axelrod *et al.*, 1941).

Note. In the course of investigating an apparent increase in riboflavin secretion in some mentally retarded children Haworth *et al.* (1971) devised a more rigorous method of removing interfering substances. The urine was first treated with zinc acetate and formalin. After centrifuging, the riboflavin in the supernatant was separated by elution chromatography using a talc column, and the eluate subjected to one-dimensional chromatography on silica gel plates in order to confirm the identity of the fluorescent spot. Then after drying the plate the riboflavin content was measured fluorimetrically by reflectance densitometry.

Vitamins 231

NICOTINIC ACID, NIACIN

Nicotinic acid, a deficiency of which leads to pellagra, is present as nicotinamide in the two important co-enzymes NAD and NADP (see

Nicotinic Acid   Nicotinamide N^1-Methylnicotinamide

Chapter 22, Vol. I) which are found in almost all cells and are required for a number of important oxidation processes. It is also present in food as the amide. Nicotinic acid can be determined colorimetrically using the reaction with cyanogen bromide and an aromatic amine. Aniline has been used. Rosenblum and Joliffe (1940) and Friedemann and Frazier (1950) used metol, Wang and Kodicek (1943) p-aminoacetophenone. Any nicotinamide is first hydrolysed to convert it to nicotinic acid.

However, nicotinic acid is also excreted as metabolites, the most important being N^1-methylnicotinamide. This is not determined by the colorimetric method for nicotinic acid referred to above. The amount excreted in the urine appears to give a better indication of nicotinic acid nutrition than does excretion of the vitamin itself. N^1-Methylnicotinamide fluoresces in alkaline solution so that it can be determined fluorimetrically after preliminary adsorption, elution and exctraction. For further information concerning other metabolites of nicotinic acid see Sebrell and Harris (1967), Vol. IV.

N^1-Methylnicotinamide also reacts in alkaline solution with ketones to give a fluorescent compound which can be converted by acid into a more stable compound whose blue fluorescence is measured. Details of this technique are given by Györgi and Pearson (1967; see also Pelletier and Campbell, 1962).

Determination of N^1-Methylnicotinamide in Urine (Johnson *et al.*, 1945; see also Hochberg *et al.*, 1945, and Huff and Perlzweig, 1947).

N^1-Methylnicotinamide is adsorbed at pH 4.5 on to a column of synthetic zeolite, eluted with potassium chloride, made alkaline and extracted with n-butanol. It is then compared fluorimetrically with standards.

Reagents. These are the same as Reagents 1-6 for thiamine in urine.

Technique. Collect urine as for thiamine, and proceed as described for thiamine up to the point of washing the Permutit or Decalso on to which the adsorption has been carried out. Whereas thiamine is firmly adsorbed, this is not so for N^1-methylnicotinamide, which is washed off relatively

232   *Practical Clinical Biochemistry*

easily. So wash only twice and adhere closely to a definite technique for test and standards. After elution with 0.5 ml potassium chloride, run 2 ml isobutanol into the tube, add 0.25 ml sodium hydroxide, stopper at once and shake up and down for about a minute (25 times). Stand to separate, or centrifuge. Transfer 1 ml of the supernatant butanol layer to a cuvette and read in the fluorimeter at 460 nm using an excitation wavelength of 360 nm. Readings should not be made earlier than 5 min after shaking with the sodium hydroxide. For the working standard a concentration of 0.1 mg/l is convenient. No blank correction is required so long as the urine concentration is below 15 mg/l.

INTERPRETATION

The daily excretion of N^1-methylnicotinamide, when adequate nicotinic acid is being taken ranges from 3 to 17 mg (Huff and Perlzweig, 1947), the average being 7 mg.

PYRIDOXINE (VITAMIN B_6)

Pyridoxine as pyridoxal phosphate is the coenzyme of several enzymes including some transaminases. It is also present in kynureninase, the enzyme which catalyses the conversion of kynurenine and 3-hydroxy-

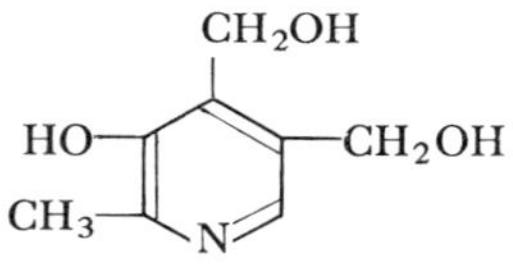

Pyridoxine 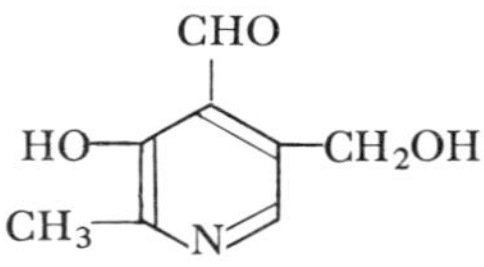   Pyridoxal

kynurenine to anthranilic acid and 3-hydroxyanthranilic acid respectively, and in other enzymes catalysing stages in one of the metabolic pathways of tryptophan. This is shown opposite with the blocks resulting from pyridoxine deficiency. For another pathway for tryptophan metabolism see Chapter 18, Vol. I.

As a result in patients with pyridoxine deficiency there is accumulation of 3-hydroxykynurenine, xanthurenic acid, 8-hydroxyquinaldic acid and kynurenine. Estimation of some of these, particularly of xanthurenic acid, has been used to detect this state, especially after giving a load of tryptophan. It should be noted that although there is a block between 3-hydroxykynurenine and xanthurenic acid an alternative pathway is available through xanthomatin.

Determination of Xanthurenic Acid

Several methods are in use, a colorimetric one using the green colour given with ferric salts in sodium bicarbonate solution, paper chromato-

Vitamins

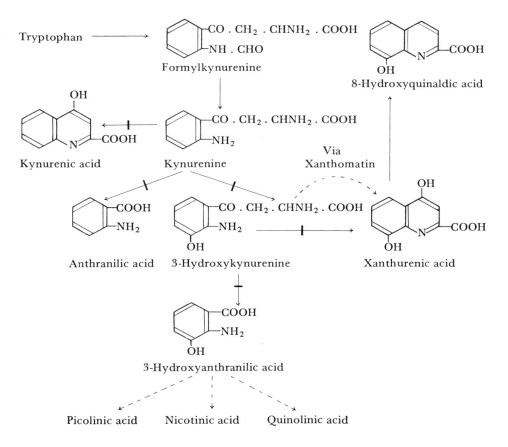

Fig. 6,1. Formation of Nicotinic Acid from Tryptophan.

graphy, and fluorimetry. For those with a fluorimeter the last-named is the method of choice.

Fluorimetric Method (Satoh and Price, 1958)

The xanthurenic and kynurenic acids are adsorbed on to a column of Dowex 50 H$^+$ form and are eluted with a large volume of water. Possible interfering substances are either not eluted by the water or only in minimal amounts. Xanthurenic acid fluoresces in alkaline solution, in which fluorescence of kynurenic acid is slight, the reverse being the case in acid solution. However, in the presence of marked excess of kynurenic acid, readings for xanthurenic are too high, but such interference is unlikely.

Reagents. 1. Dowex 50W (hydrogen form) × 8 -400 mesh.
2. Hydrochloric acid, 5 mol/l, 1 mol/l and 200 mmol/l.
3. Xanthurenic acid, 1 g/l sodium hydroxide, 100 mmol/l. Dilute 1 to 100 with water for use. This contains 10 mg/l.

234 *Practical Clinical Biochemistry*

4. Phosphate buffer, 500 mmol/l, pH 7.4, 13.00 g anhydrous potassium dihydrogen phosphate and 71.97 g of disodium hydrogen phosphate (Na_2HPO_4, $2H_2O$)/l. Check the pH and adjust if necessary.

5. Phosphate buffer, 5 mmol/l, pH 7.4. Dilute the 500 mmol/l buffer 1 to 100.

6. Sodium hydroxide, saturated solution.

Technique. Prepare several ion exchange columns, 15 cm × 1.2 cm outside diameter with a constriction near the bottom, above which there is a plug of glass wool which supports a 3 cm column of Dowex 50. Before use wash with 50 ml hydrochloric acid 5 mol/l, followed by 100 ml water. Take duplicate samples of the urine, 5 per cent of the volume of a 24 h specimen (or less down to 2 per cent for higher concentrations). To one add 1 ml of the strong standard (= 1 mg xanthurenic acid) to check the recovery. Prepare standards containing 1, 5, 10 and 20 μg xanthurenic acid by taking 0.1, 0.5, 1.0 and 2.0 ml of the standard solution and diluting to 5 ml with phosphate buffer, 5 mmol/l. Dilute all samples to 120 ml with water and add 30 ml hydrochloric acid, 1 mol/l. Mix and add each solution to one of the columns. When the liquid has passed through wash with 50 ml hydrochloric acid, 200 mmol/l, and then with 20 ml water. Then elute each with 396 ml of water, add 4 ml of phosphate buffer, 500 mmol/l, pH 7.4, making up to 400 ml. Take 1, 2, and 4 ml portions, dilute each to 5 ml with phosphate buffer, 5 mmol/l, and to each add 5 ml saturated sodium hydroxide. Mix, stand for at least 1 h, centrifuge, and read against a blank of half saturated sodium hydroxide with excitation at 370 nm and fluorescence at 525 nm

Calculation. If 5 per cent of the 24 h specimen was used and 4 ml portion of the eluate, and 10 μg of standard, then

Urinary xanthurenic acid (mg/24 h)

$$= \frac{\text{Reading of unknown}}{\text{Reading of standard}} \times \frac{100}{5} \times \frac{400}{4} \times 10 \times \frac{1}{1000}$$

$$= \frac{\text{Reading of unknown}}{\text{Reading of standard}} \times 20.$$

The suggested standards are

Xanthurenic acid (mg/24 h)	0	2	10	20	40
Standard solution (ml)	0	0.1	0.5	1.0	2.0
Phosphate buffer 5 mmol/l (ml)	5.0	4.9	4.5	4.0	3.0

Proceed as for the test. These figures are for a volume of urine 5 per cent of the specimen, and 4 ml of the eluate made to 400 ml. If either of these is varied, correct accordingly.

A recovery of 95 ± 5 per cent should be obtained.

Vitamins 235

Other Techniques

Paper chromatography. For this butanol–glacial acetic acid–water, 5/1/4, v/v, can be used as solvent. For the test spot apply 200 µl of urine and for the standards 2.5, 5, 10, and 20 µg. With a sheet size 50 × 25 cm use a descending run overnight. Remove next morning, dry, and view in ultraviolet light, activating at approximately 360 nm. A Universal UV Lamp, Camag (254, 350 nm) from Camlab, Cambridge, is convenient. A silvery blue fluorescence results. A roughly quantitative assessment can be made.

Colorimetric method. It was shown (Lepkovsky and Nielsen, 1942; Lepkovsky *et al.,* 1943) that the urine of pyridoxine-deficient rats contained a substance producing a green colour with ferric ammonium sulphate and saturated sodium bicarbonate. Bessey *et al.* (1957) used this to determine the urinary xanthurenic acid after tryptophan loading in infants suffering from infantile convulsions, and give details of this technique. It is, however, less sensitive and less specific than the above procedures.

Tryptophan Loading Test (Price *et al.,* 1965)

Collect a 24 h specimen starting at 0800 h. Then give 2 g of L-tryptophan in orange juice, or in the case of young children, 0.1 g/kg body weight up to a maximum of 2 g, and collect a further 24 h specimen of urine until 0800 h the next day. Collect the urines into 25 ml hydrochloric acid, 1 mol/l. Alternatively, since the rise in xanthurenic acid occurs in the first 12 h after taking the tryptophan, collect two 6 h specimens before and two after doing so.

INTERPRETATION

Normal persons excrete 1 to 3 mg of xanthurenic acid per day and 2 to 11 mg in the 24 h after taking a 2 g load of tryptophan. In pyridoxine deficiency there is a greater increase than this following a loading test, when up to 60 mg may be excreted in 24 h.

In infants a deficiency in pyridoxine can lead to convulsions due to a deficiency in γ-aminobutyric acid, the formation of which from glutamic acid requires pyridoxine as coenzyme. In these infants an abnormal tryptophan loading test is obtained.

FOLIC ACID

The molecule of folic acid shows three features, a pteridine group linked by *p*-aminobenzoic acid to glutamic acid, and is referred to as

Practical Clinical Biochemistry

Folic Acid

pteroylglutamic acid (PGA). PGA occurs as such in foodstuffs but is also present as various derivatives. These include molecules with further bound glutamate, namely the triglutamate and polyglutamates; also a reduced form 5,6,7,8-tetrahydrofolic acid (THF) and its derivatives may be present. In addition to being essential in human metabolism these substances are growth factors for certain micro-organisms and these have been used in determining "folate" content of foods and in the microbiological assay of red cell and serum folate. Thus *Strept. faecalis* measures PGA and THF and most derivatives of THF apart from 5-methyl-THF. The organism *L. casei* measures these substances and in addition 5-methyl THF and the triglutamate, the total often being referred to as "free folate". The polyglutamates are not available to these micro-organisms and are poorly absorbed as such. They are hydrolysed by "conjugases" and after such treatment the "total folate" content of food can be measured.

An average diet contains 160 μg "free folate" and 500 μg "total folate" per day. The daily requirement is 100 to 200 μg. Folate is stored in the body, the total stores amounting to about 15 mg, enough for 75 to 150 days. The main storage form is 5-methyl THF.

The metabolic role of folic acid is of considerable importance and largely involves THF, a molecule which has the ability to accept and donate various one-carbon fragments such as methyl ($-CH_3$), methylene ($= CH_2$), methenyl ($= CH-$), formyl ($-CH = 0$) and formimino ($-CH = NH$). This activity involves the N atoms at positions 5 and 10. The various molecules permit cyclical regeneration of THF as shown in Fig. 6,2. The main source of one-carbon fragments is serine. Four points are of special interest: 5,10-methylene THF is involved in the synthesis of thymine residues in deoxyribonucleic acid; 5-methyl THF is only effectively recycled in the presence of the appropriate methyl transferase, an enzyme which requires vitamin B_{12} as its prosthetic group; the formimino group only enters the scheme through FIGLU, a degradation product of histidine (see below) and this requires a supply of THF; the enzyme, folate reductase, which reduces dihydrofolate is antagonised by the drugs aminopterin and amethopterin which are effective cytotoxic agents on this account.

Causes of Folate Deficiency

Folate deficiency of subclinical degree is common. Body stores are inadequate to protect against long-term inadequacy of supply but are a

Vitamins

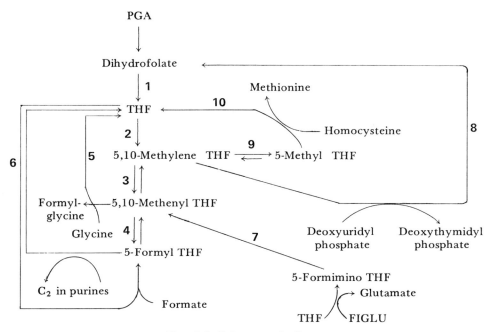

Fig. 6,2. Folate metabolism.

Enzymes. **1.** Folate reductase. **2.** Serine hydroxymethyl transferase. **3.** 5,10-Methylene THF dehydrogenase. **4.** 5,10-Methenyl THF cyclohydrolase. **5.** Glycinamide-diribonucleotide transformylase. **6.** 5-Formyl THF synthetase. **7.** 5-Formimino THF reductase. **8.** Thymidylate synthetase. **9.** 5,10-Methylene THF reductase. **10.** 5-Methyl THF methyl transferase.

buffer against transient deficiencies. Inadequate intake of foods rich in folate, especially green-leaf vegetables, is a factor as also is any malabsorption from the intestine of water-soluble materials, particularly if this involves the jejunum, the site of most folate absorption. Thus folate deficiency is often seen in chronic malabsorption syndrome. Increased needs for folate as in haemolytic anaemia but especially in pregnancy may cause deficiency when intake is barely sufficient under normal circumstances. Finally, drugs such as phenytoin and the barbiturates, have been shown to interfere with the enzymes of the folate cycle.

Consequences of Folate Deficiency

Folate deficiency leads to disordered haemopoiesis. As this also occurs in vitamin B_{12} deficiency the condition is discussed below (p. 244). The deficiency of THF leads also to a disturbance of histidine catabolism. Although this has little clinical effect the accumulation and increased excretion of the intermediary metabolite, FIGLU, is used for the chemical assessment of folate status. The relevant metabolic steps in the breakdown

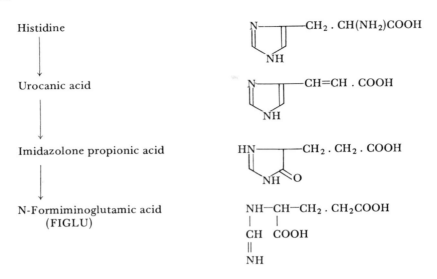

Fig. 6,3. Histidine metabolism.

of histidine are shown in Fig. 6,3). FIGLU is further metabolised to glutamate as shown in Fig. 6,2.

Sometimes, however, in cases of folate deficiency little increase is found because there is insufficient histidine in the diet. The determination of urinary FIGLU after a histidine load increases the sensitivity of the test considerably.

Assessment of Folate Deficiency

Folate deficiency may be assessed directly by determining folate itself under various conditions or indirectly by determining urinary folate, usually with histidine loading.

Methods Involving Folate Determination

Folate is determined by a microbiological method utilising the fact that it is a growth factor of *L. casei*. Assays may be done on serum or on red cells. Folate in mature red cells is in polyglutamate form and is retained in these cells until their destruction. Folate absorption from the intestine has been studied by comparison of folate levels after oral and intravenous doses of folate. The rate of clearance of administratively administered folate has been used to study folate stores.

The analytical performance of such tests leaves much room for improvement. There is wide interlaboratory variation in comparative trials and the normal ranges quoted by different workers using the same methods vary considerably. Red cell folate concentrations are about 20 times serum levels.

Vitamins 239

INTERPRETATION

Serum folate levels are sensitive to minor degrees of folate deficiency and drop within a few days of folate deprivation despite reasonable folate stores. A low serum folate is an index of negative folate balance. A more useful assessment comes from red cell folate determinations which reflect the state of the folate stores. A normal result indicates no significant degree of folate deficiency. Reduced red cell folate levels indicate clinically important deficiency and are seen in cases of malabsorption syndrome and in dietary insufficiency particularly in the elderly. In pernicious anaemia red cell folate is usually normal or even increased. In general red cell folate values show a good correlation with urinary FIGLU excretion.

For a review of folate metabolism and methods for assessing folate deficiency, see Luhby and Cooperman (1964) and Chanarin (1969).

Histidine Loading Test

This can be done either as an 8 h or 24 h test.

(*a*) *Eight-hour test.* Allow the patient nothing after midnight. Empty the bladder at 0600 h and give 15 g of L-histidine. Since this is insoluble and acid, give in orange juice. Mix well and drink quickly. Rinse the cup out two or three times to ensure that all the histidine has been taken. Collect all the urine passed up to 1400 h, emptying the bladder at that time. Place the urine into a bottle containing 2 ml concentrated hydrochloric acid and a few crystals of thymol. Breakfast can be taken after 0830 h.

(*b*) *Twenty-four-hour test.* Empty the bladder at 0800 h and discard this specimen. Give breakfast then and at 0830 h 5 g of histidine as above, then further 5 g amounts half an hour after each of the mid-day and evening meals. Collect urine as passed until 0800 h the following morning at which time the bladder is emptied. Place all the urine specimens immediately into a bottle containing acid as above.

Determination of FIGLU

Several kinds of method have been used; enzymic, chromatographic and electrophoretic, chemical, and microbiological (see Luhby and Cooperman, 1964). Electrophoresis is convenient but less sensitive than enzymic methods.

I. Cellulose Acetate Electrophoresis (Kohn *et al.*, 1961; Kohn, 1964)

Electrophoresis on cellulose acetate with a pyridine-acetic acid buffer is carried out in duplicate using a test and standard. One pair is stained directly with ninhydrin, the other pair after treatment with ammonia to liberate glutamic acid from the FIGLU present.

Reagents. 1. Pyridine—acetic acid buffer, pH 5.3. Dilute 25 ml pyridine and 10 ml glacial acetic acid to 2 litres with distilled water.

240   *Practical Clinical Biochemistry*

2. Standard. FIGLU has been added to urine, 100 μg per ml. It can be obtained as the hemibarium salt, 100 μg of which equals 67 μg of pure FIGLU. Kohn (1964) found that glutamic acid, 1 mmol/l in acetic acid (10 ml glacial acid/l in water), corresponded to 400 mg/l of the barium salt of FIGLU or 270 mg/l FIGLU itself. It is suggested that if glutamic acid is used as standard, a urine from a positive test and so containing an increased amount of FIGLU should be put up alongside the test for staining after treatment with ammonia.

3. Ammonia, sp. gr. 0.88.

4. Ninhydrin. Dissolve 200 mg ninhydrin in 6 ml ethanol and make to 100 ml with ether. Traces of ammonia should be removed if necessary (Jacobs, 1960).

Technique. Horizontal electrophoresis is used with 12 × 5 cm strips of cellulose acetate. Four spots are used, the two middle ones of the patient's urine and the other two of marker urine containing FIGLU, 100 mg/l (or one of glutamic acid, 1 mmol/l and one of a FIGLU positive urine—Kohn, 1964). Impregnate the strip with the buffer solution allowing the strip to float before submerging. Blot the strip lightly between filter papers to remove water. With the strip in place apply 6 to 8 μl volumes of the test urine and standards in the positions stated above (or 10 to 15 μl for urines containing very small amounts). Apply a constant voltage of 200 V for about half an hour. Determine the most suitable time by observation.

Remove the strip, dry at 80 to 100° C for 10 to 15 min. Cut the strip lengthwise into two halves each with one test spot. Hang one half in a closed vessel containing a layer of ammonia for about half an hour. Remove the ammonia by warming again to 90 to 100° C for a few minutes. Pass both strips slowly through the ninhydrin solution in a Petri dish and then dry them held between two sheets of filter paper kept flat between cardboard for about 5 min at 90 to 100° C. The colour takes about half an hour to develop fully.

Three spots are seen on each strip, basic aminoacids (histidine) nearer the cathode, neutral ones (glycine) near the point of application of the samples, the acidic ones with glutamic acid nearer the anode. An increase in FIGLU is shown by an increased intensity of this anodic spot. In a normal urine this is quite faint. The difference between the glutamic acid on the ammonia-treated half and that on the other gives the amount of FIGLU.

Kohn (1964) and Kohn and Feinburg (1965) eluted the spots to quantitate the procedure. Cut out the spots and divide into small pieces. Then place in 1 ml eluting fluid, prepared by mixing 95 ml ethanol (750 ml/l with water) with 5 ml copper sulphate solution (1 g/l) in water. Stopper the tubes, shake vigorously for quarter to half an hour, centrifuge hard, and read at 525 nm, using the spots from the part of the strip not exposed to ammonia as blanks. The concentration of FIGLU is then easily calculated from the ratio of the differences in extinction of the pairs of spots from the patient's urine and the standard multiplied by the concentration of the standard, provided the same volume was used.

Vitamins 241

II. Enzymic Assay (Tabor and Wyngarden, 1958; Luhby and Cooperman, 1964)

The enzymes required—FIGLU transferase and formiminotetrahydrofolate cyclodeaminase—are prepared from liver and along with folic acid, the coenzyme, added to the urine plus buffer. N^5-Formimino THF is converted to $N^5 N^{10}$-methenyl THF which is then converted to N^{10}-formyl THF (Fig. 6,2). This latter is read at 350 nm at which it has a peak absorption.

Reagents. 1. Phosphate buffer, 1 mol/l, pH 7.2. To a 1 mol/l solution of potassium dihydrogen phosphate (34.89 g of the anhydrous salt in 200 ml aqueous solution) add 1 mol/l phosphoric acid (9.8 g or 5.6 ml of the 1.75 sp. gr. acid in 100 ml solution) until the pH is 7.2.

2. Enzyme solution. Take 2 pig livers, cut up into pieces about 1 cm square and homogenise in 100 g portions for about a minute with 500 ml acetone. Filter through a Buchner funnel, break up the cake, and again homogenise with the same volume of acetone. Then break up the cake and dry overnight at room temperature. This gives about 200 g of product. Stir the dry powder with water (a litre per 100 g of powder) for a quarter of an hour at room temperature and filter through a nylon stocking. Centrifuge the filtrate in 4 portions in a large capacity centrifuge at 2 000 r.p.m. for 30 min. At this stage centrifuging in a refrigerated centrifuge is not essential but thereafter the material must be kept below 4° C.

Add 300 g of ammonium sulphate to each 1 400 ml of the supernatant and dissolve by swirling gently. Keep in a refrigerator for an hour to allow full precipitation to occur, then centrifuge in a refrigerated centrifuge for 30 min. Decant the supernatant. Combine the precipitates and keep overnight suspended in 50 ml distilled water in a refrigerator. Centrifuge next day using a high speed centrifuge at 20 000 to 30 000 g for 2 h. The precipitate now obtained contains the enzymes in comparatively pure form. Test both precipitate and supernatant for enzyme activity (see below) since sometimes considerable activity is still present in the latter. If this is so, repeat the centrifuging and pool the precipitates. (If the precipitate is stored 3 to 4 days instead of overnight as above, a better yield is obtained and it is usually not necessary to spin the supernatant again.)

Dissolve the total precipitate in 38 ml sodium acetate, 200 mmol/l, stirring gently for 2 h in a bath of iced water. Then centrifuge for 5 to 10 min, preferably in a refrigerated centrifuge. The enzymes required are in the supernatant, sufficiently purified from other enzymes which are able to break down histidine, urocanic acid, formiminoglycine and formiminoaspartate. Store in 10 ml portions in screw-topped bottles at -10 to -20° C. In this state it will keep for at least a year.

A preparation containing both enzymes is available from Sigma (London) Ltd.

3. Tetrahydrofolic acid (Sigma or Nutritional Biochemicals). Dilute with sufficient 2-mercaptoethanol, 1.1 mmol/l, to obtain a solution containing 4.4 mg per ml. Wrap in aluminium foil to keep out light.

242   *Practical Clinical Biochemistry*

4. FIGLU standard, 30 to 40 mg/l in water. This may be bought from the California Corporation for Biochemical Research, Los Angeles, and British Drug Houses supply it as the hemibarium salt.

5. Perchloric acid, 10 ml concentrated acid diluted to 100 ml with water.

Technique. Measure 0.1 ml of the urine, freshly neutralised to pH 7.0, into each of two tubes and add immediately 0.1 ml of the phosphate buffer and 0.1 ml of the THF solution. To one (the test) add 0.45 ml distilled water and 0.25 ml enzyme solution, and to the other (the urine blank) 0.7 ml of distilled water. At the same time put through two further tubes containing 0.1 ml phosphate buffer, 0.1 ml THF, 0.55 ml distilled water and 0.25 ml enzyme solution (the enzyme blank), and 0.1 ml phosphate buffer, 0.1 ml THF, and 0.8 ml distilled water (control). Shake gently to mix and incubate for 30 min at room temperature (25° C) preferably in the dark. Then add 0.3 ml perchloric acid to each, mix, and stand for 2 h at room temperature. Centrifuge at about 2 000 r.p.m. for 5 to 10 min and transfer the supernatants to the spectrophotometer cuvettes (semi-micro holding 1.0 to 1.5 ml). Read at 350 nm using a 1 cm light path. Use the control to set the instrument, then read the extinctions of the unknown and blanks.

The corrected extinction of the test is given by (Reading of unknown—Reading of urine blank—Reading of enzyme blank).

If a standard solution of FIGLU is put through a factor can be obtained to convert the extinction obtained in the test to μmol FIGLU. In the 1.3 ml volume used above, 0.01 μmol has an extinction of 0.19, so the factor is $0.01 \div 0.19$, i.e. 0.052. This should be checked with a known amount of FIGLU. A value between 0.17 and 0.20 is acceptable. If it is not obtained the volume of THF solution can be increased, the volume of water used being correspondingly decreased. If a correct factor is still not obtained an increased volume of enzyme solution can be tried. If this still fails fresh enzyme must be made.

For high values of FIGLU the urine should be diluted, for example 1 in 5 or 10 ml. The molecular weight is 174 so that the concentration of FIGLU is given by:

Urinary FIGLU (mg/l) = Corrected extinction × Factor (0.052) × dilution of urine (e.g. 10) × 174.

INTERPRETATION

Luhby *et al.* (1959), using the 24 h test found a FIGLU excretion of 0.6 to 30 mg/24 h (0.1 to 25 mg/l) in normal persons, and 185 to 2 050 mg/24 h (90 to 1 910 mg/l) in folate deficiency. For infants given 73 mg/kg, Luhby *et al.* (1962) found 0 to 24 mg/l in controls and 30 to 450 mg/l in folate deficiency. They preferred the 24 h form of test.

An increase in the excretion of FIGLU, often considerable, may be found in patients with malignant disease (Noeypatimanond *et al.*, 1966), and to a less extent in patients with pernicious anaemia. In megaloblastic

Vitamins 243

anaemia, treatment with the deficient vitamin, folate or B_{12} as appropriate, results in a fall of FIGLU to normal values.

VITAMIN B_{12}, THE COBALAMINS

The molecule of Vitamin B_{12} is a complex one. Co^+ is present in a tetrapyrrole ring and is linked through an organic base to ribose-3-phosphate. Several related cobalamins are known. The usual form has CN^- linked to Co^+ and is referred to as cyanocobalamin; where OH^- replaces CN^- hydroxycobalamin results. When CN^- is replaced by a deoxyadenosyl group the product deoxyadenosylcobalamin shows coenzyme activity. Such activity is also seen in methylcobalamin.

Important coenzyme functions of cobalamins include:
(a) Coenzyme for 5-methyl THF methyltransferase (Fig. 6,2) which allows 5-methyl THF, the storage form of folate, to enter the folate cycle;
(b) Coenzyme in the methylation of soluble RNA;
(c) Coenzyme in the conversion of methylmalonylcoenzyme A to succinylcoenzyme A (and hence succinate) by methylmalonyl CoA mutase (Fig. 6,4).

Reaction (a) involves vitamin B_{12} with folate metabolism. Both these vitamins when deficient lead to the same condition of megaloblastic anaemia. Reaction (c) is made use of in the chemical assessment of vitamin B_{12} deficiency states (see below).

Vitamin B_{12} is present in the diet in many animal tissues, especially in liver, and also in milk and eggs. The dietary intake varies from 3 to 30 μg daily. The daily needs are uncertain but are probably around 2 to 5 μg. The vitamin is stored in the liver, total stores being about 3 to 6 mg, enough for 5 years' supply. The absorption of vitamin B_{12} is confined to the terminal ileum and requires the presence of intrinsic factor, a glycoprotein secreted in gastric juice.

Causes of Vitamin B_{12} Deficiency

Dietary deficiency of vitamin B_{12} is unusual but is described in vegetarians. More important is intrinsic factor deficiency. This is typically seen in the gastric atrophy found in classical pernicious anaemia but congenital deficiency is known and acquired deficiency occurs after gastrectomy. Direct interference with absorption occurs in disease processes affecting the terminal ileum, for example, Crohn's disease. Utilisation of dietary vitamin B_{12} by bacteria colonising the small intestine reduces the amount available for absorption. This occurs in some cases of steatorrhoea particularly those associated with the "blind-loop" syndrome or in tropical sprue. Certain intestinal parasites can also remove the vitamin.

244 *Practical Clinical Biochemistry*

Whatever the cause, the liver stores protect the body from the consequences of deficiency for several years.

Consequences of Vitamin B_{12} Deficiency

Vitamin B_{12} deficiency, as does that of folate, leads to disordered haemopoiesis. Vitamin B_{12} deficiency, however, also leads to disordered function of nervous tissue recognised clinically as subacute combined degeneration of the spinal cord.

Megaloblastic anaemias. Deficiency of folate leads to disordered synthesis of DNA, deficiency of vitamin B_{12} impairs the folate cycle and again leads to impaired DNA synthesis. Cell cytoplasmic functions which depend on RNA are unaffected. There is thus delayed maturation of cell nuclei and increased cell size. In the red cell precursors in the marrow, cytoplasmic formation of haemoglobin continues but the disordered nuclear development leads to changes recognised down the microscope as conversion of the usual normoblast to a megaloblast. Similar disordered maturation occurs in precursors of leucocytes and platelets. The marrow output of red cells, polymorphs and platelets is impaired and they are reduced in peripheral blood. The red cells are larger than usual, are often distorted and are more readily haemolysed. Both folate and B_{12} deficiency thus lead to an increase in serum bilirubin, urinary urobilinogen and serum lactate dehydrogenase. In many cases serum iron is increased with even greater increase in the percentage bound to transferrin.

Assessment of Vitamin B_{12} Deficiency

Vitamin B_{12} deficiency may be assessed by studying the serum B_{12} concentration, by studying the absorption of vitamin B_{12} from the gut, by measuring liver B_{12} and, indirectly by studying the urinary excretion of methylmalonic acid especially after valine loading (compare the FIGLU test, pp. 239 to 243).

Methods Involving Vitamin B_{12} Itself

The concentration of vitamin B_{12} in serum (or liver) has usually been studied by microbiological assay methods using *L. Leichmannii* or *E. gracilis*. The methods show considerable interlaboratory variation and the normal ranges using the two organisms differ. With *E. gracilis* the lower end of the normal range is 130 to 160 ng/l and the upper end 750 to 925 ng/l with mean figures varying from 305 to 604 ng/l. Figures for *L. Leichmannii* are somewhat higher, varying from 110 to 300 ng/l to over 800 to

Vitamins 245

1 700 ng/l with means of 392 to 682. More recently radioimmunoassay and competitive protein binding methods have been introduced.

Attention has been paid to assessing the absorption of the vitamin from the gut. For this purpose radioactive B_{12} labelled with ^{57}Co or ^{58}Co is available and simplifies the procedure. This is given in doses of 0.5 to 2 μg orally and is usually combined with parenteral administration of 1 mg B_{12} (non-radioactive) to saturate binding sites in tissues and plasma proteins. Different workers have measured faecal excretion of unabsorbed vitamin, hepatic uptake, or urinary excretion. The test most used involves the latter, the Schilling test, in which normal persons excrete over one-third of the oral dose in the urine within 24 h.

INTERPRETATION

Low serum B_{12} values are seen in pernicious anaemia and in general are lower the more severe the anaemia. Figures of 10 to 110 ng/l with a mean of 38 are recorded. However, low values are also commonly seen in vegetarians, following total gastrectomy, in small gut congenital anomalies such as jejunal diverticulitis, in fish tape worm infestations and in tropical sprue, and also in regional ileitis. About half the cases of folate deficiency have reduced B_{12} levels which rise to normal on folate therapy. In general a low serum B_{12} level is suggestive of clinical deficiency of the vitamin and there is evidence of impaired B_{12} absorption, other features of pernicious anaemia, dietary history of vegetarianism or an increased excretion of methylmalonic acid. Increased serum B_{12} has been reported in liver cell necrosis presumably due to release of hepatic stores.

Tests for B_{12} absorption assess the ability of the stomach to secrete intrinsic factor, the absence of significant destruction of the B_{12}-intrinsic factor complex in the small intestine by bacteria or parasites, and the integrity of the ileal absorptive site. Impaired absorption due to the first factor can be corrected by administration of the intrinsic factor with radioactive B_{12}. Loss by the second factor can often be demonstrated by improved absorption following broad-spectrum antibiotic therapy.

Methods Involving the Urinary Excretion of Methylmalonic Acid

Propionic acid is produced in the body as a metabolite of certain amino acids, especially valine and isoleucine. It may also arise from metabolism of fatty acids with an odd number of carbon atoms. Propionate is metabolised in several steps (Fig. 6,4) to succinate, which enters the tricarboxylic acid cycle.

P.C.B.(II)−9

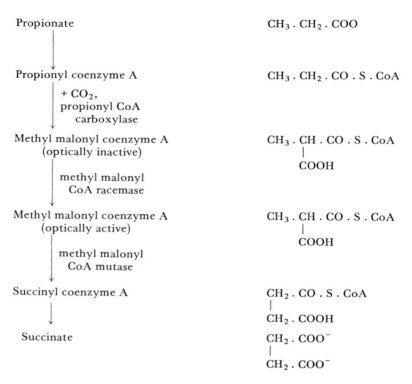

Fig. 6,4. Conversion of propionate to succinate.

Methylmalonyl CoA mutase has B_{12} as a coenzyme and in B_{12} deficiency methylmalonyl coenzyme A accumulates and is excreted as methylmalonic acid (MMA) or its salts. It is more obvious if the production of propionate increases. This is best achieved by giving oral valine in a dose of 10 g. Isoleucine or propionate orally is less effective.

Methods for determining methylmalonic acid have used gas chromatography, thin layer chromatography, and colorimetry of the green compound formed on reaction with diazotised p-nitroaniline.

Gas chromatography, the most sensitive and specific, and the only one which gives meaningful accurate results in the normal range, was used by Cox and White (1962, see also White, 1971) and Green and Pegrum (1968) who, after preliminary separation by extraction with ether and passage down a column of an anion exchange resin and elution, esterified with diazomethane before gas chromatography with polyethylene glycol adipate as stationary phase on Celite or Gas Chrom P. This was also used by Gompertz (1968) who, however, did the preliminary separation by thin layer chromatography. Hoffmann and Barboriak (1967) after preliminary separation on a Dowex column decarboxylated the acids in the injector so that gas chromatography was of the propionic acid. Gibbs et al. (1972) after a series of ether extractions carried out gas chromatography of the

Vitamins   247

trimethylsilyl esters thus avoiding the use of diazomethane which is toxic and may explode unexpectedly.

Thin layer chromatography is only semi-quantitative and so is suitable for screening purposes, visible spots being obtained only when there is an increase in methylmalonic acid. Silica gel has been used as stationary phase with either ethanol (950 ml/l in water), ammonia (250 ml sp. gr. 0.88/l in water), water, or amyl acetate, glacial acetic acid, water as mobile phase. Dreyfuss and Dubé (1967) used the former 25/4/3 staining with bromcresol green, as did Gompertz 53/13/2 with methyl red, while Bashir *et al.* (1966) used the latter 60/10/0.5 staining with bromcresol green and Gutteridge and Wright (1970) 60/20/6 with Fast Blue B.

The colorimetric method was introduced by Giorgio and Plaut (1965, see also Giorgio, 1970) has also been studied by Green (1968), Dale (1972) and Davies *et al.*, while Gawthorne *et al.* (1971) published an automated version. In this a preliminary separation is also made using an ion exchange column. There is also some background colour, to allow for which Dale used an Allen type correction and Davies *et al.*, extracted into amyl alcohol. This method too is less sensitive than gas chromatography (see below).

Colorimetric Method for Determination of Urinary Methylmalonic Acid (Davies *et al.*)

Reagents. 1. Deacidite FF (1P) 200 mesh, chloride form (Permutit Co. Ltd.). Wash three times with water (5 volumes) and then keep as an aqueous suspension in a dark bottle at room temperature.

2. Diethyl ether. Wash with approximately one-tenth its volume of sodium hydroxide, 5 mol/l, then with water until the washings are neutral. Use wet.

3. Hydrochloric acid, 10, 100 mmol/l, and the concentrated acid.

4. Sodium hydroxide solution, 3 mol/l.

5. Acetate buffer, 1 mol/l, pH 4.3, 42 ml glacial acetic acid and 21.8 g anhydrous sodium acetate/l with water.

6. Ammonium hydroxide, 5 mol/l. Dilute 250 ml ammonia, sp. gr. 0.88 to 1 litre with water.

7. Diazo reagent. Prepare the following solutions:
(a) *p*-Nitroaniline, 750 mg/l in hydrochloric acid, 200 mmol/l;
(b) Sodium nitrite, 0.5 g/l (kept at 4°C);
(c) Sodium acetate, 200 mmol/l.
Cool these to below 5°C and prepare the diazoreagent by mixing 4 volumes of the nitrite and 15 volumes *p*-nitroaniline, then add 5 volumes of the acetate, mix and keep below 5°C for not more than 12 h.

8. Stock standard solution of methylmalonic acid (Kodak), 10 mmol/l, 118.1 mg/100 ml in water. Keep at 4°C.

9. Working standard, 0.1 mmol/l. Dilute the stock standard 1 to 100 with hydrochloric acid, 100 mmol/l.

248   *Practical Clinical Biochemistry*

10. Amyl alcohol.
11. Anhydrous sodium sulphate.

Technique. Collect urine without preservative for 24 h following an oral loading dose of 10 g valine. Acidify 5 ml urine with concentrated hydrochloric acid to pH 2 and extract three times with 50 ml portions of ether, for 15 min each time. Shake each ether extract with 5 ml ammonium hydroxide for 15 min. These extractions are conveniently carried out on a mechanical shaker. Prepare a column of the resin (6 × 1.5 cm) in distilled water. Add the combined ammoniacal extracts to the column and after they have entered the resin wash with 50 ml water followed by 50 ml hydrochloric acid, 100 mmol/l. The pH of the effluent should be about 5. Allow the column to drain and then elute the methylmalonic acid with 25 ml hydrochloric acid, 100 mmol/l. The column can then be regenerated with 50 ml hydrochloric acid, 100 mmol/l, followed by 50 ml water.

Pipette 1.5 ml acetate buffer into three glass-stoppered tubes (100 × 16 mm) and add respectively 1.0 ml well mixed eluate (the test), working standard, hydrochloric acid, 100 mmol/l (the blank). Add 1.5 ml fresh diazo reagent, mix and place in a water bath at $95 \pm 1^{\circ}$ C for exactly 2.5 min. Then transfer to cold water for 1 min. To each tube add 1 ml sodium hydroxide solution and, after mixing well, 3 ml amyl alcohol and stand for 10 min. Then stopper and shake vigorously for 1 min. After the phases have separated, remove the lower aqueous solution by suction. Add approximately 0.2 g anhydrous sodium sulphate to the organic layer and shake to remove water. Centrifuge briefly, transfer to cuvettes and read against water in the colorimeter at 650 nm. The blank absorbance should be 0.02 to 0.05 and that of the standard 0.60 to 0.65 for a path length of 8 mm. If the absorbance of the test solution is too high dilute with amyl alcohol or, preferably, repeat the determination using a smaller amount of the eluate.

Recovery of methylmalonic acid can be checked by adding 0.5 ml of the stock standard to 5 ml acidified urine before carrying through the whole procedure. Recovery should be 100 ± 10 per cent.

Calculation. Urinary methyl malonic acid (mmol/l)

$$= \frac{\text{Reading of unknown}}{\text{Reading of standard}} \times \frac{25}{5} \times 0.1$$

$$= \frac{\text{Reading of unknown}}{\text{Reading of standard}} \times 0.5; \text{ or } \times 59 \text{ as mg/l.}$$

INTERPRETATION

In normal persons the excretion of MMA is 0 to 35 μmol/24 h (0 to 4 mg/24 h) for simple GLC methods (for example, Cox and White, 1962) rising to an upper level of 78 μmol/24 h (9.2 mg/24 h) if internal standards are used (Gompertz *et al.*, 1967). This is not increased after valine loading. Colorimetric methods give higher results probably being less specific.

Vitamins

Giorgio and Plaut (1965) obtained 0 to 93 μmol/24 h (0 to 11 mg /24 h) without valine loading. Green (1968) accepted up to 127 μmol/24 h (15 mg/24 h) and Davies et al., whose method is given above quote a normal range up to 0.21 mmol/24 h (25 mg/24 h) following a loading dose of 10 g valine.

In pernicious anaemia basal excretion of MMA is frequently increased, figures up to 2.5 mmol/24 h (294 mg/24 h) being seen in more severe cases (Cox and White). Milder cases may show excretion at the upper limit of the normal range but are usually unequivocally abnormal after valine loading with excretion of MMA from 0.34 to over 10 mmol/24 h (40 mg/24 h up to several g/24 h, Green and Pegrum, 1968). Following partial gastrectomy there is increased excretion of MMA in cases with reduced serum B_{12} concentration. Similarly increased excretion has been reported after total gastrectomy, in jejunal diverticulitis, after lower small gut resections and in some cases of malabsorption syndrome, tropical sprue and folate deficiency. In most cases there is a good correlation between increased MMA extretion and reduced serum B_{12} concentration. The excretion falls rapidly within 2 days on treating the deficiency of B_{12}, reaching normal values in 3 to 5 days.

Considerably increased excretion of MMA is found as a rare inborn error of metabolism in which the excretion may be as great as 50 mmol/l (6 g/24 h) (Levin et al., 1966).

ASCORBIC ACID (VITAMIN C)

There are some points concerning the chemistry of L-ascorbic acid which are important in connection with its determination. It forms white crystals which are stable in air, but it oxidizes easily in solution, especially in the presence of metallic ions such as Cu^{2+} being converted into dehydro-L-ascorbic acid. Both these are biologically active, since dehydro-L-ascorbic acid can be reduced in the body to L-ascorbic acid. The rate of oxidation of

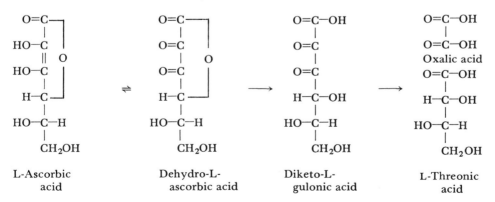

Fig. 6,5. The oxidation of ascorbic acid.

250   *Practical Clinical Biochemistry*

L-ascorbic acid increases with increasing pH, so that it is much more stable in acid solution. Dehydro-L-ascorbic acid itself undergoes further oxidation above pH 5, the ring opening to give diketo-L-gulonic acid with subsequent breakdown to oxalic acid and L-threonic acid (Fig. 6,5). With opening of the ring biological activity ceases.

One of the methods most frequently used for the determination of ascorbic acid is the titration with 2,6-dichlorophenolindophenol in acid solution. This blue compound is red in acid solution and on titration with a solution of ascorbic acid is reduced to the colourless leucobase, the ascorbic acid being oxidised to dehydroascorbic acid. It is thus seen that if a mixture of ascorbic acid and dehydroascorbic acid is present, only the former reacts

2,6-dichlorophenolindophenol
(oxidised form)

colourless leucobase
(reduced form)

with the dye, although both are biologically active. Dehydroascorbic acid, however, can be reduced back to ascorbic acid in acid solution by hydrogen sulphide, so that titration then measures all the biologically active substances present. In body fluids such as blood and urine only ascorbic acid appears to be present, so that if the determination is carried out on a fresh specimen before conversion to dehydroascorbic acid is able to occur, all the active vitamin present will be measured. However, particularly in urine, other substances may be present which react with dichlorophenolindophenol, thus impairing the reliability of the method. Attempts have been made to overcome this.

Another method suggested for the determination of ascorbic acid is to form the derivative of dehydroascorbic acid with 2,4-dinitrophenylhydrazine. When treated with sulphuric acid this gives a red product, which can be determined colorimetrically Thus it is necessary to convert all the ascorbic acid into dehydroascorbic acid by shaking with Norit and filtering. The Norit clears the liquid and oxidises the ascorbic acid. This method is given below (p. 254).

Determination of Ascorbic Acid in Urine. Method using Titration with 2,6-Dichlorophenolindophenol (Harris and Ray 1935)

Reagents. 1. Glacial acetic acid.

2. Solution of 2,6-dichlorophenolindophenol. Weigh out accurately 40 mg of the dye and dissolve in 100 ml distilled water. One ml of this

Vitamins 251

solution is equivalent to 0.2 mg ascorbic acid. Since the keeping qualities of the solution are poor, prepare freshly at frequent intervals. It should not be kept in use for more than a week. It may be more convenient to use the tablets of the dye, which can be obtained from British Drug Houses. These contain an amount of dye equivalent to 1 mg of ascorbic acid, so that when dissolved in 5 ml water the same solution is obtained.

Solutions of dye can be checked against an ascorbic acid solution of known concentration. Dissolve 40 mg pure dry ascorbic acid in 100 ml acetic acid (100 ml glacial acid diluted to 1 litre with water). Dilute 5 ml of this to 100 ml with the acetic acid. Titrate 0.5 ml of the dye with this solution. Five ml should be required to decolorise it.

Ascorbic acid itself can be standardised against iodine. Since 1 mol of ascorbic acid loses 1 mol H_2 on oxidation, it reacts with 1 mol I_2. So 1 ml iodine, 5 mmol/l (= 1.27 mg), is equivalent to 1 ml ascorbic acid, 5 mmol/l (= 0.88 mg). Or 1 mg ascorbic acid is equivalent to 1.14 ml iodine, 5 mmol/l.

Dissolve 50 mg ascorbic acid in 100 ml glass-distilled water and titrate 5 ml with iodine, 5 mmol/l, using starch as indicator. Use a microburette. Five ml contains 2.5 mg of ascorbic acid and so should require $1.14 \times 2.5 = 2.85$ ml of the iodine.

Technique. Pipette 0.5 ml dye solution into a test tube (15×2.5 cm) and add 1 ml glacial acetic acid. Run in the urine slowly, with constant shaking, until the red colour has been discharged. Note the urine volume required.

Calculation. As 0.5 ml of dye reacts with 0.1 mg ascorbic acid

$$\text{Urinary ascorbic acid (mg/l)} = \frac{0.1 \times 1000}{\text{ml urine required}}$$

$$= \frac{100}{\text{ml urine required}}$$

Alternative Technique. Mix a portion of the urine with one-ninth its volume of glacial acetic acid and determine the volume required to decolorise 0.5 ml dye. This ensures a uniform concentration of acetic acid. Then

$$\text{Urinary ascorbic acid (mg/l)} = \frac{111}{\text{ml urine required}}$$

Notes. 1. The urine must be titrated fresh, that is, within a few minutes of being passed, unless acetic acid is added immediately in the proportion of 1 part to 9 parts of urine. Such acidified urine will keep for several hours. The determination is most often done on urine specimens collected as part of saturation tests (see below) which can be titrated at once. A rather large amount of acetic acid is required to protect 24 h specimens, the determination of ascorbic acid in which is not very convenient.

252   *Practical Clinical Biochemistry*

2. Other substances particularly sulphydryl compounds which also decolorise the dye are present in urine, so that the result is inaccurate for ascorbic acid. However, these react more slowly than ascorbic acid at pH 3 so that it is sufficiently accurate for most clinical purposes. Some modifications of the method use this fact, but it is doubtful whether they are warranted. In saturation tests, because of the greater quantity of ascorbic acid often present, the effect of these interfering substances is much less important and can be ignored.

INTERPRETATION

The daily output of ascorbic acid is roughly half the intake. A usual amount is 20 to 30 mg. The daily intake of persons on a reasonably satisfactory amount of ascorbic acid is 30 to 60 mg. The minimum amount which protects against scurvy is 10 to 15 mg daily. In deficiency states urinary ascorbic acid is reduced virtually to zero. The small amounts measured by the above method are probably due to other reducing substances. The quantity of ascorbic acid excreted in 24 h is not a satisfactory method of studying the nutritional state, even apart from preservation problems.

Ascorbic Acid Saturation Tests

These widely used tests assume that if the previous intake of the vitamin has been insufficient, the tissues will take up quite large amounts when ascorbic acid is given so that little or none will be excreted in the urine. On the other hand, persons whose intake of ascorbic acid has been adequate will excrete appreciable amounts of such ingested ascorbic acid. Various dosages have been used, the ascorbic acid has been given orally and intravenously, and different times for urine collection have been used. Thus at least 200 mg should be excreted in 4 h after intravenous injection of 500 mg ascorbic acid in 5 ml distilled water. The test described is almost identical with that of Harris and Abbasy (1937).

Technique. An oral dose of 11 mg ascorbic acid/kg body weight is used, giving an average dose for adults of about 700 mg. This may be given in water either fasting or 2 to 3 h after a meal. Only one specimen of urine is collected covering the period 4 to 6 h after the dose when excretion is maximal. Thus the test might be carried out as follows:

1000 h Give the ascorbic acid dissolved in about 150 ml water.
1400 h Empty the bladder completely and discard the urine.
1600 h Empty the bladder completely and estimate the ascorbic acid content almost immediately as described above.

Repeat the test daily until a normal response is obtained.

Vitamins 253

INTERPRETATION

In a normal nutritional state for ascorbic acid an average of about 50 mg should be obtained on the first or second day. In ascorbic acid deficiency a longer time is required. In milder cases 6 to 10 days may be needed; in severe cases, in which symptoms of scurvy may be present, up to 2 to 3 weeks may be necessary. In deficiency states the excretion usually corresponds to less than 2 mg ascorbic acid, this probably being due to other reducing substances. This level is, as a rule, maintained until the deficiency has almost been made good when there is quite a quick rise to the region of 40 to 50 mg for the 2 h urine found in a normal person. With such specimens of urine containing 50 mg ascorbic acid in perhaps about 100 ml urine, a more accurate result is obtained if the urine is diluted 1 to 5 or 1 to 10 with water, before carrying out the titration. Otherwise very small amounts of urine, less than 1 ml will be required.

This test has been criticised quite considerably, but appears to be as convenient and satisfactory as anything available at present. Ascorbic acid in therapeutically useful amounts is being given whilst the test is carried out, and the effect may be visible clinically.

Determination of Ascorbic Acid in Blood

Determination of Plasma Ascorbic Acid by 2,6-Dichlorophenolindophenol Titration

Reagents. 1. Trichloracetic acid 100 g/l, *or* freshly prepared metaphosphoric acid 50 g/l.

2. Solution of 2,6-dichlorophenolindophenol. Prepare as under urine and dilute this, 5 ml to 25 ml so that 1 ml is equivalent to 40 μg ascorbic acid.

Technique. Mix equal volumes (4 ml is convenient) of plasma separated immediately after withdrawing the blood, and of the trichloracetic or metaphosphoric acid. Filter or centrifuge. Pipette 0.2 ml of the diluted dye solution into a test tube and titrate with the filtrate until the reddish colour has disappeared.

Calculation. Since 0.2 ml dye is equivalent to 8 μg ascorbic acid.

Plasma ascorbic acid (mg/l)

$$= \frac{1000}{\text{ml titration}} \times 2 \times \frac{8}{1000} = \frac{16}{\text{ml titration}}$$

Notes. 1. Whilst metaphosphoric acid has advantages over trichloracetic acid, even in the solid form it keeps poorly once the reagent bottle has been opened, so it is usually more convenient to use trichloracetic acid.

2. If the plasma cannot be separated immediately, blood can be preserved by the method used by Mindlin and Butler (1938). The blood is

254 *Practical Clinical Biochemistry*

collected into a test tube containing 1 drop each of potassium cyanide (50 g/l) and potassium oxalate (200 g/l) for 4 to 5 ml of blood.

Mindlin and Butler have also used a method in which an excess of dye is added to plasma, and the amount of unreduced dye is determined colorimetrically.

Determination of Plasma Ascorbic Acid by the 2,4-Dinitrophenylhydrazine Method (Roe and Kuether, 1943; Roe, 1961).

The ascorbic acid is converted to dehydroascorbic acid by shaking with Norit and this is then coupled with 2,4-dinitrophenylhydrazine in presence of thiourea as a mild reducing agent. Sulphuric acid then converts the dinitrophenylhydrazone into a red compound which is assayed colorimetrically.

Reagents. 1. Trichloracetic acid solution, 60 g/l.

2. 2,4-Dinitrophenylhydrazine reagent. Dissolve 2 g of the solid in 100 ml sulphuric acid (1 part of concentrated acid added to 3 parts water). Add 4 g thiourea and shake to dissolve. Filter when necessary and keep in the refrigerator. To check whether enough thiourea is present add the reagent drop by drop to 2 ml mercuric chloride solution containing 10 g/l. A copious precipitate of mercurous chloride should form after adding 2 to 5 drops.

3. Acid washed Norit. Place 200 g Norit in a large flask, add a litre of hydrochloric acid (100 ml concentrated acid plus 900 ml water), heat to boiling and filter with suction. Transfer the cake of Norit to a beaker, add a litre of water, stir thoroughly and filter. Repeat until the washings show a negative test for Fe^{3+} ions. Dry overnight at $110\text{-}120^\circ$ C (not higher). Some batches of Norit do not need this washing. If a blank using unwashed Norit treated with trichloracetic acid is the same as with trichloracetic acid alone, then washing is unnecessary.

4. Sulphuric acid. Add 900 ml concentrated acid to 100 ml water.

5. Standard solutions of ascorbic acid. Prepare a stock standard by dissolving 50 mg in 100 ml trichloracetic acid solution, 40 g/l, or oxalic acid solution, 5 g/l. For the working standard dilute 2 ml of this to 100 ml with the acid solution used. This solution contains 10 mg/l.

Technique. To 6 ml trichloracetic acid in a centrifuge tube add 2 ml plasma slowly, with constant stirring to produce a fine suspension. Stand 5 min, centrifuge, then add 300 mg Norit to the supernatant fluid, shake vigorously and filter. Place 2 ml of the filtrate into each of two test tubes. Keep one for the blank and to the other, the test, add 0.5 ml 2,4-dinitrophenylhydrazine reagent. Stopper and place in a water bath at 37° C for exactly 3 h. Remove and place both test and blank in ice-cold water and slowly add 2.5 ml sulphuric acid, drop by drop, taking about half a minute to do so, so that there is no appreciable rise in temperature. Finally add 0.5 ml dinitrophenylhydrazine to the blank. Mix well the contents of both tubes while still in iced water. Remove, and after 30 min

Vitamins 255

read at 540 nm, or using a yellow green filter against the blank. As standard treat 2 ml of the working standard in the same way as the test.

Calculation.

$$\text{Plasma ascorbic acid (mg/l)} = \frac{\text{Reading of the unknown}}{\text{Reading of standard}} \times 10.$$

A standard curve can be prepared as follows:

Plasma ascorbic acid (mg/l)	0	2.5	5.0	7.5	10.0	12.5	15.0	20.0
Standard solution, 10 mg/l (ml)	0	0.5	1.0	1.5	2.0	2.5	3.0	4.0
Trichloracetic acid, 40 g/l, (ml)	8.0	7.5	7.0	6.5	6.0	5.5	5.0	4.0

Add Norit, shake, stand, filter, take 2 ml filtrate, and proceed as described for the test.

INTERPRETATION

Plasma ascorbic acid levels are of limited value in diagnosing scurvy and subclinical conditions of ascorbic acid under-nutrition. Various levels from about 7 mg/l downwards have been stated to indicate scurvy, but while persons on an adequate intake will generally be found to have a plasma level 4 to 20 mg/l with typical values from 8 to 14, it would appear that values below this are obtained in apparently healthy persons. However, values below 2 mg/l suggest the possibility of marked ascorbic acid deficiency.

It has been shown (Crandon *et al.*, 1940; see also Butler and Cushman, 1940; Butler *et al.*, 1943) that ascorbic acid disappears more rapidly from the plasma than from the cells when a diet low in vitamin C is taken. The largest concentration of ascorbic acid is in the leucocytes and in the platelets. The white cells appear to be the last to be depleted. The fall in leucocyte ascorbic acid is more gradual than that of plasma ascorbic acid which reaches very low values much earlier. Determination of leucocyte ascorbic acid has been used as a better indication of a severe deficiency.

Determination of Leucocyte Ascorbic Acid (Denson and Bowers, 1961; Gibson *et al.*, 1966)

Blood is put into a diluent containing sodium chloride, EDTA as anti-coagulant, and dextran which brings about rouleaux formation of the red cells causing them to settle out more rapidly on standing. The white cells and platelets which remain suspended are recovered from the supernatant fluid by centrifugation and redissolved in trichloracetic acid. The ascorbic acid content is determined by the 2,4-dinitrophenylhydrazone method.

Reagents. 1. Diluent. Mix 200 ml sodium chloride solution, 8.5 g/l, 50 ml dextran, 60 g/l, and 2 ml sodium edetate, 100 g/l. Measure 12.5 ml

256 *Practical Clinical Biochemistry*

portions into Universal Containers and autoclave for 15 min at a pressure of 5 lb/in^2 (35 kPa).

2. Trichloracetic acid solution, 50 g/l.

3. Colour reagent. Mix in the proportions 20/1/1 the solutions: 2,4-dinitrophenylhydrazine, 22 g/l in sulphuric acid, 10 mol/l; thiourea 50 g/l water; copper sulphate, 6 g $CuSO_4, 5H_2O$/1 water.

4. Sulphuric acid, 650 ml/l.

5. Standard ascorbic acid solution, 10 mg/l trichloracetic acid, 50 g/l.

Technique. Collect 3 ml venous blood and add immediately to a container of diluent. Mix, and allow to stand for 30 min for the red cells to settle, most of which will have done so in this time. Take off the supernatant, mix well and centrifuge 10 ml for 15 min at 3 000 r.p.m. Discard the supernatant allowing the tube to drain for 30 sec. Add 1.3 ml trichloracetic acid to the compact button of leucocytes and platelets, homogenise thoroughly, centrifuge and transfer 1 ml of the supernatant to a test tube (7.5 × 1.3 cm). In other tubes place 1 ml trichloracetic acid (for the blank) and as standards (a) 0.5 ml standard + 0.5 ml trichloracetic acid, (b) 1.0 ml standard. To each tube add 0.3 ml colour reagent and incubate 4 h at 37° C. Cool in iced water, add 2 ml sulphuric acid, mix, and read the extinction at 520 nm zeroing with the blank.

Carry out a leucocyte count on the remainder of the original supernatant using a 1 in 50 dilution in the Coulter Counter and subtracting the background blank.

Calculation. A standard curve can be prepared by putting through the following:

Supernatant fluid (mg/l)	0	1	2	4	6	8	10
Standard (ml)	0	0.1	0.2	0.4	0.6	0.8	1.0
Trichloracetic acid (ml)	1.0	0.9	0.8	0.6	0.4	0.2	0

Ascorbic acid content of supernatant (mg/l)

$$= \frac{\text{Reading of unknown}}{\text{Reading of standard}} \times 10 \text{ for standard (b)} \quad \text{or} \times 5 \text{ for (a)}.$$

and Buffy layer (leucocyte + platelet) ascorbic acid (μg/10^8 leucocytes)

$$= \frac{\text{Supernatant ascorbic acid (mg/l)} \times 1.3}{\text{Leucocyte count}/\mu\text{l supernatant}}$$

INTERPRETATION

In normal blood the concentration of ascorbic acid in leucocytes and platelets is about the same. If the number of either of these is abnormal the buffy layer ascorbic acid level is a misleading index of leucocyte ascorbic acid concentration. Gibson *et al.* proposed a formula for deriving the leucocyte ascorbic acid value from the buffy layer result in various haematological conditions.

$$\text{Leucocyte ascorbic acid} = \frac{\text{Buffy layer ascorbic acid}}{\text{Conversion factor}}$$

Vitamins 257

When the platelet and leucocyte counts are normal the factor is 2.0 (SD 0.32). In patients with thrombocytopenia and normal leucocyte counts the value for the leucocyte layer approaches that of the buffy coat layer. The mean ratio of the buffy coat layer ascorbic acid to leucocyte ascorbic acid is 1.3 (SD 0.02). In patients with various types of leukemia with normal platelet counts but increased white cell counts the ratio is similar. In thrombocythaemic patients with a relative increase in the number of platelets over leucocytes the ratio is 3.0 (SD 0.66).

The normal range for the buffy layer is given as 21 to 57 $\mu g/10^8$ leucocytes and for the leucocytes alone 11 to 21 $\mu g/10^8$ leucocytes.

REFERENCES

Axelrod, A. E., Spies, T. D., Elvehjem, C. A. and Axelrod, V. (1941), *J. clin. Invest.*, **20**, 229.
Baker, H. and Frank, O. (1968), *Clinical Vitaminology*, Wiley, New York. p. 172.
Baker, H. and Sobotka, H. (1962), *Advances in Clinical Chemistry*, edited H. Sobotka, and C. P. Stewart, Academic Press, New York, Volume 5, p. 178.
Barnes, B. C., Wollaeger, E. E. and Mason, H. L. (1950), *J. clin. Invest.*, **29**, 982.
Bashir, H. V., Hinterbergen, H. and Jones, B. P. (1966), *Brit. J. Haematol.*, **12**, 704.
Bessey, O. A., Adams, D. J. B and Hauser, A. E. (1957), *Pediatrics*, **20**, 33.
Bessey, O. A., Lowry, O. H., Brock, M. J. and Lopez, J. A. (1946), *J. biol. Chem.*, **166**, 177.
Braybrooke, J., Lloyd, B., Nattrass, M. and Alberti, K. G. M. M. (1975), *Ann. clin. Biochem.*, **12**, 252.
Brin, M. (1962), *Ann. N.Y. Acad. Sci.*, **98**, 528.
Brin, M. (1964), *J. Amer. med. Ass.*, **187**, 762.
Brin, M. (1965), *Amer. J. clin. Nutr.*, **17**, 240.
Brin, M. (1967), *Newer Methods of Nutritional Biochemistry*, Vol. 3, edited A. Albanese, Academic Press, New York and London, p. 407.
Brin, M., Tai, M., Ostashever, A. S. and Kalinski, H. (1960), *J. Nutr.*, **71**, 273.
Bueding, E., Stein, M. H. and Wortis, H. (1941), *J. biol. Chem.*, **137**, 793.
Butler, A. M. and Cushman, M. (1940), *J. clin. Invest.*, **19**, 459.
Butler, A. M., Cushman, M. and MacLachen, E. A. (1943), *J. biol. Chem.*, **150**, 453.
Campbell, D. A. and Tonks, E. L. (1949), *Brit. med. J.*, **2**, 1499.
Chanarin, I. (1969), *The Megaloblastic Anaemias*, Blackwell, Oxford.
Cheldelin, V. H., Bennett, M. J. and Kornberg, H. A. (1946), *J. biol. Chem.*, **166**, 779.
Cox, E. V. and White, A. M. (1962), *Lancet*, **2**, 853.
Crandon, J. H., Lund, C. C. and Dill, D. B. (1940), *New Eng. J. Med.*, **223**, 353.
Dale, H. (1972), *Clin. chim. Acta*, **41**, 141.
Davies, G., Kennedy, J. H. and Westwood, A. To be published.
Denson, K. W. and Bowers, E. F. (1961), *Clin. Sci.*, **21**, 157.
Dreyfuss, P. M. and Dubé, V. E. (1967), *Clin. chim. Acta*, **15**, 525.
Dugan, R. E., Frigerio, N. A. and Siebert, J. M. (1964), *Anal. Chem.*, **36**, 114.
Friedemann, T. E. and Frazier, A. N. (1950), *Arch. Biochem.*, **26**, 361.
Friedemann, T. E., and Haugen, G. E. (1943), *J. biol. Chem.*, **147**, 415.
Friedemann, T. E., and Kmieciak, T. C. (1942-3), *J. Lab. clin. Med.*, **28**, 1262.
Gawthorne, J. M., Gabor, J. and Stockstad, E. L. R. (1971), *Anal. Biochem.*, **42**, 555.
Gibbs, B. F., Itiaba, K., Marner, O. A., Crawhall, J. C. and Cooper, B. A. (1972), *Clin. chim. Acta*, **38**, 447.
Gibson, S. L. M., Moore, F. M. L. and Goldberg, A. (1966), *Brit. med. J.*, **1**, 1152.
Giorgio, A. J. (1970) in *Methods in Enzymology*, edited McCormick, D. B. and Wright, L. D., Academic Press, Vol. 18, Part C, p. 103.

258 *Practical Clinical Biochemistry*

Giorgio, A. J. and Plaut, G. W. E. (1965), *J. Lab. clin. Med.*, **66**, 667.
Gloster, J. A. and Harris, P. (1962), *Clin. chim. Acta*, **7**, 206.
Gompertz, D. (1968), *Clin. chim. Acta.*, **19**, 477.
Gompertz, D., Jones, J. H., and Knowles, J. P. (1967), *Clin. chim. Acta*, **18**, 197.
Green, A. (1968), *J. clin. Path.*, **21**, 221.
Green, A. E. and Pegrum, G. D. (1968), *Brit. med. J.*, **3**, 591.
Gutteridge, J. M. C. and Wright, E. B. (1970), *Clin. chim. Acta*, **27**, 289.
György, P. and Pearson, W. N., editors (1967), *The Vitamins*, Volumes VI and VII. Academic Press.
Haig, C. and Patek, A. J. (1942), *J. clin. Invest.*, **21**, 377.
Harris, L. J. and Abbasy, M. A. (1937), *Lancet*, **2**, 1429.
Harris, L. J. and Ray, S. N. (1935), *Lancet*, **1**, 71, 462.
Haworth, C., Oliver, R. W. A. and Swaile, R. A. (1971), *Analyst*, **96**, 432.
Hochberg, M., Melnick, D. and Oser, B. L. (1945), *J. biol. Chem.*, **158**, 265.
Hoffmann, N. E. and Barboriak, J. J. (1967), *Anal. Biochem.*, **18**, 10.
Huff, J. W. and Perlzweig, W. A. (1947), *J. biol. Chem.*, **167**, 157.
Jacobs, S. (1960), *Analyst*, **85**, 257.
Johnson, R. E., Sargent, F., Robinson, P. F. and Consolazio, F. C. (1945), *Ind. Eng. Chem., Anal. Ed.*, **17**, 384.
Kagan, M., Thomas, E. M., Jordan, D. A. and Abt, A. F. (1950), *J. clin. Invest.*, **29**, 141.
Karmarker, G. and Rajagopal, K. (1952), *Curr. Sci.*, **21**, 193.
Kaser, M. and Stekol, J. A. (1943), *J. Lab. clin. Med.*, **28**, 904.
Kimble, M. S. (1938-9), *J. Lab. clin. Med.*, **24**, 1055.
Kleeberg, J. and Gitelson, S. (1954), *J. clin. Path.*, **7**, 116.
Krebs, H. A. (1950), *Ann. Rev. Biochem.*, **19**, 420.
Krebs, H. A. and Hume, E. M. (1949), Medical Research Council Special Report Series, No. 264.
Kohn, J. (1964), *J. clin. Path.*, **17**, 466.
Kohn, J. and Feinberg, J. G. (1965), *Electrophoresis on Cellulose Acetate*, Shandon Monographs on Scientific Techniques, No. 11, p. 12.
Kohn, J., Mollin, D. L. and Rosenbach, L. M. (1961), *J. clin. Path.*, **14**, 345.
Lancet (1974), Leading article, **2**, 26.
Lepkovsky, S. and Nielson, E. (1942), *J. biol. Chem.*, **144**, 135.
Lepkovsky, S., Roboz, E. and Haagen-Smit, A. J. (1943), *J. biol. Chem.*, **149**, 195.
Levin, B., Oberholzer, V. G., Burgess, E. A. and Young, W. F. (1966), *Lancet*, **2**, 1415.
Lindquist, T. (1938), *Acta med. Scand.*, **97**, Suppl., p. 1.
Luhby, A. L. and Cooperman, J. M. (1964), *Advances in Metabolic Disorders*, edited R. Levine and R. Luft, Academic Press, New York, Volume 1, p. 262.
Luhby, A. L., Cooperman, J. M. and Teller, D. N. (1959), *Proc. Soc. exper. Biol. and Med.*, **101**, 350.
Luhby, A. L., Cooperman, J. M., MacIver, J. E. and Montgomery, R. D. (1962), *Proc. Soc. Pediat. Res.*, p. 84.
Mason, H. L. and Williams, R. D. (1942), *J. clin. Invest.*, **21**, 247.
Meiklejohn, A. P. (1937), *Biochem. J.*, **31**, 1441.
Melnick, D. (1942), *J. Nutrition*, **24**, 139.
Melnick, D. and Field, H., Jr. (1942), *J. Nutrition*, **24**, 131.
Mindlin, R. L. and Butler, A. M. (1938), *J. biol. Chem.*, **122**, 673.
Najjar, V. A. (1941), *J. biol. Chem.*, **141**, 355.
Najjar, V. A. and Holt, L. E., Jr. (1940), *Bull. Johns Hopk. Hosp.*, **67**, 107.
Najjar, V. A. and Holt, L. E., Jr. (1941), *Science*, **93**, 20.
Najjar, V. A. and Wood, R. W. (1940), *Proc. Soc. exper. Biol.*, **44**, 386.
Noeypatimanond, S., Watson-Williams, E. J. and Israëls, M. C. G. (1966), *Lancet*, **1**, 454.
Paterson, J. C. S. and Wiggins, H. S. (1954), *J. clin. Path.*, **7**, 56.
Pearson, W. N. (1967), in Gyorgy and Pearson above, Vol. VI, p. 87.

Vitamins 259

Pelletier, O. and Campbell, J. A. (1962), *Anal. Biochem.*, 3, 60.

Price, J. M., Brown, R. R. and Yess, N. (1965), *Advances in Metabolic Disorders*, edited R. Levine and R. Luft, Academic Press, New York, Volume 2, p. 159.

Quaife, M. L., Scrimshan, N. S. and Lowry, O. H. (1949), *J. biol. Chem.*, 80, 1229.

Roe, J. H. (1961), *Standard Methods of Clinical Chemistry*, Volume III, edited David Seligson, Academic Press, New York, p. 35.

Roe, J. H. and Kuether, C. A. (1943), *J. biol. Chem.*, 147, 399.

Rosenblum, L. A. and Joliffe, N. (1940), *J. biol. Chem.*, 134, 137.

Sammons, H. G., Harding, V. and Frazer, A. C. (1961), *Proc. Ass. clin. Biochem.*, 1, 70.

Sarett, H. P. and Cheldelin, V. H. (1944), *J. biol. Chem.*, 171, 617.

Satoh, K. and Price, J. M. (1958), *J. biol. Chem.*, 230, 781.

Sebrell, W. H., Jr. and Harris, R. S., editors (1967), *The Vitamins*, Volumes I-V, Academic Press.

Sinclair, H. M. (1938), *Biochem. J.*, 32, 2185.

Sinclair, H. M. (1939), *Biochem. J.*, 33, 2027.

Sinclair, H. M. (1947), *Recent Advances in Clinical Pathology*, edited S. C. Dyke, 1st edition, p. 180, Churchill, London.

Slater, E. C. and Morell, D. B. (1946), *Biochem. J.*, 40, 644, 652.

Sobel, A. E. and Snow, S. D. (1947), *J. biol. Chem.*, 152, 445.

Tabor, H. and Wyngarden, L. (1958), *J. clin. Invest.*, 37, 824.

Wang, Y. L. and Kodicek, E. (1943), *Biochem. J.*, 37, 530.

Wenger, J., Kirsner, J. B. and Palmer, W. L. (1957), *Amer. J. Med.*, 22, 373.

White, A. M. (1971), in *Methods in Enzymology*, Vol. 18, Part C, edited McCormick, D. B. and Wright, L. D., Academic Press, p. 101.

Williams, R. D., Mason, H. L., Power, M. H. and Wilder, R. M. (1943), *Arch. int. Med.*, 71, 38.

Yudkin, S. (1941), *Biochem. J.*, 35, 551.

CHAPTER 7

DRUGS AND POISONS

THIS chapter describes the detection and, in some cases, the quantitation of a number of drugs and poisons. The publication "Hospital Treatment of Acute Poisoning" (HM (68) 92, Department of Health and Social Security, HMSO, London, 1968) required hospital laboratories to be capable of determining salicylate, barbiturates and iron in blood or gastric aspirates; ethanol and carboxyhaemoglobin in blood. Screening tests for phenothiazines in urine were also required. Such methods are covered here but in view of the large number of drugs, perhaps as many as 6 000, currently used the range has been extended to include groups which the clinical biochemist may also be asked to investigate.

Several aspects of the subject require consideration. Firstly there are differences in the rate of metabolism of many drugs between individuals (Vesell and Passananti, 1971). For long term treatment of chronic disorders it is important to maintain the plasma concentration of a drug between certain limits for optimal activity. Individual adjustment of dose to match the rate of metabolism is needed to avoid low concentrations with inadequate control, or abnormally high ones with the possibility of toxic effects. The situation may be complicated by the simultaneous use of other drugs which can modify the metabolism of the drug under consideration; this is sometimes due to enzyme "induction". This is also seen after the administration of a drug has been continued for several days and is part of the development of "tolerance" whereby a patient is able to take much larger doses of a drug and to tolerate much higher drug levels than is the case for acute ingestion of the same agent. The need for monitoring of drug therapy often requires the development of sensitive and specific quantitative methods.

Secondly a number of drugs are taken in large doses for their effects on the mental state. Although some of these drugs such as alcohol, caffeine and nicotine, may be socially acceptable under defined circumstances, others are carefully controlled as drugs of abuse under the Misuse of Drugs Act. Their intake causes drug dependence or addiction and the detection of these substances may be required. The methods are most often qualitative.

Thirdly, drugs may be taken in large doses in acute poisoning. Most of these cases are of self-poisoning, not done with suicidal intent but in an effort to attract attention to problems which loom large in the mind of the patient. A minority are true suicidal attempts and a similar number may be accidental or homicidal poisonings. Death may occur in self-poisoning and in all cases is more likely the larger the dose of the poison. In many cases there will be no specific therapy but proper management, in an intensive care unit for the more serious cases, is assisted by recognition of the poison. This can involve examination of blood, urine and gastric aspirate. It is often

Drugs and Poisons 261

sufficient to perform qualitative analyses, but in a few cases actual determination of drug concentration is necessary.

With the introduction and wide prescription of a variety of potentially lethal drugs these have become much commoner agents in acute poisoning than household chemicals or coal gas. The commonest drugs taken in such circumstances are barbiturates, then come the tranquillisers, non-barbiturate hypnotics and anti-depressants. All these may be prescribed for mentally disturbed patients. Aspirin and paracetamol are also fairly commonly taken and are readily available. The relative incidence of the different drugs used varies with age, sex, geographical area and prescribing fashions. There is an increasing tendency to take several different drugs, and in about a third of cases, at least in Edinburgh, alcohol is one of these. Not all drugs are equally toxic and barbiturates are involved in over half the fatal cases due to solids or liquids (Table 7,1 and 7,2). In fatal cases due to solid or liquid poisons only 64 per cent are attributable to a single poison. In the rest an average of 2.1 poisons is used. Deaths due to gases or vapours are becoming less common. Of these the great majority are due to carbon monoxide either from piped gases or from car exhaust fumes or faulty heaters.

Fourthly, increasing concern about environmental pollution has particularly involved such toxic metals as lead and mercury and to a lesser extent, cadmium. Their quantitative measurement, often at low concentrations, is often mandatory for certain employees in industry, but monitoring members of the general public thought to be exposed to environmental contamination may be requested.

In this chapter the various drugs and poisons are dealt with alphabetically either individually or as groups with similar actions. Qualitative and quantitative methods appear within this scheme. In most cases it has been decided to use mass concentration rather than molar concentration, as drugs are prescribed and dispensed in mass units.

For a comprehensive account of techniques for the determination and detection of drugs see Stolman and Stewart (1960, 1961), Curry (1969a), Clarke (1969, 1975), and Sunshine (1969). Simple qualitative tests are described by Meade *et al.* (1972). Several useful papers will also be found in the Special Issue on Toxicology of the Annals of Clinical Biochemistry (1971) and the Special Issue — "Toxicology and Drug Assay", of Clinical Chemistry (1974).

Details of a large number of drugs including composition, uses, doses, metabolism, etc., are given in Martindale (1972). An up to date list of ethical drugs is published monthly as the Monthly Index of Medical Specialties (MIMS) produced by Haymarket Publishing Ltd., London.

Some General Considerations Concerning Methods

Several types of technique are available. The choice will depend partly on the knowledge as to which drugs are likely to be present, whether

TABLE 7,1

Deaths by Poisoning[1], England and Wales, 1973
(Adapted from Pharm. J., 214, 260, (1975).)

1—Deaths by suicide; 11—Deaths by accidental poisoning; 111—Deaths by poisoning undetermined whether accidentally or purposely inflicted. (Figures in parentheses are cases in which other poisons were simultaneously involved).

	1	11	111	Total	
A. Hypnotics [1062 + (1605) = 2667]					
(i) *Barbiturates* [971 + (1418) = 2389]					
Amylobarbitone[2]	179	35	72	286	905
	(348)	(136)	(135)	(619)	
Quinalbarbitone[2]	35	8	8	51	627
	(330)	(124)	(122)	(576)	
Pentobarbitone	111	28	45	184	273
	(53)	(13)	(23)	(89)	
Butobarbitone	108	21	28	157	205
	(33)	(7)	(8)	(48)	
Phenobarbitone	37	12	16	65	103
	(18)	(8)	(12)	(38)	
Other (barbitone, cyclobarbitone	13	—	6	19	23
heptabarbitone, hexobarbitone	(2)	(1)	(1)	(4)	
sodium, thiopentone)					
Unspecified barbiturate	107	50	52	209	253
	(30)	(10)	(4)	(44)	
(ii) *Non-barbiturates* [91 + (187) = 278]					
Nitrazepam	21	6	5	32	77
	(36)	(5)	(4)	(45)	
Methaqualone[3]	—	1	1	2	74
	(45)	(14)	(13)	(72)	
Carbromal[4]	—	—	—	—	50
	(36)	(7)	(7)	(50)	
Glutethimide	13	2	6	21	30
	(3)	(—)	(6)	(9)	
Chloral and related compounds	7	1	10	18	26
	(3)	(4)	(1)	(8)	
Others (ethchlorvynol,	4	1	2	7	9
methyprylone, paraldehyde)	(2)	(—)	(—)	(2)	
Unstated hypnotics	4	5	2	11	12
	(—)	(1)	(—)	(1)	

(1) Alcohol is excluded as a contributory factor. The Annual Report of the Registrar-General for 1971, suggests that it is a contributory factor in nearly 10 per cent of poisonings of this type.
(2) Tuinal (amylo- and quinalbarbitones) accounts for most of the figures in parentheses.
(3) Almost entirely as Mandrax (methaqualone and diphenhydramine).
(4) All as Carbitral (carbromal and pentobarbitone).

Drugs and Poisons

TABLE 7,1 (continued)

	1	11	111	Total	
. Analgesics [281 + (159) = 440]					
Aspirin, salicylic acid, salicylamide	150 (44)	22 (5)	22 (9)	194 (58)	252
Paracetamol	44 (33)	11 (6)	11 (8)	66 (47)	113
Dextropropoxyphene	1 (15)	— (4)	4 (7)	5 (26)	31
Phenacetin	1 (11)	1 (3)	— (2)	2 (16)	18
Others (dipipanone, methadone, pentazocine, pethidine, phenazocine, phenylbutazone, methyl salicylate)	6 (8)	3 (3)	5 (1)	14 (12)	26
, Antidepressants [174 + (138) = 312]					
(i) *Dibenzazepines* [47 + (30) = 77]					
Imipramine	20 (15)	6 (1)	8 (2)	34 (18)	52
Trimipramine	6 (5)	2 (1)	1 (2)	9 (8)	17
Others (clomipramine, desipramine, opipramol)	2 (3)	1 (—)	1 (1)	4 (4)	8
(ii) *Dibenzocycloheptenes* [100 + (83) = 183]					
Amitriptyline	64 (50)	17 (12)	15 (13)	96 (75)	171
Nortriptyline	1 (7)	1 (—)	2 (1)	4 (8)	12
(iii) *Dibenzthiepins &-oxepins* [19 + (7) = 26]					
Dothiepin	7 (1)	2 (—)	3 (—)	12 (1)	13
Doxepin	1 (2)	4 (1)	2 (3)	7 (6)	13
(iv) *MAO inhibitors* [8 + (18) = 26]					
Phenelzine	3 (3)	1 (4)	1 (1)	5 (8)	13
Other (iproniazid, tranylcypromine, unspecified)	3 (7)	— (—)	— (3)	3 (10)	13
Tranquillisers [50 + (147) = 197]					
(i) *Benzodiazepines* [17 + (93) = 110]					
Diazepam	5 (40)	4 (10)	1 (8)	10 (58)	68
Chlordiazepoxide	5 (13)	2 (10)	— (5)	7 (28)	35

Practical Clinical Biochemistry

TABLE 7,1 (continued)

	1	11	111	Total	
Others (lorazepam, medazepam, oxazepam)	— (4)	— (—)	— (3)	— (7)	7
(ii) *Phenothiazines* [23 + (54) = 77]					
Chlorpromazine	12 (12)	2 (8)	2 (8)	16 (28)	44
Trifluoperazine	— (14)	1 (1)	— (4)	1 (19)	20
Others (fluphenazine, perphenazine, prochlorperazine, thiethylperazine, thioridazine)	2 (6)	2 (1)	2 (—)	6 (7)	13
(iii) *Other types or unstated* [10]					
(Haloperidol, hydroxyzine, meprobamate)	5 (—)	2 (—)	3 (—)	10 (—)	10
E. Antihistamines [2 + (80) = 82]					
Diphenhydramine[3]	— (47)	— (13)	— (12)	— (72)	72
Antazoline, cyclizine, pheniramine & promethazine	— (3)	1 (3)	1 (2)	2 (8)	10
F. Alkaloids [36 + (29) = 65]					
Morphine, heroin & unspecified narcotics	9 (2)	9 (2)	4 (1)	22 (5)	27
Codeine	4 (16)	— (1)	1 (2)	5 (19)	24
Dihydrocodeine	2 (1)	2 (1)	— (1)	4 (3)	7
Ergotamine, nicotine, quinine, strychnine	3 (1)	1 (1)	1 (—)	5 (2)	7
G. Alcohols[1] [57 + (0) = 57]					
Ethanol	—	50	1	51	51
Methanol preparations	1	4	1	6	6
H. Anticonvulsants [10 + (10) = 20]					
Chlormethiazole	3 (2)	3 (—)	3 (—)	9 (2)	11
Phenytoin, primidone	— (6)	— (1)	1 (1)	1 (8)	9
I. CNS stimulants [0 + (15) = 15]					
Caffeine	— (6)	— (2)	— (4)	— (12)	12
Amphetamine	— (—)	— (3)	— (—)	— (3)	3

Drugs and Poisons 265

TABLE 7,1 (continued)

	1	11	111	Total	
J. Other drugs [75 + (34) = 109]					
Orphenadrine	11	1	3	15	31
	(10)	(4)	(2)	(16)	
Cardiac glycosides	3	5	2	10	12
	(1)	(—)	(1)	(2)	
Insulin	6	1	—	7	7
	(—)	(—)	(—)	(—)	
26 others	5	11	2	18	32
	(7)	(6)	(1)	(14)	
Unspecified drugs	15	2	8	25	27
	(1)	(1)	(—)	(2)	
K. Chemicals [123 + (3) = 126]					
Corrosive poisons (phenolics, acids, alkalis)	29	4	2	35	36
	(—)	(—)	(1)	(1)	
Inorganic—cyanides	20	—	5	25	
Cd, Fe, Pb, Mn	—	8	—	8	37 (2)
Other	3	1	—	4	39
	(1)	(—)	(1)	(2)	
Weedkillers—Paraquat	10	4	4	18	
Chlorate	2	2	2	6	37
Other	9	0	4	13	
Solvents (various)	6	3	1	10	
Other household chemicals	—	4	—	4	
TOTAL POISONS	1118	370	382	1868	
	(1336)	(438)	(446)	(2220)	
TOTAL DEATHS	1741	579	594	2914	

TABLE 7,2

Deaths by Poisoning, England and Wales, 1973

1—Deaths by suicide; *11*—Deaths by accidental poisoning; *111*—Deaths by poisoning undetermined whether accidentally or purposely inflicted. (Figures in parentheses are cases in which other poisons were simultaneously involved).

	1	11	111	Total
Drugs, medicaments, other solids and liquids	1741	579	594	2914
Gases or vapours	426	197	31	654
(1971 figures)	(613)	(297)	(37)	(947)

(Compiled from Quarterly Returns of the Registrar-General)

266 *Practical Clinical Biochemistry*

qualitative or quantitative methods are required, the equipment and time available, and the nature of the material for analysis.

Material for Analysis

Most investigations are carried out on blood, urine, vomit, or gastric aspirate, the stomach contents removed before gastric lavage commences. Occasionally tablets, capsules etc., may be submitted. In the latter case identification is aided by published lists categorising preparations by size, colour and manufacturer's markings (The Chemist and Druggist. Tablet and Capsule Identification Guide. Mark 2. Morgan Brothers (Publishers) Ltd., 28 Essex Street, Strand, London, WC2.)

Gastric aspirate if removed within an hour or two of ingestion of the poisoning agent often contains this in relatively high concentration and in chemically unchanged form. Sometimes tablet residues or characteristic odours can aid identification. Separation from other gastric contents usually requires extraction procedures (see opposite).

Blood can usually be obtained and is best anticoagulated so that the maximum volume can be extracted if necessary. Some drugs are rapidly removed from the circulation by the tissues making identification or quantitation more difficult. The blood concentration is often important for therapeutic monitoring but is less essential for the treatment of poisoning. Extraction procedures are usually needed, the extracts being relatively free from interfering substances. The simpler qualitative tests are not usually applicable but more elaborate quantitative or qualitative methods are available. Metabolites of the drug are sometimes present in the circulation but this is usually less of a problem than with urine.

Urine has the advantage that it is often available in large quantities. A number of drugs are not excreted as such and the urine may contain several metabolites some of which can be detected by simple qualitative tests. Extraction procedures and more elaborate methods for detection and quantitation are possible but variable metabolism between individuals may make interpretation difficult. One advantage is that drugs can usually be detected in the urine, often as metabolites, for some time after they have become undetectable in blood.

Extraction Methods (Clarke, 1975)

In many cases, and particularly when the nature of the drug or poison is unknown, preparation of suitable extracts, fractionated according to simple chemical properties, is invaluable. The following methods are suitable for general use. If the nature of the agent is known they may be modified or simplified.

In the case of urine or gastric aspirate limitation of volume is rarely a problem and the extracts separate strongly acidic, weakly acidic, neutral and basic drugs all of which are soluble in organic solvents (Table 7,3). The

Drugs and Poisons

TABLE 7,3
Extraction of Urine, Gastric Aspirate or Blood (if sufficient)

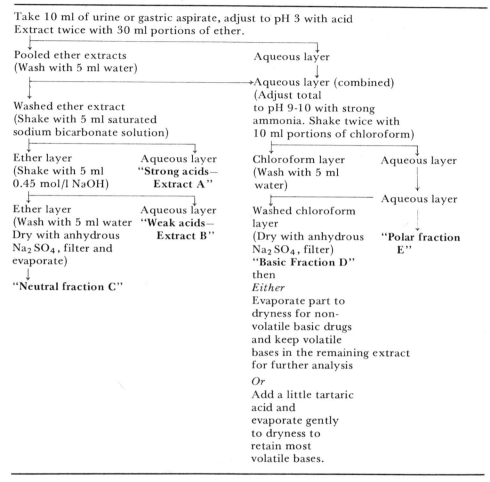

polar fraction E contains toxic anions such as bromide, chlorate and oxalate; organic anions such as paraquat, bretylium and, for gastric aspirates, water-insoluble materials. The same technique can be used for blood if enough is available. Otherwise a modified technique (Table 7,4) is used to conserve material but at the expense of less clear cut separation.

The commoner drugs occur in these fractions as follows:

Extract A. Important members are salicylic acid and aspirin. Some phenytoin may be extracted.

Extract B. This includes anticonvulsants such as phenytoin and some primidone (much in E); hypnotics such as barbiturates and glutethimide (some); analgesics such as paracetamol and its metabolite *p*-aminophenol,

TABLE 7,4
Extraction of Blood

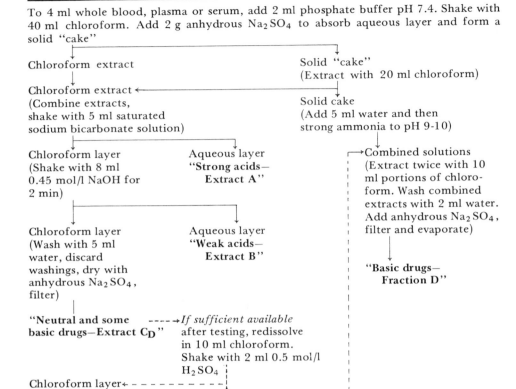

If enough blood still available, adjust to pH 9-10 with strong ammonia. Extract twice with 10 ml portions of chloroform. Add anhydrous Na₂SO₄, filter and evaporate. "**Basic and some neutral drugs—Extract Dc**".

phenylbutazone and salicylamide; tranquillisers such as the lactam of chlordiazepoxide.

Extract C. This includes anticonvulsants such as methoin, ethotoin, ethosuximide, methsuximide, phensuximide, paramethadione and troxidone; hypnotics such as carbromal (gastric aspirate only), ethchlorvynol, ethinamate, glutethimide, methyprylone; analgesics such as paracetamol (part), phenacetin and phenazone; tranquillisers such as meprobamate, and antidepressants such as amitriptyline (part).

Extract C_D includes in addition the hypnotic methaqualone and tranquillisers of the benzodiazepine group.

Drugs and Poisons

Extract D. Many drugs contain one of a relatively small number of basic side chains and are found in this group. These include many of the tranquillisers, antidepressants, alkaloids and volatile amines.

Simple Colour Tests.

These may be used on the extracts prepared above or in some cases directly on urine and occasionally on gastric contents and even serum. Details are given below for particular substances.

Chromatographic Methods

These are applied to suitably purified extracts for further characterisation.

Paper chromatography is much less used than previously. For an account and details of methods see Fox (1969, 1975).

Thin-layer chromatography (TLC) has largely replaced paper for qualitative work in view of its speed, high resolution, sensitivity, and suitability for more corrosive detecting agents. Curry (1969b, 1975) discusses several solvent systems for use with silica gel plates for different classes of compounds, and specific and general purpose detecting agents.

Gas-liquid chromatography (GLC) has been increasingly used to investigate extracts. The high resolving power, speed, and use for quantitation are important. For a general review see Leach (1969, 1975).

Spectroscopic Methods

Many drugs show characteristic absorption spectra, sometimes altering with pH, which are helpful in the examination of extracts.

Ultra-violet absorption spectroscopy is convenient as equipment is widely available. The position of the absorption peaks and their shift with pH help identification and the intensity is used under certain conditions to determine drugs. For details of spectra see Clarke (1969, 1975).

Infra-red absorption spectroscopy provides much more characteristic absorption peaks over the wavelength range 2.5 to 15.4 μm (frequency 4 000 to 650 cm^{-1}) and particularly so in the "fingerprint region" 6.25 to 15.4 μm (1 600 to 650 cm^{-1}). Such spectra provide a highly selective method for characterising drugs. The structure of their metabolites can also often be determined by such methods. The main problem for routine use is that the sample for analysis must be as pure as possible and often 50 μg is required. This implies a further careful purification of the original extract. Gas chromatography offers the best method of separation from other components but the technique of collection from the column effluent and further handling are only applicable to specialised laboratories. An atlas of infra-red spectra is given by Clarke (1969, 1975).

270 *Practical Clinical Biochemistry*

Mass spectroscopy has been used increasingly lately. The instrument can conveniently be combined with a gas chromatograph so that the emerging peak from the column can be examined directly by mass fragmentation. The spectra are usually highly specific and are applicable to the identification of the structure of drug metabolites.

AMPHETAMINES AND OTHER STIMULANT OR ANORECTIC AMINES

dl-Amphetamine, its *d*-isomer dexamphetamine, and its methyl derivative methylamphetamine, are examples of volatile basic drugs obtained by the usual extraction methods. When such extracts are evaporated, even at room temperature, serious losses can occur. These drugs, which cause stimulation of the CNS, are addictive and their use is controlled by the Misuse of Drugs Act. The volatile amine, propylhexedrine, is used as a vasoconstrictor in nasal inhalers. Other volatile amines include the appetite-suppressant or anorectic drugs, fenfluramine, phentermine and chlorphentermine, the alkaloid nicotine, and the addictive base, pethidine.

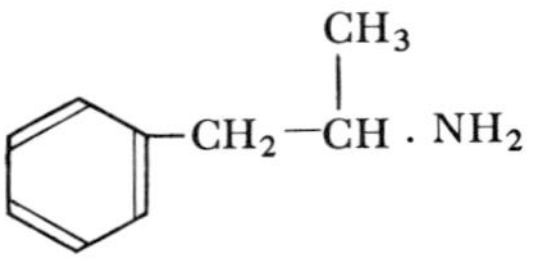

amphetamine*, dexamphetamine*
(Dexamed, Dexedrine, Durophet)

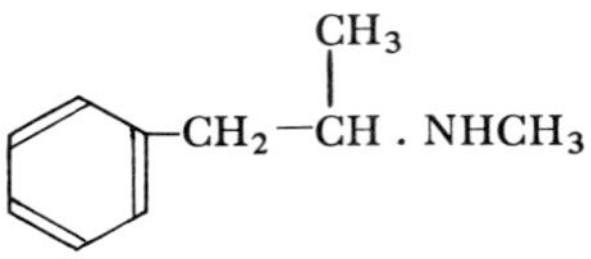

methylamphetamine*
(Methedrine)

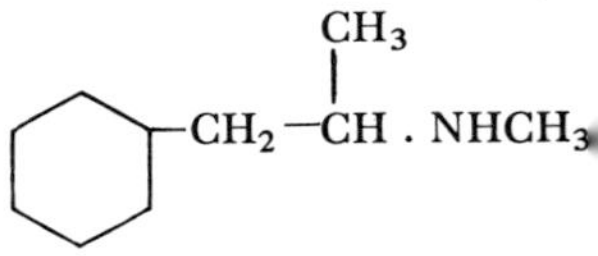

propylhexedrine
(Benzedrex)

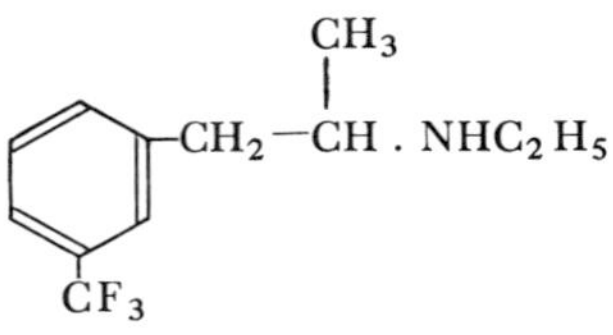

fenfluramine
(Ponderax)

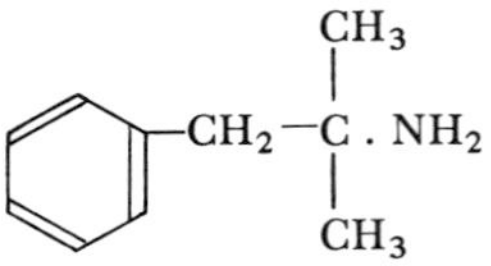

phentermine
(Duromine, Ionamine)

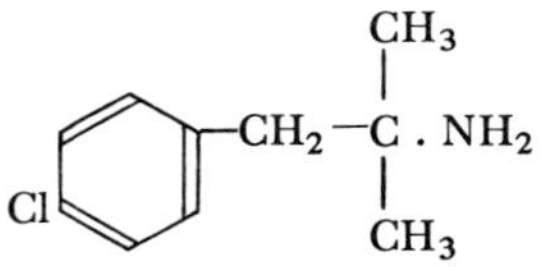

chlorphentermine
(Lucophen)

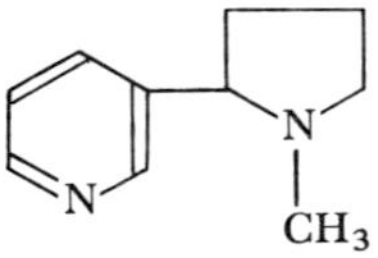

nicotine

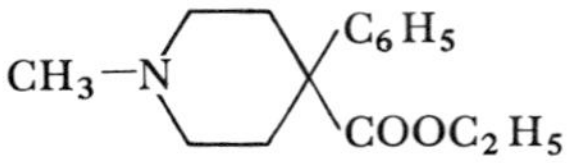

pethidine*

Drugs and Poisons 271

Other less volatile basic drugs used for similar purposes are the CNS stimulants:

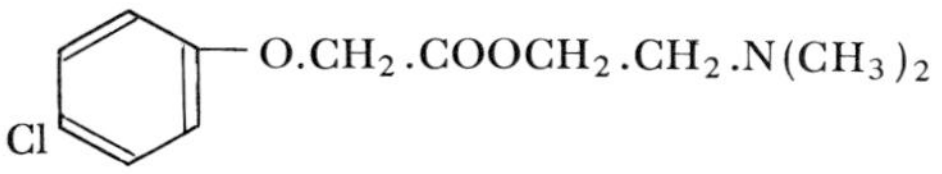

meclofenoxate
(Lucidril)

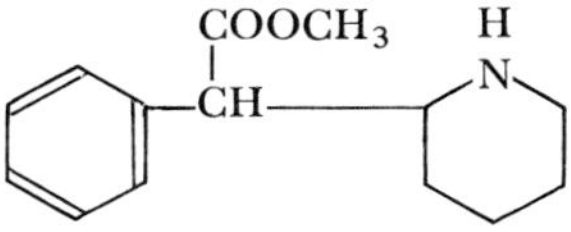

methylphenidate*
(Ritalin)

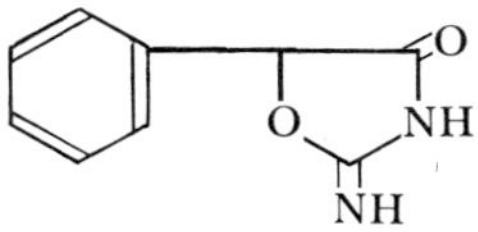

pemoline
(Kethamid, Ronyl, Volital)

and the anorectics:

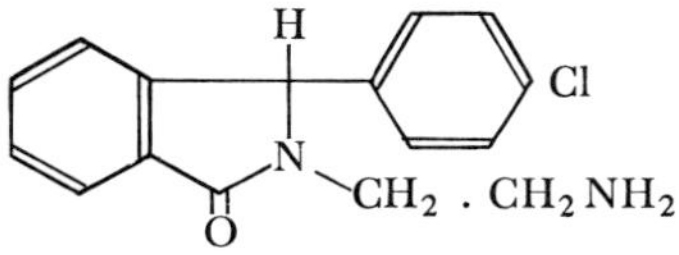

mazindol
(Teronac)

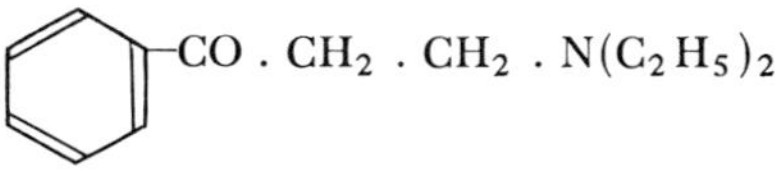

diethylpropion
(Apisate, Tenuate)

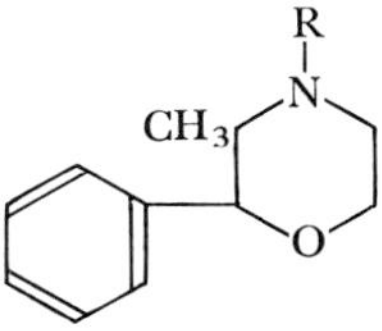

phenmetrazine* (R = H)

phenbutrazate (R = $\begin{smallmatrix} C_6H_5 \\ \\ C_2H_5 \end{smallmatrix}$ CH . COO . $(CH_2)_2$)

(Filon = phenmetrazine + phenbutrazate)

The drugs marked * are potentially addictive and are controlled under the Misuse of Drugs Act.

Amphetamines and many basic drugs combine with sulphonic acids to form salts soluble in organic solvents. Thus Connell (1958) formed a coloured complex with methyl orange. A more sensitive but similarly non-specific test uses metanil yellow which is diazotised 3-aminobenzene-sulphonic (metanilic) acid (Golbey, 1971). Negative results in this screening test indicate that basic drugs are unlikely to have been taken recently. Positive results may be caused by many substances. The method avoids concentration by evaporation so reducing greatly the losses referred to above.

272   *Practical Clinical Biochemistry*

A Simple Screening Test for Amphetamine in Urine (Golbey, 1971)

Amphetamine is extracted from alkaline solution with dichloromethane, shaken with metanil yellow, and the coloured complex extracted back into dilute acid.

Reagents. 1. Sodium hydroxide solution, 2.5 mol/l.

2. Dichloromethane, redistilled.

3. Potassium dihydrogen phosphate solution, 5 g KH_2PO_4/l in water.

4. Metanil yellow solution. Dissolve 100 mg in 100 ml phosphate solution.

5. Hydrochloric acid, 1 mol/l.

6. Stock amphetamine solution containing 750 μg free base/ml. Dissolve 130 mg amphetamine sulphate in water and make to 100 ml.

7. Working standard, 7.5 mg/l. Dilute 1 ml stock standard to 100 ml with water as required.

Technique. Collect urine specimens in bottles containing 1 to 2 ml glacial acetic acid as preservative. Samples may be kept at least a week at 4°C. To 2 ml urine in a 15 ml stoppered centrifuge tube add 0.5 ml sodium hydroxide solution and 5 ml dichloromethane, stopper and shake for 2 to 3 min. Centrifuge and discard the upper aqueous layer. Filter the solvent into a clean stoppered tube, add 1 ml metanil yellow reagent, stopper, shake vigorously for 30 s, centrifuge, and discard the upper aqueous layer. Carefully remove 3 ml of the solvent layer to another tube making certain that none of the aqueous dye solution is transferred, and shake with 3 ml hydrochloric acid. This extracts the dye back into the aqueous layer as a purple solution which is read at 540 nm against the reagent blank. Carry the working standard through the procedure to check the spectrophotometer reading which should be about 0.6.

Samples from patients known to be taking amphetamines (10 to 20 mg/day) and volunteers taking 10 mg amphetamine sulphate/day, analysed by the method give extinctions ranging from 0.6 to 2.3. All urines contain substances which extract from alkaline solution into organic solvents and react with metanil yellow, but cannot easily be removed so allowance must be made for them. Golbey found only 1 per cent of 170 "normal" urines gave an extinction above 0.2. So for screening purposes a value above 0.2 indicates the need for further investigation.

Additional information on the nature of the substance(s) causing the positive test may involve spectroscopy or GLC.

Spectroscopic Identification of Amphetamines and Related Amines

This is suitable if large doses have been taken. Adjust the urine to pH 11 with sodium hydroxide and extract 20 ml twice with 20 ml volumes of chloroform. Wash the combined extracts once with 3 ml water and then extract the amines by shaking with 3 ml sulphuric acid, 100 mmol/l. Scan the spectrum from 200 to 300 nm against a sulphuric acid blank. Details of the absorption peaks of the relevant amines are given in Table 7,5.

Drugs and Poisons

TABLE 7,5
Absorption Spectra of Amphetamine and Related Substances

Substance			
Amphetamine	252 (0.55)	257 (1.5)	263 (0.8)
Chlorphentermine	259	265	274
Diethylpropion	253 (58)		
Fenfluramine	259 (1.59)	264 (2.18)	271 (1.95)
Meclofenoxate	225 (34.5)	277 (4.0)	283 (inflection)
Methylamphetamine	252 (0.8)	257 (1.0)	263 (0.8) 266 (infl)
Methyl phenidate	247 (0.5)	251 (0.6)	257 (0.8) 263 (0.6)
Nicotine	260 (49)		
Pemoline	250 (1.8)	256 (1.8)	262 (1.7) 268 (1.15)
Pethidine	252 (0.6)		263 (0.61)
Phenmetrazine	250 (0.78)	256 (1.06)	261 (0.94) 267 (0.58)
Phentermine	252 (1.33)	258 (1.88)	281 (2.38)
Propylhexedrine	insignificant		

(Figures are wavelengths of maxima (nm) and in parentheses, the extinction of a solution containing 1 mg in 1 ml).

It will be apparent that definitive identification of amphetamine cannot be achieved by spectroscopy.

Method Using Gas-Liquid Chromatography

Amphetamines are extracted from alkaline urine into a minimal amount of chloroform containing N,N-diethylaniline (NNDEA) as internal standard. An aliquot of the extract is examined directly by GLC thus avoiding possible evaporation losses.

Reagents. 1. Sodium hydroxide solution, 5 mol/l (20 g/100 ml).

2. Chloroform.

3. N,N-Diethylaniline, supplied as a liquid b.p. 215.5°C. Distil before use collecting the fraction 212 to 214.5°C. A minor component in the NNDEA may still be found to migrate in the dexamphetamine region of the GLC trace but for practical purposes this does not seriously interfere with the sensitivity.

4. Extraction solution containing internal standard. Add 200 μl NNDEA to each ml chloroform as required.

5. Standard solution of amphetamine, 150 mg/l. Dilute the stock standard (Reagent 6, p. 272) 1 to 5 with water.

6. Standard solution of methyl amphetamine, 150 mg/l. Dissolve 18.7 mg methylamphetamine hydrochloride in water and make to 100 ml.

7. Mixed standard containing equal volumes of reagents 5 and 6.

Technique. To 2 ml urine, or 0.2 ml mixed standard made up to 2 ml with water, in a conical stoppered centrifuge tube add 0.2 ml sodium hydroxide solution. Add 100 μl NNDEA solution in chloroform and mix on a rotary mixer for 30 s. Centrifuge vigorously for 1 min, then inject 5 μl

274 *Practical Clinical Biochemistry*

of the chloroform layer onto the GLC column. The column is a mixture of 10 per cent apiezon L and 10 per cent potassium hydroxide on chromosorb G, A.W. DMCS operating at 160°C with nitrogen flow at 50 ml/min. The detector flow rates are: air 500 ml/min, and hydrogen 50 ml/min. The order of elution from the column is amphetamine, fenfluramine, methylamphetamine, NNDEA. Nicotine and phenmetrazine have retention times about 2 and 3 times that of NNDEA and the other amines are eluted still later.

Calculation. Measure the peak heights of the unknown and standard traces. The NNDEA serves as an internal standard and

Urinary amphetamine or methylamphetamine (mg/l)

$$= \frac{\text{Reading of unknown/Reading of NNDEA}}{\text{Reading of standard/Reading of its NNDEA}} \times 15.$$

INTERPRETATION

Amphetamines are not usually implicated in fatal poisoning (Table 7,1) but they are taken for their stimulant action on the brain. Addiction to amphetamine, methylamphetamine, and certain anorectics is sufficient of a problem to bring them within the Misuse of Drugs Act. As many patients deny taking them, a method for their detection is helpful.

Dependence on any drug usually increases the tolerance of the body to high doses. Thus the normal dose of amphetamine of up to 40 mg/24 h may be considerably exceeded and intakes of between 1 and 3 g/24 h have been recorded. Thirty-fold increases have been recorded for the other amines in this section. Many of these amines are excreted in the urine unaltered at least in part. The rate of excretion is markedly pH dependent, being much more rapid in acid urines.

Amphetamine and methylamphetamine are detectable in urine up to 48 h after an average dose but may take 6 days to disappear following very large doses. Methylamphetamine is partly demethylated to amphetamine. Fenfluramine is detectable for 48 h and is excreted unchanged and as the N-dealkylated product in similar quantities. Nicotine is mainly oxidised but some unchanged amine is present and up to 0.5 mg may appear in the urine during 24 h following smoking two cigarettes. Chlorphentermine and phentermine are mainly excreted unchanged with a half-life of 8 h. About 5 per cent of pethidine is excreted unchanged within 24 h. Diethylpropion is metabolised to over 20 products but some unchanged material is excreted. Tolerant patients may ingest over 2 g/24 h. Propylhexedrine is unlikely to be present in urine unless it has been taken orally and not intra-nasally.

Drugs and Poisons

ANALGESICS

These pain-relieving drugs are in many cases, readily available to the general public. They are in common use and form an important group of drugs associated with fatal poisoning (Table 7,1). Those most frequently encountered in overdose are the various forms of salicylates and paracetamol.

Aspirin and Other Salicylates

The salicylate most often employed therapeutically is acetyl-salicylic acid, aspirin. It is rapidly hydrolysed to salicylic acid so the acetylated compound is rarely found in appreciable concentration in plasma later than 3 h after ingestion. A few preparations contain salicylamide which is also rapidly hydrolysed to salicyclic acid

Salicylic acid   Aspirin   Salicylamide

A number of proprietary preparations contain aspirin in combination with other analgesics, purines, alkaloids or other drugs (Table 7,6). Aspirin tablets are also often taken with other drugs both therapeutically and in suicidal attempts. The finding of salicylate should not deter one from

TABLE 7,6

Aspirin Combinations with Other Drugs

Proprietary Names	Other Components
Anadin, Phensic	salicylamide, caffeine, quinine
Antoin, Hypon	caffeine, codeine
Codis	codeine
Onadox	dihydrocodeine
BPC preparation	phenacetin
BPC preparation	phenacetin, caffeine
Analgin; BP preparation	phenacetin, codeine
Dexocodene*	phenacetin, codeine, dexamphetamine
Daprisal*	phenacetin, amylobarbitone, dexamphetamine
Doloxene	phenacetin, dextropropoxyphene
Safapryn	paracetamol
Veganin	paracetamol, codeine
Zactirin	ethoheptazine
Equagesic	ethoheptazine, meprobamate
Equaprin	meprobamate
Dolasan, Napsalgesic	dextropropoxyphene
Tercin	butobarbitone

* = controlled drug under the Misuse of Drugs Act.

276 *Practical Clinical Biochemistry*

investigating the possibility of other drugs having been taken. These may increase the risk of a fatal outcome (Brown, 1971). In young children the accidental ingestion of aspirin is important and shares the top place with iron tablets as the most frequent drug involved. The mortality rate varies from 1 to 7 per cent over the whole age group but is greatest in children under 5 and in late middle age.

In adults, moderately severe poisoning occurs following an intake of 50 or more 300 mg aspirin tablets. Unlike poisoning with many other agents, the patient is normally mentally alert but is usually restless and may complain of tinnitus and abdominal pain. Hyperventilation as a result of drug stimulation of the respiratory centre lasting several hours is usually obvious. The body temperature is increased and sweating occurs. Many patients vomit. The combined extra losses of salt and water may result in dehydration with a reduction in urinary volume and rate of salicylate excretion, (Brown, 1971). Changes in potassium metabolism occur with passage of potassium ions from extracellular into intracellular fluid. This and the increased urinary excretion of potassium salicylate accounts for the hypokalaemia seen. The blood pH is usually normal or slightly increased as the respiratory alkalosis is compensated for by a metabolic acidosis due to increased metabolism and the acid nature of the drug. The Pco_2 falls to below 25 mm Hg (3.3 kPa) with a base deficit of over 6 mmol/l in half the cases of moderately severe poisoning.

More severe poisoning in adults leads to shock, intravascular haemolysis, reduced prothrombin levels and the possibility of acute renal failure. The metabolic acidosis may be exacerbated by inadequate tissue perfusion and the blood pH falls sometimes to as low as 7.10. This is often associated with drowsiness, a bad prognostic sign. In such severe poisoning there is a danger of pulmonary oedema or sudden respiratory or cardiac arrest. The toxic effects are related to the circulating salicylate concentration but the clinical signs are not always so closely correlated. An important part of the assessment of such a patient is thus an early determination of serum salicylate.

The clinical picture in children is somewhat different in that the metabolic acidosis is usually marked and persistent and of greater degree than the initial respiratory alkalosis. The blood pH falls and the child may be very drowsy or even unconscious. Hypokalaemia may be less marked but hypoglycaemia sometimes occurs. Again it is important to know the serum salicylate level early to assess therapy.

The principles of treatment are the removal of residual drug in the stomach, the correction of water and electrolyte deficiencies, correction of low blood pH if present and the rapid elimination of salicylate by the kidney. For the latter purpose in the more severe cases of aspirin poisoning, forced alkaline diuresis is often used provided renal function is satisfactory. Otherwise some form of dialysis is needed. In either case the laboratory is involved in the monitoring of serum salicylate and electrolyte concentrations and in the assessment of acid-base status.

Drugs and Poisons 277

The Determination of Serum Salicylate

The simplest methods rely on reactions of the phenol group. Brodie *et al.,* (1944), Keller (1947) and Trinder (1954) used the reaction with ferric salts while Smith and Talbot (1950) used the Folin-Ciocalteu reagent. Trinder's method is preferred as it gives the lowest results (under 10 mg/l) for sera containing no salicylate (cf. Keller, 40 to 50 mg/l; Smith and Talbot, 45 to 95 mg/l). The method is unsatisfactory for post-mortem blood, however, for which the method of Brodie *et al.,* is preferable. Then salicylate is extracted from acidified blood into dichloroethane and re-extracted as "strong acids" into bicarbonate before the colour reaction.

Salicylate in extracts may be determined spectrophotometrically. After acidifying the sample to pH 3.5 for the extraction into organic solvent, salicylate is re-extracted into sodium hydroxide, 450 mmol/l. The absorption maximum at 300 nm then shown by salicylic acid differs from that for acetylsalicylic acid, a property used by Routh *et al.* (1967) to estimate the latter in the presence of the former. This helps to determine the approximate time of aspirin ingestion.

For most purposes concerned with salicylate overdose the simpler technique of Trinder is adequate.

Method of Trinder (1954)

Serum is diluted with a ferric chloride-mercuric chloride mixture in acid solution, the precipitated protein centrifuged off and the colour of the supernatant read at 540 nm.

Reagents. 1. Colour reagent. Dissolve 40 g mercuric chloride in 850 ml water, add 120 ml hydrochloric acid, 1 mol/l, and 40 g ferric nitrate, $Fe(NO_3)_3, 9H_2O$. When this has dissolved make to 1 litre with water.

2. Stock standard solution of salicylic acid (1.5 g/l) or sodium salicylate. Dissolve 150 mg salicylic acid or 172 mg sodium salicylate in water and make up to 100 ml. Add a few drops of chloroform.

3. Standard for use. Dilute 20 and 40 ml stock standard to 100 ml to give standards equivalent to 300 and 600 mg/l as salicylic acid and treat as the test. Alternatively a standard curve can be produced by diluting 0.1, 0.2, 0.4, 0.6, and 0.8 ml of the stock standard to 2 ml with water and then taking 0.5 ml of these as for the test. These are equivalent to 75, 150, 300, 450 and 600 mg/l.

Technique. To 0.5 ml serum add 4.5 ml colour reagent with shaking. Mix thoroughly and centrifuge at high speed. Prepare a standard using 0.5 ml of the 300 mg/l working standard and a blank with 0.5 ml water. Read unknown and standard against blank at 540 nm.

Calculation.

$$\text{Serum salicylate (mg/l)} = \frac{\text{Reading of unknown}}{\text{Reading of standard}} \times 300$$

P.C.B.(II)—10

Notes. 1. This method gives a low blank equivalent to about 10 mg/l but the use of a pool of serum known to contain no salicylate will assess such interference and it may be allowed for if necessary. As results below about 50 mg/l are unreliable and of dubious practical significance, any blank contribution can usually be ignored.

2. Low concentrations may not be detected in gastric aspirate unless the pH of the fluid is first adjusted to 8-9 by careful addition of sodium hydroxide, 4 mol/l.

INTERPRETATION

When salicylates are used for their anti-inflammatory effect in rheumatic disorders the desirable serum concentration is about 350 mg/l. Lower figures are usual when aspirin is taken intermittently as an analgesic. In adults following deliberate overdosage, serum salicylate concentrations over 500 mg/l are found in moderate or severe poisoning and indicate the desirability of starting alkaline diuresis treatment. This may be continued until the concentration falls below 350 mg/l. In very severe overdosage the level may be in excess of 1 000 mg/l. In children moderate salicylate poisoning requiring the possibility of alkaline diuresis occurs at concentrations of 300 mg/l and above.

When the blood sample is collected more than 12 h after ingestion, the serum salicylate concentration may be relatively low and a better indication of the toxic effects is obtained from the potassium concentration and acid-base investigations.

Paracetamol and Phenacetin

Paracetamol, *p*-acetylaminophenol, is the pharmacologically active metabolite of phenacetin and acetanilide. It has been introduced as a safer drug than phenacetin which has a cumulative toxic effect on the kidney. Phenacetin itself replaced the earlier and still more toxic acetanilide.

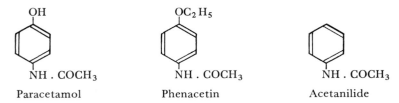

Paracetamol is an analgesic like aspirin but avoids some of the undesirable gastric irritant effects of the latter. It has become readily available to the public and is increasingly employed in attempted self-poisoning. Like aspirin (Table 7,6) both paracetamol (Table 7,7) and phenacetin (Table 7,8) are available in proprietary preparations in

Drugs and Poisons

TABLE 7,7

Paracetamol Combinations with Other Drugs

Proprietary Names	Other Components
Safapryn	aspirin
Veganin	aspirin, codeine
Cafadol, Para-Seltzer	caffeine
Parahypon, Paralgin, Pardale, Solpadeine Medocodene, Neurodyne, Panadeine	caffeine, codeine
Paracodol, Parake	codeine
Paramol	dihydrocodeine
Distalgesic	dextropropoxyphene
Fortalgesic	pentazocine
Budale, Dolalgin	butobarbitone, codeine
Gerisom	amylobarbitone, chlormezanone
Antidol, Delimon, Gevodin, Saridone, Zactipar	other mixtures

TABLE 7,8

Phenacetin Combinations with Other Drugs

Proprietary Name	Other Components
BPC preparation	aspirin
BPC preparation	aspirin, caffeine
Analgin; BP preparation	aspirin, codeine
Doloxene	aspirin, dextropropoxyphene
Daprisal*	aspirin, dexamphetamine, amylobarbitone
Dexocodene*	aspirin, dexamphetamine, codeine
Edrisal*	aspirin, amphetamine

* = controlled drug under the Misuse of Drugs Act.

combination with other drugs. A combination particularly involved in overdose cases is Distalgesic (Table 7,1).

Paracetamol is excreted in the urine partly in conjugated form as the phenolic sulphate or glucosiduronate. Both the free and the conjugated forms may also undergo hydrolysis of the acetylamino group liberating the amine. Excretion is rapid and paracetamol is quickly cleared from the circulation with a half life of about 4 h. Accumulation in the body is thus unlikely with the usual therapeutic doses.

In deliberate overdosage the main hazard is the development of hepatic necrosis several days later. Many patients recover satisfactorily but the degree of liver damage is related to the dose taken and the plasma concentrations of the drug during the first 12 h or so after ingestion (Proudfoot and Wright, 1970; Prescott *et al.*, 1971; Stewart and Simpson, 1973). The overall mortality rate is about 1 per cent and it is claimed that the administration of cysteamine to the more severely poisoned cases

280   *Practical Clinical Biochemistry*

within 10 h of ingestion has a protective action (Prescott and Matthew, 1974; Prescott *et al.*, 1974) but is questioned by Douglas *et al.* (1976). As cysteamine is not without its own toxic side-effects and as many cases of paracetamol overdosage are relatively mild it is desirable to be able to carry out the detection of paracetamol ingestion and the plasma concentration achieved as an emergency investigation.

Screening Tests for Paracetamol in Urine

Paracetamol after hydrolysis to *p*-aminophenol can be detected by two main colour reactions (Meade *et al.*, 1972). Diazotisation of the amino group and coupling with 1-naphthol gives a red-coloured product. However, other substances containing a primary aromatic amino group give similar colours and these include the sulphonamides. The latter also give coloured products when N-1-naphthylethylenediamine replaces 1-naphthol as coupling agent (p. 347) but *p*-aminophenol does not. A more specific reaction involves the indophenol reaction given by *p*-aminophenol with *o*-cresol and ammonia. The method of Meade *et al.* (1972) is rather slow and the shorter and more sensitive version devised by Simpson and Stewart (1973) is preferred.

Method of Simpson and Stewart (1973)

Paracetamol is hydrolysed by hot acid before forming an indophenol with *o*-cresol and ammonia.

Reagents. 1. Concentrated hydrochloric acid.

2. *o*-Cresol solution. Dissolve 1 g *o*-cresol in 100 ml water.

3. Ammonium hydroxide solution, 4 mol/l. Dilute 28 ml ammonia, sp. gr. 0.88, to 100 ml with water.

Technique. To 5 drops of urine in a test tube add 2 drops hydrochloric acid and one anti-bumping granule. Boil carefully over a small flame for 10 to 15 s during which time the urine colour may darken. Cool, add 1 ml *o*-cresol solution, 2 ml ammonia and mix. A blue colour developing in 1 to 2 min indicates a positive reaction. The sensitivity may be improved by using a larger sample and correspondingly more acid.

INTERPRETATION

The method is sufficiently sensitive to detect paracetamol in urine up to 24 h after a therapeutic dose of 1 g. A deep ink-blue colour, developing rapidly is consistent with an overdose and the plasma concentration should then be measured. Simpson and Stewart found no false negative or false positive results with a variety of other drugs investigated.

Drugs and Poisons

Determination of Serum Paracetamol

Brodie and Axelrod (1948) extracted the drug into ether, hydrolysed it to *p*-aminophenol and then diazotised and coupled with 1-naphthol. A simpler colorimetric method (Glynn and Kendal, 1975) is given below. The UV absorption spectra of paracetamol, acetylsalicylic acid and salicylic acid in bicarbonate solution differ in that the former shows a peak at 266 nm whereas the other two show a trough (Routh *et al.*, 1968). Gibson (1972) used a sodium hydroxide solution at 266 nm and compared the absorption with that at a pH of less than 3 to correct for non-specific absorption. Paracetamol may also be determined by gas-liquid chromatography (Grove, 1971; Prescott, 1971; Stewart and Willis, 1975).

Method of Gibson (1972)

Serum or plasma is saturated with sodium chloride, the paracetamol is extracted into ether, and then re-extracted into dilute alkali. The difference in the absorption curves at pH 2 and pH 12 is recorded in the UV and the value at 266 nm used to calculate the paracetamol concentration.

Reagents. 1. Sodium chloride, solid.

2. Diethyl ether.

3. Sodium hydroxide solution, 50 mmol/l.

4. Hydrochloric acid solution, 100 mmol/l.

Reagents 1-4 should be of analytical grade.

5. Stock standard paracetamol solution, 1.5 g/l. Dissolve 15 mg paracetamol in 10 ml water.

6. Working serum paracetamol standard, 150 mg/l. Dilute 1 ml stock standard to 10 ml with pooled serum. To obtain a standard curve this standard can be further diluted with serum to give standards containing 30, 60, 90 and 120 mg/l.

Technique. To 1 ml each of test serum, serum standard and serum blank in 10 ml glass stoppered centrifuge tubes, add 0.5 g sodium chloride and shake gently until no more dissolves. Add 5 ml ether, shake for about 3 min on a mechanical shaker and centrifuge. Pipette 2.5 ml sodium hydroxide into similar tubes and add 4 ml of the ether extracts. Shake for about 3 min, centrifuge and discard the ether layer. Into separate silica cuvettes place 1 ml sodium hydroxide and 1 ml hydrochloric acid and to each then add 1 ml of alkaline extract. Mix thoroughly and scan the spectrum of the alkaline solution against the acid between 225 and 350 nm preferably using a double beam UV spectrophotometer. Check that the spectrum is characteristic of the differential absorption of paracetamol with a peak at 266 nm and a shoulder at 300 nm. Calculate the paracetamol concentration from the extinction at 266 nm compared with that obtained for the standard serum reading.

Calculation

Serum paracetamol, (mg/l) =

$$\frac{\text{Reading of unknown at pH 12} - \text{reading of unknown at pH 2}}{\text{Reading of standard at pH 12} - \text{reading of standard at pH 2}} \times 150$$

Note. The efficiency of extraction of paracetamol from serum into ether varies. Inadequate shaking gives poor recoveries and too vigorous shaking can produce intractable emulsions. It is therefore important to use a standard in serum and to carry all tubes through *exactly* the same mixing and shaking procedure. Under good conditions about 80 per cent of the paracetamol can be extracted.

Method of Glynn and Kendal (1975). Modified.

This method is based on the finding of Chefetz *et al.* (1971) that nitrous acid will introduce a nitro group into the nucleus of paracetamol. The resulting nitrophenol is coloured deep yellow in alkaline solution.

Phenacetin and *p*-aminophenol do not react.

Reagents. 1. Trichloracetic acid solution, 100 g/l.

2. Hydrochloric acid, 6 mol/l.

3. Sodium nitrite solution, 100 g/l. Make freshly each time by dissolving 1 g in 10 ml water.

4. Sulphamic acid solution, 150 g/l.

5. Sodium hydroxide solution, 100 g/l.

6. Standard paracetamol solution, 300 mg/l in water. Stable in the dark at 4°C.

Technique. Add 1 ml serum to a 25 ml stoppered centrifuge tube containing 2 ml trichloracetic acid and mix thoroughly for 10 s. Centrifuge for 2 min. Prepare similarly a standard and blank using 1 ml standard solution or water. Transfer 1 ml supernatant fluid into a test tube and add 0.5 ml hydrochloric acid followed by 1 ml sodium nitrite. Mix and allow to stand 2 min and then carefully add 1 ml sulphamic acid solution. Mix and after frothing stops add 1 ml sodium hydroxide. Read in the colorimeter at 430 nm against the reagent blank.

Calculation. As the mean recovery of paracetamol from serum is 93 per cent.

$$\text{Serum paracetamol (mg/l)} = \frac{\text{Reading of unknown}}{\text{Reading of standard}} \times 300 \times \frac{100}{93} \text{ or } \times 323$$

Drugs and Poisons 283

Notes. 1. Any conjugates of paracetamol present in serum do not react. The method seems to be specific for paracetamol in that a range of 28 drugs did not interfere at a concentration of 50 mg/l. These included tranquillisers, barbiturates and other hypnotics, tricyclic antidepressants, antihistamines and other analgesics.

2. If preferred, a standard solution of paracetamol in serum, 300 mg/l, can be used. The recovery correction is then omitted.

3. A kit based on this method is available from Winthrop Laboratories, Surbiton upon Thames, Surrey.

INTERPRETATION

Liver damage can be expected if paracetamol is detectable in the serum 24 h after ingestion. The prognosis is serious for concentrations in excess of 300 mg/l at 4 h or 50 mg/l at 12 h but patients with levels less than 120 mg/l at 4 h are unlikely to be greatly affected. The selection of cases for cysteamine therapy during the first 10 h is based on the concentration and time.

The degree of liver damage can be followed most satisfactorily using enzyme determinations. Suitable enzymes are aspartate aminotransferase (AST), alanine aminotransferase (ALT) and γ-glutamyltranspeptidase (γGT). The determination of prothrombin is also important in the more severe cases. In the acute phase the increase in AST usually exceeds that in ALT. In the authors' experience the AST result may be in excess of 10 000 IU/l at its peak even in patients who show little clinical evidence of extensive liver damage. Such patients have recovered satisfactorily with return of AST results to the normal range. Other toxic effects of paracetamol include pancreatitis with a raised serum amylase and acute renal failure with its typical biochemical features.

ANTICONVULSANTS

The commoner anticonvulsant drugs used in various forms of epilepsy are hydantoins, succinimides, oxazolidines and barbiturates. These and other anticonvulsants have similarities as follows:

Hydantoins:

	R_1	R_2
phenytoin (Epanutin, Epiphen)	H	C_6H_5
ethotoin (Peganone)	C_2H_5	H
methoin (Mesontoin)	CH_3	C_2H_5

Succinimides:

	R_1	R_2	R_3
ethosuximide (Emeside, Zarontin)	H	CH_3	C_2H_5
methsuximide (Celontin)	CH_3	CH_3	C_6H_5
phensuximide	CH_3	H	C_6H_5

284 — Practical Clinical Biochemistry

Oxazolidones:

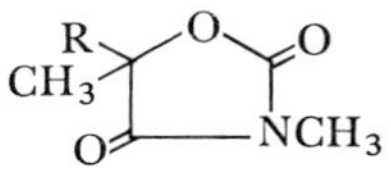

paramethadione (Paradione) $R = C_2H_5$
troxidone (Tridione) $R = CH_3$

Barbiturates and relatives:

phenobarbitone (Gardenal, Luminal)
methylphenobarbitone (Prominal) $\Big\}$ see Table 7,9.

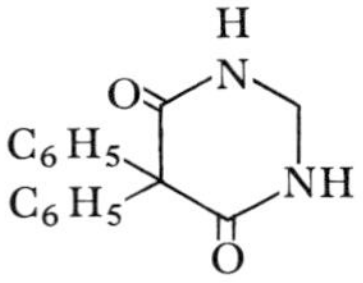

primidone (mysoline)

These drugs are often used in combination. Other anticonvulsants are:

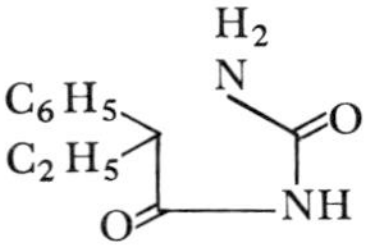

pheneturide (Benuride, Trinuride)   cf. methoin.

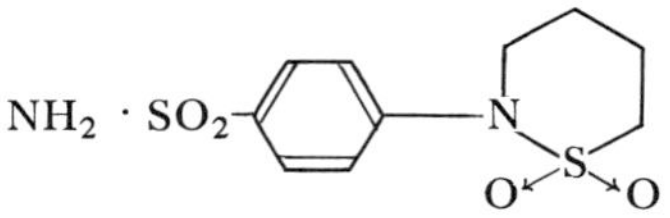

$NH_2 \cdot SO_2$— sulthiame (Opsolot) cf. sulphonamides (Table 7,19).

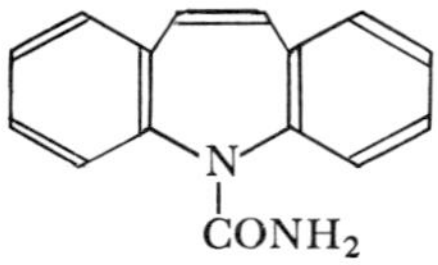

carbamazepine (Tegretol)
cf. tricyclic antidepressants

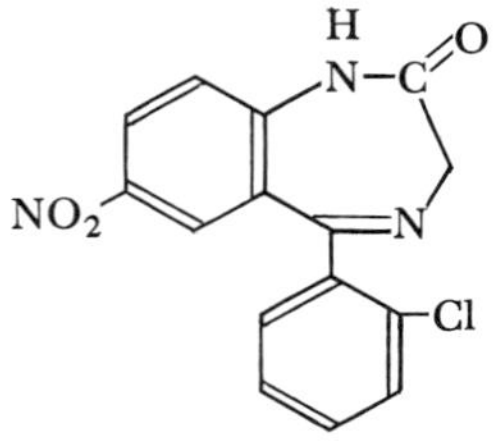

clonazepam (Rivotril)
cf. benzodiazepines

$CH_3CH_2CH_2$
$>CHCOONa$
$CH_3CH_2CH_2$
   sodium valproate (Epilim)

$C_6H_5 \cdot CH_2NHCOCH_2CH_2Cl$
   beclamide (Nydrane)

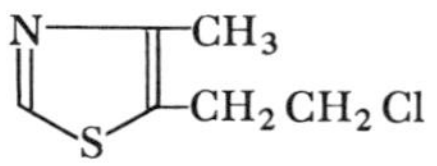

chlormethiazole (Heminevrin)

Phenytoin, phenobarbitone and primidone, which act by conversion to phenobarbitone are the most commonly used drugs for the treatment of attacks of grand mal and are often used in combination. The succinimides and oxazolidones are mainly used to control petit mal attacks. Some of the other drugs probably act by modifying the metabolism of the major anticonvulsants.

Drugs and Poisons   285

Phenytoin is metabolised and inactivated by oxidation to *p*-hydroxy-phenytoin by a specific hepatic hydroxylase. The enzyme is not induced to any great degree by administration of phenytoin or phenobarbitone and the hydroxylation of phenytoin is rate limiting. This is important in regulating the plasma concentration of phenytoin itself. The concentration of enzyme varies between individuals and the enzyme is inhibited by the other anticonvulsants sulthiame and pheneturide (Richens, 1974) and by chloramphenicol and isoniazid. Phenobarbitone is capable of inducing the synthesis of many enzymes including those responsible for its own metabolism. Carbamazepine metabolism is stimulated by phenobarbitone and phenytoin with reduction of its plasma concentration (Christiansen and Dam, 1973). Phenytoin also induces the enzyme system responsible for the oxidation of primidone to phenobarbitone (Fincham *et al.,* 1974).

These interactions, the frequent use of combined therapy with anticonvulsants and the toxic effects of unduly high plasma concentrations particularly of phenytoin have led to the development of methods of monitoring the levels in individual patients. Anticonvulsants do not seem to be involved in fatal poisonings to any great extent (Table 7,1). The chemical similarity of many anticonvulsants presents problems for their individual estimation. With UV methods similar to that for barbiturates, mutual interference occurs between phenytoin and phenobarbitone unless some form of partition is used. In one of the earlier methods for determining phenytoin Svensmark and Kristensen (1963) extracted into chloroform and partitioned between chloroform and buffer at pH 8.8. The slightly more acidic phenobarbitone passes into the buffer leaving most of the phenytoin in the chloroform, and achieving about 90 per cent separation. The chloroform layer was washed with buffer and then extracted with alkali, followed by spectroscopic quantitation at 240 and 260 nm.

Phenytoin can be oxidised to benzophenone which has a characteristic spectrum peaking at 247 nm. At the same time phenobarbitone is converted to a non-absorbing product. Wallace *et al.* (1965) first used alkali and bromine for this, then potassium permanganate (Wallace, 1966). In earlier methods the benzophenone was steam distilled and extracted into an organic solvent. Later, oxidation and extraction were carried out simultaneously by refluxing in the presence of *n*-heptane (Wallace, 1969). The phenytoin was originally extracted from serum into chloroform but this interfered with the oxidation unless completely removed by vacuum distillation. Dill *et al.* (1971) avoided this by using dichloroethane instead of chloroform and then extracted into *iso*-octane which is cheaper than *n*-heptane.

Determination of Serum Phenytoin. Method of Dill *et al.* (1971)

The phenytoin is extracted from buffered serum or plasma into dichloroethane and back extracted into sodium hydroxide. It is then

286   *Practical Clinical Biochemistry*

oxidised by permanganate to benzophenone which is extracted into *iso*-octane and read at 247 nm.

Reagents. 1. Phosphate buffer, 1 mol/l, pH 6.8, 67.44 g KH_2PO_4 and 140.2 g $Na_2HPO_4,2H_2O$ in 1 litre.

2. Dichloroethane, specially purified reagent. Stand over concentrated sulphuric acid, wash well with alkali and then water, dry over anhydrous sodium sulphate and distil.

3. Sodium hydroxide solution, 1 mol/l.

4. Saturated sodium hydroxide solution. Dissolve 50 g sodium hydroxide pellets in 50 ml water. Allow to cool and settle. Siphon off the clear, carbonate-free solution.

5. Saturated aqueous potassium permanganate solution.

6. *iso*-Octane, 2,2,4-trimethylpentant. Purify for use by percolating through layers of equal parts of acid and basic alumina.

7. Stock standard phenytoin solution, 1 g/l. Dissolve 100 mg phenytoin in a minimal amount of 100 mmol/l sodium hydroxide and dilute to 100 ml with water.

8. Working standard in serum, 20 mg/l. Add 100 μl stock standard to 4.9 ml pooled serum.

Technique. To 2 ml serum or heparinised plasma, 2 ml pooled serum plus standard, and 2 ml water for the reagent blank, contained in suitable glass-stoppered tubes (16 × 150 mm) add 0.2 ml phosphate buffer and 10 ml dichloroethane. Shake for 10 min, centrifuge, transfer 8 ml of the dichloroethane layers to a second set of glass-stoppered tubes containing 3 ml sodium hydroxide, 1 mol/l, shake for 5 min and centrifuge. Transfer 2 ml of each sodium hydroxide extract to a third glass-stoppered centrifuge tube and add 1.5 ml saturated sodium hydroxide solution, 4 ml *iso*-octane and 0.5 ml permanganate solution. Insert the tubes in a steam bath through a close fitting gasket of aluminium foil so that only the aqueous phase is exposed to the steam while the upper *iso*-octane layer is air-cooled. Heat for 30 min with the tubes loosely stoppered, cool to room temperature and shake mechanically for 5 min to complete extraction of the benzophenone. Read the extinction of the *iso*-octane extracts of test and standard against the reagent blank at 247 nm.

Calculation.

$$\text{Serum phenytoin (mg/l)} = \frac{\text{Reading of unknown}}{\text{Reading of standard}} \times 20.$$

Notes. 1. Some batches of dichloroethane may require an undesirably large amount of permanganate and so need to be purified. Interference may also be removed by washing the alkali layer with *n*-heptane before the oxidation.

2. The calibration is linear up to the equivalent of 25 mg/l for 2 ml samples but falls away with greater amounts of phenytoin because of incomplete oxidation. The permanganate colour shows the presence of excess reagent. Complete decoloration shows the presence of reducing

Drugs and Poisons

contaminants which can be removed by adding solid permanganate to the reaction mixture. High drug levels can be determined by reducing the volume of sample taken or by increasing the volume of saturated sodium hydroxide to 2 ml and permanganate to 1 ml. Then linearity can extend to 50 mg/l.

3. Recovery is the same from serum or water and a 20 mg/l standard should read about 0.36 when 2 ml is used.

4. Wallace *et al.* (1974a) pointed out that permanganate should be added to the alkali just before use in the oxidation otherwise decomposition products are formed which cause undesirable side reactions in the phenytoin oxidation. They reduced the amount of permanganate to 200 mg and sodium hydroxide, 8 mol/l, to 15 ml. They still used heptane (see Note 1) but carried out the final estimation by GLC. Mullen (1974) stated that although the alkaline solution should be added through a funnel, splashing can occur resulting in fusion of the ground glass joints of the condenser unless a polytetrafluorethylene sleeve is inserted.

GLC Separation of Anticonvulsants

The technique of GLC is suitable for the separation of anticonvulsants and has been used both for the separation and determination of primidone, phenobarbitone and phenytoin (see p. 301) and for the development of methods for the newer anticonvulsants which are not easily measured by other techniques.

INTERPRETATION

Introduced in 1938, *phenytoin* is one of the most frequently prescribed drugs for convulsive disorders. Its mode of action is unknown but it appears to inhibit the accumulation of sodium in nerve cells thus stabilising hyperexcitable cell membranes. It has a half life of 18 to 24 h so that two doses/day should produce a fairly constant blood level. The dose needs to be adequate to control seizures but not be high enough to cause toxic side effects. The response to treatment varies from patient to patient, in some giving complete relief from seizures, in others reducing the frequency of attacks. Adequate blood levels have been given as 10 to 20 mg/l but some workers (see Toseland *et al.*, 1972) found satisfactory control at values between 3 and 17 mg/l. It seems to be agreed that side effects appear between 25 and 30 mg/l and become severe over 30 mg/l. Definite criteria are difficult to establish as phenytoin is seldom given alone and results may be influenced by the technique used.

The relationship between phenytoin dose and plasma concentration is significantly non-linear unlike that of phenobarbitone (Bochner *et al.*, 1972; Richens, 1974). Once the hydroxylating enzyme is saturated, a small increment in the dose produces a marked increase in plasma concentration

288 *Practical Clinical Biochemistry*

with the possibility that toxic levels will be reached. As there are marked variations in enzyme activity due to genetic factors and the presence of other drugs, measurement of plasma phenytoin is important in establishing adequate therapy. For an individual the permitted variation in dose will be small and occasional omission of a tablet may be significant. See also Mawer *et al.* (1974). Marks *et al.* (1973) believe that isolated phenytoin determinations are only helpful in detecting gross overdosage or underdosage. Repeated monitoring is needed to establish the optimal plasma concentration initially and to check its maintenance during long term therapy.

The value of monitoring other anticonvulsant drugs is less well established. As *primidone* has a comparatively short half life of 10 to 12 h closer attention needs to be paid to the time of collection in relation to time of dosage than is the case with phenytoin. It is still not certain whether control of seizures is due to the phenobarbitone formed or to the native primidone. Plasma levels less than 10 mg/l are usually considered safe but Toseland *et al.* (1972) found therapeutic values between 2 and 22 mg/l.

Phenobarbitone, the oldest of the drugs used in anticonvulsant therapy, has a half life of about 3 days and plasma levels correlate fairly well with daily dose. Toseland *et al.* (1972) found plasma phenobarbitone concentrations of 4 to 50 mg/l in 240 patients receiving primidone or phenobarbitone. A further 25 patients with values above 50 mg/l (range 54 to 101) showed side effects. This is in agreement with earlier observations that toxicity rarely occurs with values below 50 mg/l.

Marks *et al.* (1973) concluded that monitoring blood phenytoin is valuable in the management of patients with epilepsy, but the value of such monitoring is not established for other anticonvulsant drugs.

BARBITURATES

Barbiturates are widely used as hypnotics, some as tranquillisers. Phenobarbitone and methylphenobarbitone have been described under "anticonvulsants". The very short acting barbiturates are used in the induction of anaesthesia. Their preponderance as the cause of death by poisoning (Table 7,1) emphasises their availability by prescription to mentally disturbed patients and the high toxicity of these substances when an overdose is taken. Barbiturates create dependence in the patient with the development of tolerance so that high doses in such cases have much less effect than in the normal person. Barbiturates are drugs of addiction and are sometimes taken intravenously in large doses.

A feature of barbiturate overdosage is that it is often not due to a single substance (Table 7,1). A number of proprietary preparations contain other drugs (Table 7,9) and ingestion of several different types of tablet is common in barbiturate poisoning. The finding of a barbiturate should therefore cause suspicion that another drug may also be present.

Drugs and Poisons 289

Most barbiturates are derived from barbituric acid by substituting the two hydrogen atoms on the C-5 methylene group by various alkyl or aryl groups. A few also contain a methyl group on the N-1 atom or are thiobarbiturates in which the oxygen atom on C-2 is replaced by a sulphur atom. Their mode of action can be classified into three main groups, long acting, very short acting and an intermediate group, the latter comprising most of those commonly used as hypnotics. Barbiturates in current use in the United Kingdom are listed in Table 7,9. Several are available both as the acid or its sodium salt but are not separately listed.

Determination of Barbiturates

Methods available for detecting and estimating barbiturates include colorimetry, UV spectrophotometry, and thin layer or gas-liquid chromatography. The early colorimetric methods using cobalt salts which gave a purple colour with barbiturates (for example, see Levvy, 1940) had poor specificity and precision.

Barbiturates complex with mercury to form a product extractable into chloroform or dichloromethane. The amount of mercury is estimated by means of dithizone or diphenylcarbazone. Several screening methods based on this principle are used to detect the presence of barbiturates (Lubran, 1961; Baer, 1965; Garvey and Bowden, 1966 and Watson and Dillion, 1973). The last named studied the efficiency of extraction using different solvent to water ratios of chloroform and dichloromethane and obtained most consistent results using dichloromethane at a ratio of at least 80 : 1. Similar extinctions were then obtained with all the 5,5'-disubstituted barbiturates which was not the case with earlier methods, but the N-1 substituted barbiturates gave values only half as great. Diphenylcarbazone, stable indefinitely when prepared in isopropanol, was the most satisfactory colour reagent. A micro version is given below.

The most widely established method for identification and estimation of the barbiturates uses UV spectroscopy. Ionisation of the molecule at a pH above 9.5 gives the enol forms. In borate buffer at pH 10.0 all barbiturates show an absorption maximum at 240 nm. This corresponds to enolisation of the ketone group on C-4. The absorption values of Stevenson (1961) correspond to millimolar extinction coefficients under these conditions of 8.9 to 10.0 (Table 7,10). At pH 13.4 the absorption maximum shifts to about 255 nm for the 5,5'-disubstituted barbiturates following enolisation of the ketone group on C-6 (Fig. 7,1). In the N-1 substituted derivatives this cannot occur so they lack this characteristic shift. The difference between the absorption curves at pH 10 and 13.4 (or lack of it in the N-1 substituted) is useful for detecting the presence of barbiturates and for their quantitation, the difference in reading at 260 nm at which wavelength and at 236 nm there is the greatest difference between the two curves. In acid solution the molecule is un-ionised and shows no absorption peak. All barbiturates can therefore be determined by reading the difference at

TABLE 7,9

Barbiturates

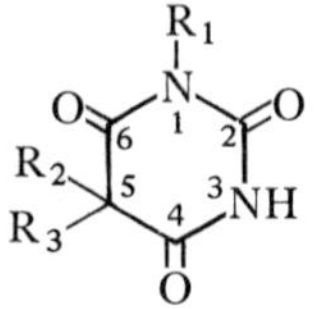

	R_1	R_2	R_3	
Long acting	H	C_2H_5	C_2H_5	barbitone
	H	C_2H_5	C_6H_5	phenobarbitone (Gardenal, Luminal)
	CH_3	C_2H_5	C_6H_5	methylphenobarbitone (Prominal)
Intermediate acting				
	H	C_2H_5	$(CH_2)_2 CH(CH_3)_2$	amylobarbitone (Amytal)
	H	C_2H_5	$(CH_2)_3 . CH_3$	butobarbitone (Soneryl)
	H	C_2H_5	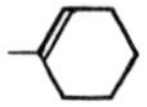	cyclobarbitone (Phanodorm, Rapidel)
	H	C_2H_5	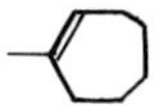	heptabarbitone (Medomin)
	CH_3	CH_3	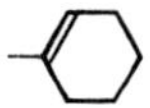	hexobarbitone
	H	C_2H_5	$-CH . (CH_2)_2 . CH_3$ / CH_3	pentobarbitone (Nembutal)
	H	$CH_2-CH=CH_2$	$-CH . (CH_2)_2 . CH_3$ / CH_3	quinalbarbitone (Seconal)

Drugs and Poisons

Very short acting (used as sodium salts intravenously)

CH_3 . CH_2 . $CH=CH_2$	$-CH$. $C{\equiv}C$. C_2H_5 $\;\mid\;$ CH_3	methohexitone (Brietal)
H	C_2H_5	$-CH$. $(CH_2)_2$. CH_3 $\;\mid\;$ CH_3	thiopentone (Intraval, Pentothal) [also has S replacing O at C-2]

The following mixed preparations are important

"Proprietary" name

	Evidorm	hexobarbitone/cyclobarbitone
	Tuinal	quinalbarbitone/amylobarbitone
	Protamyl	amylobarbitone/promethazine (anti-histamine)
	Sonergan	butobarbitone/promethazine
CD	Drinamyl	amylobarbitone/dexamphetamine
	Amylozine	amylobarbitone/trifluoperazine (a phenothiazine)
	Carbrital	pentobarbitone/carbromal (a hypnotic)
	Budale, Dolalgin	butobarbitone/paracetamol/codeine
	Gerison	amylobarbitone/paracetamol/chlormezanone (a tranquilliser)
	Sonalgin	butobarbitone/phenacetin/codeine
CD	Daprisal	amylobarbitone/aspirin/phenacetin/dexamphetamine
	Doloxytal	amylobarbitone/dextropropoxyphene (an analgesic)
	Tercin	butobarbitone/aspirin

CD – controlled drug under the Misuse of Drugs Act.

292   *Practical Clinical Biochemistry*

240 nm for solutions at pH 10 and pH 2. The method described below is that of Broughton (1956). The barbiturates should be exposed to the alkaline solution for as short a time as possible to minimise hydrolysis and subsequent fall in extinction value. The different barbiturates have been categorised by their differential resistance to hydrolysis in alkaline solution, the long acting being the least stable and the short acting most stable.

Determination of Blood Barbiturate Using the Mercury Reaction. Method of Watson and Dillion (1973)

The sample is placed on a cellulose disc and extracted with dichloromethane. Mercuric nitrate is added and after separation the amount of barbiturate-mercury complex is determined by adding diphenylcarbazone.

Reagents. 1. Cellulose paper discs, Whatman No. 3MM 30 mm diameter.

2. Dichloromethane, analytical reagent grade. Check each batch by adding 0.15 ml diphenylcarbazone reagent to 8 ml. The extinction at 555 nm in 1 cm cells should not exceed 0.05.

3. Stock mercuric nitrate solution. Dissolve 2 g mercuric nitrate in water containing 0.1 ml concentrated nitric acid/100 ml and make to 100 ml with this.

4. Phosphate buffer, 100 mmol/l, pH 7.0. Dissolve 15.6 g $Na_2HPO_4,2H_2O$ in about 800 ml water, adjust to pH 7.0 with sodium hydroxide, 5 mol/l, and make to 1 litre.

5. Mercuric reagent. To 85 ml phosphate buffer add 15 ml stock mercuric nitrate solution dropwise with constant stirring. Store at room temperature in a clear glass bottle and discard when a precipitate forms.

6. Phenylcarbazone reagent. Dissolve 200 mg phenylcarbazone in 100 ml warm isopropanol, analytical reagent grade.

7. Aqueous isopropanol diluent. Mix 85 ml isopropanol with 15 ml water.

8. Stock standard solution of phenobarbitone, 100 mg in 100 ml reagent 7.

9. Working standard, 100 mg/l. Dilute 10 ml stock standard to 100 ml with reagent 7.

10. Control serum. Burrough's Wellcome "Wellcomtrol" containing amylobarbitone (free acid), 50 mg/l.

Technique. Dispense 8 ml dichloromethane into acid-washed glass-stoppered tubes (23 ×100 mm) for the standard, control sera and duplicate tests. Apply 100 μl barbiturate standard to the centre of one cellulose disc, wait 10 s, partially fold using forceps and drop into the corresponding extraction tube. Repeat using control serum and the patient's serum or plasma. Wet each stopper with two drops of water, stopper and invert the tubes repeatedly by hand for 2 min and remove the cellulose discs with forceps. Add 0.5 ml mercuric reagent to each tube, stopper and shake hard

Drugs and Poisons 293

for 15 to 20 s. Allow the layers to separate and, using a fine tipped Pasteur pipette, remove as much as possible of the top aqueous layer. Into clean tubes, 100 × 16 mm, calibrated at 10 ml, filter the separated organic layer through a 7 cm Whatman No. 31 paper contained in a small glass funnel. After filtration wash the paper with dichloromethane to make the volume to 10 ml. At the same time set up a blank of 10 ml dichloromethane. Add 0.15 ml diphenylcarbazone reagent to each tube, mix and protect from direct sunlight. Read in 2 cm cuvettes against the blank at 555 nm.

Calculation. Serum barbiturate (mg/l as phenobarbitone)

$$= \frac{\text{Reading of unknown}}{\text{Reading of standard}} \times 100$$

Notes. 1. The quality of the dichloromethane is of the utmost importance. Watson and Dillion report contamination by tin caused by a damaged screw-cap foil of a stock bottle.

2. The method is about ten times more sensitive than the UV method of Broughton given below with which it shows fair agreement. It is not recommended to replace that but provides a useful technique capable of proving unequivocally the absence of clinically significant amounts of barbiturate in a short time.

3. At non-toxic levels the benzodiazines do not interfere. Equimolar concentrations of glutethimide give slightly less colour than barbiturate. The hydantoin drugs also interfere.

Method Using Ultraviolet Spectrophotometry (Broughton, 1956)

The barbiturates are extracted first into chloroform then into alkali and identified by studying the absorption curves at pH 10 and pH 13.4 over the range 227 to 265 nm. They can be determined by using the difference in extinction at these two pH's at 260 nm. An indication as to the type of barbiturate present can be obtained by studying the rate of hydrolysis.

Reagents. 1. Chloroform.

2. Sulphuric acid, 1 mol/l.

3. Sodium hydroxide, 450 mmol/l.

4. Phosphate buffer, 500 mmol/l, pH 7.4. Mix 80.8 ml $Na_2HPO_4, 2H_2O$ (89.07 g/l) and 19.2 ml KH_2PO_4 (68.085 g/l).

5. Boric acid-potassium chloride solution, 600 mmol/l. Dissolve 37.1 g boric acid and 44.7 g potassium chloride in water and make up to a litre.

6. Borate blank solution. Mix equal volumes of the sodium hydroxide and boric acid-potassium chloride solutions.

7. Stock standard solution of butobarbitone or amylobarbitone. Dissolve 100 mg in chloroform and make up to 100 ml.

8. Working standard. Dilute the stock standard 5 ml to 100 ml with chloroform.

Technique. For *whole blood* extract 5 ml three times with about 30 ml chloroform. Filter the combined extracts through an 11 cm Whatman

No. 31 paper into a dry separating funnel, washing the paper with a little chloroform. Extract the barbiturates by shaking vigorously with 10 ml sodium hydroxide. Clarify by centrifuging.

Take two 2 ml portions of the extract and to one add a further 2 ml sodium hydroxide, to give pH 13.4, and to the other 2 ml boric acid-potassium chloride, to give pH 10. Read from 227 to 265 nm using the sodium hydroxide as blank for the former at pH 13.4 and the borate blank for readings at pH 10. Read the borate solution first diluting if necessary with borate blank to bring the extinction at 240 nm to between 1.0 and 1.5. Dilute the sodium hydroxide solution to the same extent with sodium hydroxide before reading.

As standard, extract 10 ml of the working standard containing 0.5 mg of the barbiturate with the sodium hydroxide.

For the detection of barbiturates all the criteria referred to on p. 289 and shown in Fig. 7,1 must be present, that is a maximum at 238 to

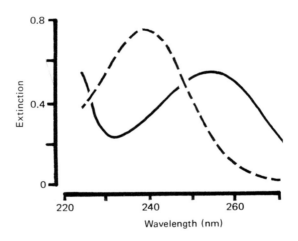

Fig. 7,1. Absorption spectra of barbitone in borate buffer, pH 10 (— — — — —) and in 450 mmol/l sodium hydroxide, pH 13.4 (————). (After Broughton, 1956).

240 nm at pH 10, a maximum at 252 to 255 and a minimum at 234 to 237 nm at pH 13.4, isosbestic points at 227 to 230 and at 247 to 250 nm, and greatest difference between the two curves at 236 and 260 nm. In dilute solutions some of these may not be given; also some other compounds, for example salicylic acid and sulphanilamide may give some of them. It is not then sufficient to find a difference in extinction at 260 nm. The full absorption curve must be studied.

Drugs and Poisons   295

Calculation. Blood barbiturate (mg/l) =

$$\frac{\Delta E_{260} \text{ for the unknown}}{\Delta E_{260} \text{ for the standard}} \times \frac{\text{Final volume if diluted before reading}}{4}$$

$$\frac{\times 0.5 \times 1\ 000}{5} \qquad \text{that is, } \times 100$$

where ΔE_{260} is the reading in sodium hydroxide—the reading in borate.

This result will be in terms of the particular barbiturate used as standard. For discussion of the relative behaviour of different barbiturates see below, Note 2.

For *urine* or *gastric contents* take 10 to 25 ml, acidify with sulphuric acid, extract with chloroform as above but wash twice with 5 ml phosphate buffer before filtering and extracting into the sodium hydroxide. Some loss of barbiturate results from shaking with phosphate and can be corrected for by putting the standard through the same procedure. In the calculation substitute the volume taken for the 5 ml used for blood.

Notes. 1. *Identification of the type of barbiturate.* Absorption curves of individual barbiturates are similar and cannot be used to identify them. Partial identification can be achieved by studying the rate of decomposition with alkali.

Heat the solution in alkali obtained in the above method in a boiling water bath for 15 min and read at 260 nm using the sodium hydroxide as blank. The ratio of ΔE_{260} after heating to that before heating, when multiplied by 100 gives the percentage barbiturate remaining after alkaline hydrolysis. This was found by Broughton to be over 90 per cent for cyclobarbitone, quinalbarbitone, and pentobarbitone (short acting barbiturates) 56 per cent for amylobarbitone and 50 per cent for butobarbitone (intermediate acting), 43 per cent for barbitone and 32 per cent for phenobarbitone (long acting).

2. Jamieson and Frew (1973) further studied the above method with a view to shortening and standardising the procedure. Using the same reagents as Broughton, their technique is as follows. Shake 2 ml whole blood, serum or plasma with 10 ml chloroform in a glass-stoppered conical flask for exactly 3 min. This should cause intimate mixing without forming an emulsion which hinders separation of the layers and decreases recovery. Decant the chloroform extract carefully through a 7 cm Whatman No. 41 filter paper into a 150 × 20 mm glass-stoppered tube of 25 ml capacity and add 4 ml sodium hydroxide solution. Stopper and shake again for 3 min to ensure intimate mixing of the two phases. Transfer the contents of the tube to a 110 × 16 mm tube and centrifuge at 2 000 rpm for 2 min.

To determine the type of barbiturate present transfer 2 ml of the sodium hydroxide extract to a 10 ml graduated tube, stopper loosely and place in a rapidly boiling water bath for exactly 15 min, cool rapidly and adjust the volume to 2 ml with water. Prepare alkali and borate solutions for the

TABLE 7,10
Extinction Coefficients, Recoveries and Calibration Factors for Barbiturates

	Mol. wt.	Borate buffer pH 10* 240 nm		$\dfrac{E_{1cm}^{1\%}\ \text{in NaOH}}{E_{1cm}^{1\%}\ \text{in borate}}$ 260 nm		Per cent recovery		Coefficient of variation	Factor F
		ϵ	$E_{1cm}^{1\%}$	A	B	A	B	%	
Amylobarbitone	226	9 580	424	240	132	"good"	72	2.1	211
Barbitone	184	9 900	538	267	147	90	66	1.9	210
Butobarbitone	212	9 600	453	258	140	"good"	68	1.5	211
Cyclobarbitone	236	9 980	423	224	140	"good"	66	2.2	215
Pentobarbitone	226	9 290	411	208	121	"good"	72	0.9	231
Phenobarbitone	232	10 000	431	229	129	"good"	60	3.4	258
Quinalbarbitone	238	8 900	374	210	109	"good"	70	1.1	264

* = Stevenson (1961); A = Broughton (1956); B = Jamieson and Frew (1973).

Drugs and Poisons 297

heated and unheated extracts as described in the Broughton method using 0.6 ml for each solution instead of the 2 ml given above. Transfer the final solutions to 1 ml semi-micro cuvettes of 1 cm path and scan against the appropriate blank solutions over the range 225 to 300 nm.

The results for alkaline hydrolysis are similar to those of Broughton. Some differences exist in recoveries and extinction coefficients. The results of Stevenson (1961), Broughton (1956) and Jamieson and Frew (1973) are compared in Table 7,10. Stevenson's figures refer to absorption at 240 nm in the borate buffer and show that the specific extinction coefficients $(E_{1\,cm}^{1\,\%})$ vary more than the molar extinction coefficients (ϵ). Figures for the difference in specific extinction coefficients at 260 nm in borate buffer and 450 mmol/l sodium hydroxide, are calculated from the data of Broughton and of Jamieson and Frew. Published absorption curves suggest that this difference is approximately half that of the single value at 240 nm. Broughton's figures agree with this but those of Jamieson and Frew are low. As might be expected from the simplified extraction procedure, there is a difference in the per cent recoveries. Broughton found almost complete recovery except for barbitone which is no longer used. Jamieson and Frew's recoveries, calculated from their observed extinction coefficients and based on 50 determinations for each drug are appreciably lower for all barbiturates and this has to be allowed for. The coefficient of variation of the extraction step is listed in the Table. The method of Jamieson and Frew thus requires an individual calibration factor (F) to convert the observed ΔE_{260} into the barbiturate concentration. F is calculated from the mean observed ΔE_{260} for blood containing 100 mg/l of added barbiturate as:

$$F = \frac{\text{concentration of barbiturate (mg/l)}}{\Delta E_{260}} = \frac{100}{\Delta E_{260}}$$

so that for the unknown sample
$$\text{Blood barbiturate (mg/l)} = \Delta E_{260} \times F$$

3. Drugs which may interfere include bemegride (Megimide), β-methyl-β-ethyl-glutarimide, which has been given to patients with barbiturate intoxication, so if possible blood for barbiturate determination should be taken before bemegride is given. It can,, however, be removed by incubating with sodium hydroxide, 450 mmol/l, for 2 h, in fact a considerable proportion is removed in 30 min. Glutethimide (see p. 320) also interferes but is rapidly hydrolysed at room temperature in alkaline solution.

As we have seen (p. 284) phenytoin is often given with phenobarbitone. It does not cause serious interference. At a level of 40 mg/l it gives an apparent barbiturate reading of 10 per cent of its concentration.

4. Phase-separating paper must not be used to separate the aqueous and organic phases as it causes marked interference (Jamieson and Frew).

298   *Practical Clinical Biochemistry*

INTERPRETATION

Broughton *et al.* (1956) studying acute barbiturate poisoning found blood concentrations of over 100 mg/l for long acting barbiturates, of over 70 mg/l for butobaritone and amylobarbitone, and of over 30 mg/l for cyclobarbitone, pentobarbitone and quinalbarbitone, were compatible with death from barbiturate poisoning but were not completely diagnostic. Determination of blood levels gave a much better correlation with the degree of coma than did urine levels. Recovery of consciousness was associated with blood concentrations of about 70 mg/l for long-acting barbiturates, 23 to 29 mg/l for amylo- and butobarbitones, and 13 to 17 mg/l for cyclo- and pentobarbitones. Curry (1963) gave similar figures.

These figures however are open to considerable individual variation. Some patients found dead following ingestion of barbiturates only, may have blood concentrations around that normally associated with recovery of consciousness. Others who have developed tolerance to the drug may be conscious with a blood level which would normally cause coma or even death.

The determination of blood barbiturates is thus not helpful for assessing the progress in poisoning by these agents although it aids in the diagnosis of barbiturate ingestion. The management of the patient depends on clinical and not biochemical assessment. For this reason, it seems reasonable to restrict the measurement of barbiturates to normal laboratory hours. The identification of the particular drug or drugs involved is of forensic interest but also has clinical implications in that phenobarbitone remains in the circulation for a long time and its elimination is aided by forced alkaline diuresis. Most other barbiturates are relatively rapidly removed from the plasma and are not amenable to removal by increased urinary excretion to any significant degree.

The role of the laboratory in acute barbiturate poisoning is in the assessment of the adequacy of respiration and tissue perfusion, by blood gas analysis (Chap. 24, Vol. I) and in monitoring electrolyte balance during diuretic therapy (Chap. 23, Vol. I).

Chromatographic Methods for Separating Barbiturates

Barbiturates can be separated quickly by chromatography. Several workers have used paper (see Wright, 1954; Jackson, 1960; Curry, 1961, 1969a). The thin layer technique is particularly suitable.

Thin-layer Chromatography of Barbiturates (Lehmann and Karamustafoglu, 1962; Sunshine, 1963; Walker and Wood, 1965)

Reagents. 1. Silica gel G.
2. Hydrochloric acid, 1 mol/l.
3. Chloroform.

Drugs and Poisons 299

4. Ethanol, 800 ml diluted to 1 litre with water.

5. Standards. Prepare stock solutions containing 100 mg per 100 ml chloroform of phenobarbitone, butobarbitone, pentobarbitone, quinalbarbitone and hexobarbitone. Pool one volume of each of these, evaporate to dryness and dissolve the residue in 10 volumes of ethanol (reagent 4).

6. Solvent system, chloroform/acetone, 9/1, v/v.

7. Mercuric sulphate, 50 g/l in sulphuric acid, 200 ml concentrated acid diluted to a litre with water. Dilute 1/1 with water for use.

8. Diphenylcarbazone, 5 mg in 50 ml methanol. Prepare freshly for use.

9. Potassium permanganate solution, 1 g/l.

10. Concentrated sulphuric acid.

Technique. Use 20×10 cm glass plates coated with a 250 μm layer of silica gel G. Activate by heating at $110°$C for 30 to 60 min.

To obtain a suitable amount of test sample for applying to the plate, determine the barbiturate concentration by Broughton's method, then pool the two alkaline extracts and neutralise with hydrochloric acid (a drop of BDH. Universal indicator can be used). About 0.5 ml is required. Then re-extract the barbiturate into about 5 ml chloroform, shaking well. Centrifuge, suck off the aqueous layer and filter the chloroform layer into a dry, chloroform-cleaned small evaporating dish, and evaporate to dryness under a current of warm air. Take up the residue in 0.2 ml ethanol, reagent 4.

Apply approximately 5 μg barbiturate. If x ml of the original fluid was taken for the determination and the concentration was y mg/l, then 1 000/xy μl of the ethanol solution would contain 5 μg barbiturate except for the small losses in its preparation. This quantity contains sufficient barbiturate to show minor components and not enough to overload the chromatogram.

Apply two such samples as small spots 3 cm apart, 2 cm from the bottom edge of the plate, and, alternating with these, three 2 μl spots of the composite standard. Place the plate in a hot air oven at 135 $°$C for 10 min. Remove, place a drop of concentrated sulphuric acid on to one of the two sample spots. Deliver the acid from a fine glass capillary so as just to cover the sample spot. Excess of acid causes local deformation of the solvent front and retards the solute. Replace the plate in the oven for a further 5 min. The times are not critical; the reaction goes to completion within 1 min at 135 $°$C. If the acid is added to the cold plate with subsequent heating, however, variable reactions result.

Remove the plate from the oven, allow to cool for 5 min and then place in the developing tank until the front has travelled 15 cm. One to 2 h is needed. Use the smallest tank which will accommodate the plate. Saturation of the atmosphere is important to keep R_f's low and to obtain clear separation. Remove the plate from the tank and dry under a current of warm air. Spray first with mercuric sulphate. The Shandon Spray Gun is convenient but its metal nozzle soon disintegrates with this reagent. It is best replaced by a length of capillary bore glass tubing the upper end of

300 *Practical Clinical Biochemistry*

which is ground to a conical profile. Many barbiturates can be seen as white spots against a grey background. Hexobarbitone of the commonly used ones does not show in this way. After spraying, dry under hot air until the white spots just disappear. Then spray with diphenylcarbazone. This produces a uniform violet background which fades rapidly to show the barbiturates as purple or blue spots. The spots fade slowly during the next two to three hours. Some non-barbiturate substances in the extracts also give violet spots but these are well away from the standards and soon fade.

Table 7,11 lists the behaviour towards the different spraying agents of several common barbiturates and the R_f values with and without sulphuric

TABLE 7,11

Chromatography of Barbiturates

Barbiturate	White spot	Violet or blue	Yellow with $KMnO_4$	Rf Cf. barbitone = 1.0	After H_2SO_4
Barbitone	W	V	—	1.0	1.0
Phenobarbitone	W	V	—	1.0	1.0
Butobarbitone	W	V	—	1.3	1.3
Cyclobarbitone	—	V	Y	1.3	0.2
Pentobarbitone	W	V	—	1.4	0.1
Amylobarbitone	W	V	—	1.4	1.4
Heptabarbitone	W	V	Y	1.4	0.2
Quinalbarbitone	W	B	Y	1.6	0.1
Hexobarbitone	—	V	Y	1.9	0.1

acid treatment. The standard resolves into four spots. Phenobarbitone is the slowest; next butobarbitone and pentobarbitone form an oval violet spot; then a blue round spot of quinalbarbitone follows, with finally hexobarbitone the fastest. Cyclo- and heptabarbitone give distinctive blue spots after acid treatment with pento-, quinal-, and hexobarbitone only just clear the halo of acid, appearing as crescents at its upper margin. Spraying with aqueous permanganate can also be used. This gives a yellow colour with some but not with others.

It will be seen that in general long, intermediate, and short acting barbiturates have low, intermediate and high R_f values.

If an ultra-violet lamp emitting at 254 nm such as the Universal U.V. Lamp of Camag, marketed by Camlab (Glass) Ltd, of Cambridge is available, barbiturates on such a plate show up as black spots against a fluorescent background. MN silica gel G, HR/UV_{254} is designed for this purpose.

Drugs and Poisons

The Use of a Single Gas-Liquid Chromatographic Column of OV-17 on Gas Chrom Q for Barbiturates, Anticonvulsants and Basic Drugs

Several columns are available for investigating the various groups of drugs likely to be present. Leach (1969, 1975) gives a combination of systems covering most circumstances, and Leech and Jones (1971) describe chemical methods for separating them into groups of drugs, types of column to use, and retention times for a comprehensive series of most of the drugs. For screening and monitoring at least for barbiturates and anticonvulsant drugs, and for screening for basic drugs in serum the single column of OV-17 on Gas Chrom Q is very useful. Brief examples of its use are given below.

Barbiturates

The barbiturates, weakly acid substances, can be extracted into organic solvents from neutral or weakly acid solution, concentrated, and injected directly onto the column. Comparison of retention times and peak heights with those of a mixed standard similarly injected is used for identification and quantitation respectively.

Reagents. 1. Saturated solution of potassium dihydrogen phosphate.

2. Diethyl ether.

3. Chloroform.

4. Stock standard solution containing 1 g/l of each of the following: barbitone, butobarbitone, amylobarbitone, pentobarbitone, quinalbarbitone, hexobarbitone, phenobarbitone and cyclobarbitone. Dissolve 100 mg of each of these in chloroform, pool, and make to 100 ml with chloroform.

5. Working standard, 200 mg/l of each of the above. Dilute 20 ml stock standard to 100 ml with chloroform.

Technique. To 200 μl blood, serum or plasma in a 10 ml glass-stoppered centrifuge tube add 200 ml saturated potassium dihydrogen phosphate solution and 600 μl water. Mix, add 5 ml ether, stopper, and shake for 30 s. Centrifuge for 1 min to separate the phases. Pipette 3 ml of the ether extract into a glass-stoppered conical centrifuge tube and evaporate under a stream of nitrogen or air in a water bath at 40 to 50°C. Add 200 μl of chloroform washing down the sides of the tube, mix on a vortex mixer and again evaporate the contents to dryness. This concentrates the residue into the tip of the tube. Immediately prior to injection add 30 μl chloroform to take up the residue.

Gas chromatography. Silanise and pack a 2 m × 4 mm glass column with 3 per cent OV-17 on Gas Chrom Q. Operate isothermally at 180 to 190°C with gas flow rates of 50 ml/min for nitrogen and hydrogen and 500 ml/min for air. Inject 5 μl of the sample extract. As no internal standard is used a correction has to be applied for the average recoveries of the barbiturates concerned. This is 87 per cent for phenobarbitone an 80 per cent for the others.

302   *Practical Clinical Biochemistry*

Calculation. Provided the quantities are as above, 5 μl of extract is equivalent to 20 μl of blood. If x is the height of the standard peak and y that of the test, then:

$$\text{Blood barbiturate (mg/l)} = \frac{y}{x} \times 200 \times \frac{100}{\text{Per cent recovery}}$$

Note. Watson and Kalman (1972) used a similar column to this but preferred dichloromethane to ether because it extracted less interfering material which ran late on the column. In the absence of this the samples could be injected at a higher rate. In addition they used an internal standard of barbitone, the use of which they considered justifiable as it is rarely used clinically now, and it could still be detected by the increase in height of the test sample.

Anticonvulsants

The extraction is as described above. An internal standard of 5-*p*-methylphenyl-5-phenylhydantoin (MPPH) is added to the sample and also included in the standard.

$$CH_3 . C_6H_4 \diagdown \; \overset{\displaystyle H}{\underset{\displaystyle C_6H_5}{}}$$

MPPH

Reagents. 1, 2, 3, as above.

4. Internal standard, 50 mg/l. Dissolve 5 mg MPPH in about 2 ml sodium hydroxide, 100 mmol/l and dilute to 500 ml with water. MPPH can be obtained from the Aldrich Chemical Co. Ltd.

5. Stock standard solution containing 1 g/l each of phenytoin, primidone, and phenobarbitone and MPPH. Dissolve 100 mg of each of these in chloroform, pool in a 100 ml volumetric flask and dilute to the mark with chloroform.

6. Working standard, 200 mg/l of each. Dilute 20 ml stock solution to 100 ml with chloroform.

Technique. To 500 μl serum or blood (preferably serum for monitoring, either for overdose) add 500 μl MPPH and 500 μl saturated phosphate solution. Mix, add 5 ml ether, shake manually for 30 s and centrifuge about 1 min. Pipette 3 ml ether extract into a conical test tube and evaporate to dryness in a water bath at 40 to 50°C under a gentle stream of air. Concentrate the residue in the tip of the tube by dissolving in 200 μl chloroform, agitating for 20 s on a rotary mixer and again evaporating to dryness under a stream of air in a warm water bath. Immediately before injecting dissolve in 30 μl chloroform.

Drugs and Poisons 303

Gas chromatography. Use a column as above and programme from 180 to 280°C at 8°C/min for phenobarbitone and phenytoin. Inject 5 µl (1 mg) standard followed by 7.5 µl sample extract. Order of elution is phenobarbitone, primidone, phenytoin and MPPH.

Calculation. Calculate the ratios of peak heights for each component, for example:

$$\frac{\text{MPPH peak height (standard)}}{\text{Phenytoin peak height (standard)}} = \text{A}.$$

$$\frac{\text{Phenytoin peak height (unknown)}}{\text{MPPH peak height (unknown)}} = \text{B}.$$

Then Serum phenytoin (mg/l) = A × B × 40/3.

Basic Drugs

These are extracted from alkaline solution into organic solvents, concentrated, and injected into the column.

Reagents. 1. Sodium hydroxide solution, 500 mmol/l (20 g/l).
2. Diethyl ether.
3. Chloroform.
4. A suitable mixed standard contains 100 mg of each drug in 100 mg chloroform. Dilute to give 200 mg/l so that 5 µl contains 1 µg of each.

Technique. To 500 µl blood, serum, plasma, or urine in a stoppered tube, add 500 µl sodium hydroxide and 5 ml ether, shake for 30 s and centrifuge. Transfer 3 ml extract to a tapered centrifuge tube and evaporate to dryness under a stream of air in a warm water bath. Add 200 µl chloroform and agitate on a vortex mixer for 20 s. Evaporate again and immediately before injecting dissolve in 30 µl chloroform.

Gas chromatography. Prepare the column as above and operate isothermally at 240°C. Inject 5 µl extract and compare with 5 µl standard.

Order of elution is amitriptyline, nortriptyline, methaqualone, protriptyline, codeine, diazepam, chlordiazepoxide. Nitrazepam can be included by programming to 280°C. These drugs can be quantitated by comparing with a suitable standard using 1 µg for injecting although only an overdose of amitriptyline can be detected, not therapeutic concentrations.

BENZODIAZEPINES

The benzodiazepine group of drugs is widely prescribed. Some are mild tranquillisers, particularly chlordiazepoxide, diazepam, lorazepam, medazepam, oxazepam, and potassium chlorazepate. Some are employed as hypnotics, in particular nitrazepam and flurazepam. The use of clonazepam as an anticonvulsant has already been mentioned while diazepam may he

304   *Practical Clinical Biochemistry*

employed in treating status epilepticus. A feature of all these drugs is the possession of a relatively unstable seven-membered ring. The structures are as follows:

chlordiazepoxide (Librium, Tropium)

R_1	R_2	R_3	
Cl	CH_3	H	diazepam (Atensine, Valium)
NO_2	H	H	nitrazepam (Mogadon)
NO_2	H	Cl	clonazepam (Rivotril)
Cl	$-(CH_2)_2NEt_2$	F	flurazepam (Dalmane).

$R = H$ oxazepam (Serenid)
$R = Cl$ lorazepam (Ativan)

medazepam (Nobrium)   potassium chlorazepate (Tranxene)

Being widely available to disturbed patients these drugs are often taken in deliberate overdose sometimes with other agents. As Table 7,1 shows they are not often fatal but are by no means innocuous. Nitrazepam has been replacing the barbiturates as a hypnotic and it is claimed that dependence is much less of a problem.

The clinical effects of overdosage with the benzodiazepines taken alone are usually mild. Gastrointestinal absorption is slow and peak concentrations in the blood may not occur for several hours. Even after taking many times the therapeutic dose, the only effect may be drowsiness. There is, however, a marked additive effect if ethanol, barbiturates, or antidepressant drugs are also taken. It is therefore helpful to know if the benzodiazepines are involved in a patient who can be shown to have taken one of these other drugs. As a group they are only slowly metabolised and the products

Drugs and Poisons 305

are excreted in the urine for several days. Less than 5 per cent is excreted unchanged in 24 h. Chlordiazepoxide and diazepam are partly metabolised to oxazepam which is excreted as its glucosiduronate. Nitrazepam and clonazepam undergo reduction of the nitro group to an amino or acetylamino group as the main pathway. Several simple tests have been described for the qualitative investigation of urine.

Screening Tests for Benzodiazepines in Blood or Urine

A. Acid hydrolysis, diazotisation and coupling.

Under acid conditions the diazepine ring is cleaved with the formation of a substituted 2-aminobenzophenone. When the amino group is unsubstituted it can be diazotised and coupled with N-(1-naphthyl) ethylenediamine.

Reagents. 1. Ammonium hydroxide solution, sp. gr. 0.88.
2. Chloroform.
3. Hydrochloric acid, 6 mol/l. Mix equal volumes of the concentrated acid and water.
4. Sodium nitrite solution, 1 g/l.
5. Ammonium sulphamate solution, 5 g/l.
6. N(1-Naphthyl)ethylenediamine dihydrochloride solution, 5 g/l.

Technique. Adjust 5 to 10 ml plasma or urine to pH 10 with ammonium hydroxide and extract twice with 10 volumes of chloroform. Wash the combined extracts with 2 ml water, add 5 ml hydrochloric acid and shake for 5 min. Remove the chloroform layer and drive off the last traces of chloroform with gentle heat. Heat in an autoclave or in an oil heating bath at 125 °C for 30 min with the tube stoppered. Cool, make the volume to 5 ml with water, add 0.5 ml nitrite solution and stand for 3 min. Add 0.5 ml ammonium sulphamate, mix, and stand for 3 min. Finally add 0.5 ml of the coupling agent. A purplish mauve colour develops gradually (Table 7,12).

This test is given by benzodiazepines with an unsubstituted N-1 atom and most of their metabolites and also by other drugs or metabolites which possess a free arylamino group.

TABLE 7,12

Colour Reactions of Benzodiazepines

	Diazotisation + NNED	Reduction, diazotisation
Chlordiazepoxide	purple	—
Diazepam	—	—
Nitrazepam	purple-red	purple
Clonazepam	purple-red	purple
Oxazepam	pink-purple	—
Lorazepam	pink	—
Medazepam	—	—
Potassium chlorazepate	pale purple	—

B. Reaction for Nitrazepam and Clonazepam in Urine

The 7-nitro group is reduced to an amino group which is then diazotised and coupled as in the last test. Their 7-amino metabolites can be detected without prior reduction.

Reagents. 1. Ammonium hydroxide solution.
2. Sodium dithionite.
3. Dichloromethane, redistilled.
4. Ethyl acetate.
5. Sodium borate solution, 50 g/l.
6. Hydrochloric acid solution, 200 mmol/l.
7. Sodium nitrite solution, 4 g/l.
8. Ammonium sulphamate solution, 20 g/l.
9. N(1-Naphthyl) ethylenediamine dihydrochloride, 4 g/l.

Technique. (a) *For unchanged drug.* To 5 ml urine add ammonium hydroxide until alkaline (pH 10) and shake for 30 s. Add 250 mg dithionite, shake for 10 min and then heat at 50°C for 60 min. Cool, add 10 ml of a mixture of equal volumes of dichloromethane and ethyl acetate and shake for 10 min. Wash the solvent layer with 10 ml borate solution and extract with 5 ml hydrochloric acid. Cool 4 ml of the acid phase on ice and add 0.2 ml nitrite, mix and stand for 5 min, add 0.2 ml ammonium sulphamate, mix well and stand for a further 5 min. Add 0.2 ml coupling reagent and allow the colour to develop. A pinkish mauve colour with maximum at 555 nm indicates the presence of nitrazepam or clonazepam (Table 7,12).

(b) *For metabolites.* Proceed as above but omitting the reduction with dithionite.

The test is also given by other drugs containing an aromatic amino group.

C. Fluorimetric Reaction (Valentour *et al.*, 1975)

Acid cleavage of the diazepine ring yields a 2-amino benzophenone as in A above. This is converted on heating in alkaline solution with lead dioxide to a fluorescent 9-acridanone.

Drugs and Poisons

The metabolites react in many cases and the reaction can be used for measurement of the mixture of unchanged drug and its derivatives.

Reagents. 1. Extraction solvent. Mix 1.7 ml isoamyl alcohol with 98.3 ml n-hexane.

2. Sulphuric acid 1.8 mol/l.
3. Sulphuric acid, concentrated.
4. Dichloromethane.
5. Sodium hydroxide solution, 2 mol/l.
6. Lead dioxide reagent. Dissolve 10 g lead tetracetate in 30 ml glacial acetic acid in a screw-capped tube. Add 30 ml water, cap and shake vigorously while holding the tube in a stream of warm tap water. Centrifuge and aspirate the liquid phase. Add 50 ml water, shake at room temperature, centrifuge and re-aspirate. Repeat the process three more times and then mix the lead dioxide slurry with 30 ml water. The product is active for several months.

Technique. *Blood or gastric contents.* Place 4 ml sample and 10 ml extraction solvent in screw-capped tubes. (Teflon-lined caps) and place on a roller extractor for 15 min. Centrifuge 5 min, remove the upper, organic phase with a pipette and filter it. Place 1 ml sulphuric acid, 1.8 mol/l, in a clean screw-capped tube and add 8 ml filtrate. Cap and rotate for 15 min before centrifuging for 5 min and removing most of the upper organic phase. Transfer the uncapped tubes to a boiling water bath for 30 min for hydrolysis to occur. Cool, add 3 ml sodium hydroxide and 4 drops lead dioxide slurry. Heat the tubes in a boiling water bath for 45 min and then cool to room temperature. Centrifuge for 5 min. Either examine the fluorescence with the naked eye using a 365 nm source, or preferably, transfer the supernatant fluid to a fluorimeter cuvette and record the emission spectrum from 400 to 480 nm with excitation at 270 nm. For semi-quantitative work set up also appropriate standards and blanks. For blood use a standard in blood and a known negative blood. For gastric contents use an aqueous standard and blank.

Urine. Place 4 ml urine and 0.5 ml concentrated sulphuric acid in screw-capped tubes (Teflon-lined cap). Cap and heat in a boiling water bath for 30 min before cooling to room temperature. Add 5 ml dichloromethane, re-cap and rotate for 15 min. Centrifuge for 5 min before removing the upper layer. Add 2 ml sodium hydroxide, seal, shake for 1 min and centrifuge. Again aspirate the upper aqueous layer. Filter the dichloromethane layer into a clean test tube and evaporate in a warm water bath. To the residue add 4 ml sodium hydroxide, 4 drops lead dioxide slurry and heat in a boiling water bath for 45 min. Cool, centrifuge and examine as before.

308　　　　　　　　　　　　　　　　　　　*Practical Clinical Biochemistry*

The reaction which seems to be rather specific, is given by several benzodiazepines and their metabolites some of which are therapeutically active. Under the above reaction conditions the greatest fluorescence is given by chlordiazepoxide, diazepam, oxazepam, and potassium chlorazepate which all give a blue fluorescence. The maximum fluorescence is at 460 nm for diazepam and at 450 to 455 and 475 to 480 nm for the others. Lorazepam gives a weaker, bluish-green fluorescence but nitrazepam, clonazepam, flurazepam and medazepam give no visible fluorescence with therapeutic concentrations. Peaks in the fluorescent spectrum are apparent with somewhat higher concentrations at similar wavelengths with the exception of nitrazepam and clonazepam which give a single peak at 465 nm.

D. Sulphuric acid-formol reaction (Meunier *et al.*, 1970)

Details of the extraction and test procedure are given later (pp. 343, 345). The benzodiazepines give only faint colours or fluorescence with the exception of oxazepam which gives an orange fluorescence turning to blue on dilution with water.

E. Phosphoric acid–lead dioxide reaction (Meunier *et al.*, 1970)

This reaction is mainly used for the tricyclic antidepressants and details are given later (p. 355). Only chlordiazepoxide gives a colour reaction, namely purple. Fluorescence is seen more often: chlordiazepoxide, diazepam, oxazepam and lorazepam (green), potassium chlorazepate (blue-green) and medazepam (blue).

Spectroscopic Identification of Benzodiazepines in Blood, Urine or Gastric Aspirate

Basic drugs are extracted into ether and their absorption spectrum determined in acid and alkaline conditions.

Reagents. 1. Phosphate buffer, 1 mol/l, pH 7.0. Dissolve 15.6 g $Na_2HPO_4,2H_2O$ in about 80 ml water, adjust to pH 7.0 with sodium hydroxide, 5 mol/l and make to 100 ml.

2. Diethyl ether.
3. Sodium hydroxide solution, 100 mmol/l.
4. Sulphuric acid solution, 50 mmol/l.
5. Strong ammonia solution.
6. Standards of selected benzodiazepines.

Technique. To 10 ml urine, 5 ml blood or a suitable aliquot of gastric contents add an equal volume of phosphate buffer to bring the pH near to neutral. Extract twice with 10 ml ether, shaking for 5 min each time. Wash the combined extracts twice with 2 ml sodium hydroxide and twice with 2 ml water. Add 3 ml sulphuric acid and shake for 10 min. Separate the acid

Drugs and Poisons   309

TABLE 7,13

Absorption Maxima (nm) of Benzodiazepines

	In acid	In alkali
Chlordiazepoxide	*246*, 307	244-252 (plateau), *262*
Diazepam	*241*, 285	*229, ca.* 250 (inflection)
Nitrazepam	*264, ca.* 300 (inflection)	*264, ca.* 300 (inflection)
Chlorazepam	*264*, 302	*364*, 310
Medazepam	*253, ca.* 285 (inflection)	*229, ca.* 330

The major peak is in italics.

layer and read the UV spectrum over the range 200 to 400 nm and compare with standards. Then make alkaline with ammonia and rescan.

Many basic drugs are extracted and show absorption peaks. The characteristic peaks for some benzodiazepines are given in Table 7,13. Oxazepam, lorazepam and potassium chlorazepate are not extracted into the acid layer. If several other drugs are present, particularly the tricyclic antidepressants and the phenothiazines, identification may be difficult.

Other Tests

The use of a simple GLC method for the determination of therapeutic concentrations of medazepam and diazepam in blood and for somewhat higher levels of nitrazepam is described by Greaves (1974).

INTERPRETATION

The tests are capable of detecting benzodiazepines at the therapeutic dose level. In overdosage the tests should be positive in the urine for several days. The therapeutic dose is usually in the range 5 to 100 mg daily whereas the minimum lethal dose may be as high as 100 to 500 mg/kg.

BROMIDE

Excessive doses of bromide produce a state of intoxication with various abnormal mental manifestations. Determination of serum bromide provides a means of confirming that such a condition is present. The use of inorganic bromides as a sedative is now uncommon but carbromal in its combination with pentobarbitone as Carbrital is still in use (Table 7,1). This substance is hydrolysed with release of bromide ions and an increased serum bromide concentration is a feature of acute and chronic overdosage.

P.C.B.(II)—11

310 *Practical Clinical Biochemistry*

Determination of Serum Bromide (Barbour *et al.,* 1936)

After precipitating the proteins with trichloracetic acid, bromide is estimated by the brown colour of gold bromide formed on adding gold chloride.

Reagents. 1. Trichloracetic acid solution, 20 g/l.

2. Gold chloride ($AuCl_3$, $HCl,3H_2O$) solution, 5 g/l.

3. Stock solution of sodium bromide. Dissolve 1.49 g pure, dry, sodium bromide in water and make to a litre.

Technique. To 2 ml serum add 4 ml water followed by 1.2 ml trichloracetic acid. Shake well and centrifuge or filter through a 7 cm No. 1 Whatman paper. To 4 ml filtrate add 0.8 ml gold chloride solution. Read the resulting colour at 470 nm and compare with a standard curve prepared as follows:

Serum bromide (mmol/l)	0	2.5	5.0	10	15	20	25	30	35
Stock standard (ml)	0	0.25	0.50	1.00	1.50	2.00	2.50	3.00	3.50
Water (ml)	5.0	4.75	4.50	4.00	3.50	3.00	2.50	2.00	1.50

Add 1 ml gold chloride solution and 1 ml trichloracetic acid

Calculation. The standard bromide solution is made of this strength so as to correct for an error due to absorption of some bromide in the protein precipitate.

Note. Iodide interferes with the test since it gives a similar colour with gold chloride, so that when a positive result is obtained it is advisable to check that the patient has not been taking iodide.

INTERPRETATION

Bromide and chloride ions are handled similarly by the body. If bromide is ingested it will replace some of the chloride. The therapeutic and toxic effects depend on the extent of this replacement and its effect on the brain metabolism. Normal plasma contains only traces of bromide, less than 0.3 mmol/l which does not show any colour with the above test. Symptoms of intoxication appear when the serum bromide is between 10 and 20 mmol/l. There are considerable personal variations. With increasing bromide the symptoms become increasingly severe until, with values over 30 mmol/l, the patient becomes demented. When there is about 50 per cent replacement death is said to occur, that is at a serum bromide over about 45 mmol/l. On stopping the drug and giving sodium chloride, 10 to 15 g daily and enough fluid to produce a daily urine flow of 3 litres, the serum bromide falls steadily. The symptoms of the intoxication disappear in two or three days and the serum bromide may become normal again in a fortnight.

Drugs and Poisons

CARBON MONOXIDE

Carbon monoxide has 200 times the affinity for haemoglobin than does oxygen. So air containing carbon monoxide in a concentration of 0.1 per cent will convert half the haemoglobin into carboxyhaemoglobin if breathed for an hour. At twice this concentration, death may supervene within a few hours. Carbon monoxide is implicated in fatal poisoning either accidentally or with deliberate intent (Table 7,2). Town gas now contains much less carbon monoxide than 20 years ago and in many areas is entirely natural gas, virtually free from carbon monoxide. The latter is, however, formed when carbonaceous matter is burnt in oxygen-poor conditions. Car exhaust fumes liberated in a closed garage or leakage from the flue of a solid-fuel stove are examples.

Methods for the determination of carboxyhaemoglobin in blood are given in Chap. 27, Vol. 1. In the absence of anaemia, toxic effects such as headache and lassitude appear at about 20 per cent saturation with carbon monoxide. More severe symptoms with muscular weakness, giddiness, fainting attacks and dyspnoea develop as the saturation increases to 50 per cent. Loss of consciousness occurs at 50 to 80 per cent saturation with a fatal outcome if exposure continues, the length of time shortening at the higher concentrations. Removal from the carbon monoxide atmosphere allows fairly rapid breakdown of carboxyhaemoglobin with reformation of oxyhaemoglobin. The important irreversible effects on cerebral function depend on the degree and duration of impaired oxygenation of the brain.

Samples of blood for analysis should be taken with minimum delay after removal from the toxic atmosphere and should be anticoagulated and stored under oil to avoid loss of carbon monoxide.

CHLORATE

Sodium and potassium chlorate are occasionally encountered in toxicology. They are components of weed killers, mouthwashes and throat lozenges. Accidental or deliberate ingestion may occur. They are strong oxidising agents, a fact made use of in their detection. Oxidation of haemoglobin to methaemoglobin and lysis of red cells occurs. Methaemoglobin is detectable in blood or sometimes plasma by spectroscopic means (Chap. 27, Vol. 1). It may also occur in the urine and if excessive is often associated with the development of anuria. Gastro-intestinal irritation and liver damage are features of chlorate poisoning.

The best chance of detecting the poison is in gastric contents. Although present in blood or urine the concentration is less and some has been lost by interaction with organic matter.

312   *Practical Clinical Biochemistry*

Screening Tests for Chlorate (Higgins and Leach, 1975)

These are based on the oxidising properties of chlorate in acid solution.

A. Diphenylamine test for oxidising agents

Reagent. Diphenylamine, 1 g/l in concentrated sulphuric acid.
Technique. Filter or centrifuge gastric contents. To 2 drops of the fluid add 1 drop of reagent and mix. The instantaneous formation of a deep blue colour indicates the presence of an oxidising agent. Faint blue colours are caused by organic matter. Preserved meats containing nitrates and nitrites also give a positive reaction. If a blue colour is obtained a more specific test should be carried out.

B. Aniline—sulphuric acid test

Reagents. 1. Aniline.
2. Concentrated sulphuric acid.
3. Ammonium sulphate, solid.
4. Ammonium hydroxide solution, sp. gr. 0.88.
5. Methanol.
Technique. Saturate 50 ml gastric contents with ammonium sulphate, make alkaline with ammonia and heat, with frequent shaking, in a boiling water bath for 10 min. Cool and filter. Bulky precipitates are washed with 25 ml saturated ammonium sulphate solution made slightly acid with sulphuric acid. Acidify the filtrate(s) with sulphuric acid and add methanol to precipitate all the ammonium sulphate; usually 200 ml suffices. Filter, make the solution strongly alkaline with ammonia and evaporate to dryness. If ammonium sulphate crystals are present dissolve in a little water, add methanol to precipitate, filter and re-evaporate to dryness. Dissolve the residue in 3 ml water and filter if necessary.

To 1 ml filtrate add 1 drop aniline and 1 ml concentrated sulphuric acid in such a way as to form a lower layer. Chlorate is recognised by a blue ring at the interface.

Note. The final colour test can be applied directly to 5 ml urine or to deproteinised blood. Mix equal volumes of blood and 200 g/l trichloracetic acid, centrifuge and use 2 ml supernatant fluid.

INTERPRETATION

Serious and sometimes fatal poisoning occurs with the ingestion of 15 g of sodium or potassium chlorate. The more severe cases are accompanied by well marked haemolysis and methaemoglobin is easily detected. Biochemical evidence of hepatic and renal damage should be sought. The haemolytic process usually causes an increase in serum potassium.

Drugs and Poisons

313

ETHANOL

This is one of the commonest agents affecting cerebral function and is readily available. Although death from acute alcohol poisoning itself is uncommon, alcohol is often taken with other drugs and potentiates their effects sometimes with fatal results. Alcohol ingestion is also important at sub-lethal levels from a medico-legal point of view, particularly in relation to the Road Traffic Acts. The clinical biochemist may require to detect alcohol in urine as part of screening tests for a variety of poisons or to determine its concentration in body fluids.

A relatively non-specific method is to distil, aerate, or allow the alcohol to diffuse into acid potassium dichromate solution. Primary alcohols are oxidised to the corresponding acids with reduction of the dichromate. The dichromate remaining is determined iodimetrically or colorimetrically. Many substances which interfere give rise to severe poisoning or death at apparent ethanol concentrations of less than 500 mg/l. Acetone only interferes at temperatures well above 37° C.

A more specific method uses alcohol dehydrogenase with NAD as coenzyme. Acetaldehyde is formed and may be bound by adding semicarbazide

$$CH_3 CH_2 OH + NAD \rightarrow CH_3 CHO + NADH_2$$

The formation of $NADH_2$ is determined from the increase in extinction at 340 nm. Reagents are commercially available. Propanol, n-butanol, allyl alcohol and ethylene glycol are also attacked, but methanol, other butanols and pentanols with branched chains are not. The enzyme is inhibited by several drugs including disulphiram, allopurinol and metronidazole. For the usual method 0.5 to 1 ml deproteinised blood is needed to give a coefficient of variation of 1 to 2 per cent.

Gas chromatography is being increasingly used as a sensitive and specific method for the determination of ethanol particularly for medico-legal purposes.

Ethanol is excreted by the lungs at a rate of 0.5 per cent of the total body alcohol content per hour. The concentration in expired air is about 1/2100 that in blood. The Breathalyser test involves passing one litre of alveolar air through a tube packed with silica gel impregnated with acid dichromate. The extent of the reduction, noted by the colour change, is proportional to the expired alcohol concentration.

If blood is analysed for medico-legal purposes certain precautions are needed. Collect the specimen as soon after the incident as possible using an anticoagulant such as potassium oxalate and sodium fluoride. Allow sterilising fluid to evaporate from the skin fully before puncturing the surface. Use a dry syringe for intravenous specimens. Divide the specimen into at least two portions and place in dry, sterile, sealed containers. Label these carefully and keep careful records of the analysis. Analyse within as short a time as possible.

314 *Practical Clinical Biochemistry*

Rapid Screening Test for Alcohols in Urine (Clarke, 1975)

Place 1 ml urine in a glass-stoppered tube. Apply to a strip of glass fibre paper one drop of acid dichromate solution. Prepare this by adding 50 ml concentrated sulphuric acid to about 40 ml water containing 2.5 g potassium dichromate, cool and make to 100 ml. Place the glass fibre strip in the upper part of the tube and seal with the stopper. Heat the tube in a boiling water bath for 2 min. Volatile alcohols produce a green colour on the strip.

To distinguish methanol from ethanol place 1 ml urine in a test tube and add 1 drop of acid dichromate solution. After leaving 5 min at room temperature add one drop of ethanol, a few mg of chromotropic acid and concentrated sulphuric acid to form a lower layer. Look for a purple zone at the interface. This is due to formaldehyde formed from methanol or occasionally present in the urine.

Determination by the Dichromate Method

A convenient form of this method is to use the Conway unit (see Chap. 27, Vol. I, and Conway, 1957).

Reagents. 1. Potassium dichromate, 5 mmol/l in 5 mol/l sulphuric acid. Dissolve 1.47 g potassium dichromate in water, add 266 ml concentrated sulphuric acid slowly while cooling and make to 1 litre with water.

2. Potassium carbonate, saturated solution.

3. Potassium iodide solution, 200 g/l.

4. Sodium thiosulphate, 50 mmol/l containing 50 mg sodium carbonate/l to stabilise it.

5. Starch solution, 10 g/l.

Technique. Pipette 1 ml dichromate-sulphuric acid reagent into the inner chamber and into the outer one run about 0.5 ml potassium carbonate solution. Place the lid in position with a suitable fixative. For this Conway used liquid paraffin. Other fixatives are a mixture prepared by melting 40 to 50 g paraffin wax m.p. about 40°C with 80 ml pure liquid paraffin and then cooling, or a silicone stopcock grease. Slide back the lid a little and place 100 μl of the sample into another part of the outer chamber, replace the lid in position and by tilting mix with the carbonate. Set aside for about 2 h at room temperature. Then remove the lid, add 1 ml potassium iodide to the dichromate, and titrate the liberated iodine immediately with thiosulphate using a Conway burette, adding a drop of starch solution when the solution becomes light yellow-green. The final disappearance of the blue colour to leave a light blue-green is quite abrupt. Carry out a blank using 100 μl water instead of the sample.

Calculation. As 1 molecule of dichromate in acid solution provides 3 atoms of oxygen:

$$K_2 Cr_2 O_7 + 4H_2 SO_4 \rightarrow K_2 SO_4 + Cr_2 (SO_4)_3 + 3O + 4H_2 O$$

Drugs and Poisons 315

and 2 atoms of oxygen are required to oxidise 1 molecule of ethanol

$$CH_3 CH_2 OH + 2O \rightarrow CH_3 COOH + H_2 O$$

1 molecule dichromate $\equiv$ 1.5 molecule ethanol
with an overall reaction:

$$2K_2 Cr_2 O_7 + 3CH_3 CH_2 OH + 8H_2 SO_4 \rightarrow$$

$$2K_2 SO_4 + Cr_2 (SO_4)_3 + 3CH_3 COOH + 11H_2 O$$

Furthermore 1 atom of oxygen oxidises 2 molecules of potassium iodide

$$2KI + O + H_2 SO_4 \rightarrow K_2 SO_4 + I_2 + H_2 O$$

1 molecule dichromate $\equiv$ 6 atoms of iodine

the overall reaction being:

$$K_2 Cr_2 O_7 + 7H_2 SO_4 + 6KI \rightarrow 4K_2 SO_4 + Cr_2 (SO_4)_3 + 3I_2$$

And finally, since

$$2Na_2 S_2 O_3 + I_2 \rightarrow 2NaI + Na_2 S_4 O_6$$

1 molecule thiosulphate $\equiv$ 1 atom iodine

So 1 molecule dichromate $\equiv$ 6 molecules thiosulphate $\equiv$ 1.5 molecules ethanol that is: 1 molecule thiosulphate $\equiv$ 0.25 molecules ethanol. So, if B = titration of blank in ml, and U = titration of the unknown in ml, and the thiosulphate solution is 50 mmol/l, and 100 μl blood were taken:

$$\text{Blood ethanol (mmol/l)} = (B - U) \times \frac{0.25 \times 50}{1\,000} \times \frac{10^6}{100} = (B - U) \times 125$$

Or blood ethanol (mg/l) = $(B - U) \times 125 \times 46 = (B-U) \times 5\,750$.

Notes. 1. The above method is suitable for ethanol concentrations above 200 mg/l.

2. If blood is not examined immediately place in a well sealed container and keep cool. Sodium fluoride, 2 to 5 mg, may be added as preservative.

3. *Modifications.* A technique using larger quantities is as follows. Use 0.5 ml 66.7 mmol/l dichromate in 5 mol/l sulphuric acid and 0.25 ml blood in severe intoxication, 0.5 ml in moderate intoxication, and 1 ml in other cases. Stand at room temperature overnight, or 6 h at 37°C. Then to the dichromate add 0.5 ml water and 0.75 ml potassium iodide and titrate from a 2 ml microburette with 100 mmol/l thiosulphate to a pale green, add starch, and complete the titration. Then if B and U are as above:

$$\text{Blood ethanol (mg/l)} = (B - U) \times \frac{1\,150}{\text{volume of specimen (ml)}}$$

Sunshine and Nenad (1953), Conway (1957), and Harger (1961) read in an absorptiometer. These workers used 3 ml acid dichromate (4.26 g dichromate in 100 ml water plus 500 ml concentrated sulphuric acid added

316 *Practical Clinical Biochemistry*

slowly while cooling), 500 μl of the specimen, and 1 ml sodium carbonate (200 g/l). Diffusion was for 20 min at 90°C after which the dichromate was removed, washing out twice with water and then making to 25 ml. This was read at 450 nm. A calibration curve was prepared by putting through a series of ethanol standards up to 4 000 mg/l.

The Widmark flask has been much used with dichromate methods. Widmark's own technique was given by Harger (1961) and Lundquist (1959) and was used by Cavett (1938).

4. The precision of the method is poorer than that of the enzymic method and the coefficient of variation is about 5 per cent. Non-ethanolic substances give an apparent ethanol concentration of 50 to 100 mg/l.

Determination by Gas Chromatography (Cooper, 1971)

In the simplest method for blood ethanol by GLC, whole blood is diluted with an internal standard of n-propanol and injected directly into the GLC column (Payne *et al.,* 1967). The blood, however, may coagulate and block the syringe needle on entry into the injection port. Also deposition of protein on the first few cm of the column necessitates frequent repacking of this part of the column. Cooper (1971) eliminated these problems by precipitating proteins with tungstate. This is the method given.

Reagents. 1. n-Propanol internal standard. A suitable concentration of n-propanol for use with blood ethanol levels ranging from 500 to 2 500 mg/l is 100 mg/l which can be obtained as follows. The specific gravity of n-propanol is 0.7859. Dilute 5 ml to 100 ml with water to give a solution containing 39.3 g/l. Dilute 12.72 ml of this solution (500 mg n-propanol) to 100 ml to give a solution containing 5 g/l. Make a further dilution of 2 ml to 100 ml with water to get the solution containing 100 mg/l for use.

2. Sodium tungstate, 100 g/l.

3. Sulphuric acid, 330 mmol/l.

4. Standard ethanol solution, 800 mg/l. Weigh 80 mg ethanol and dilute to 100 ml with water.

Technique. To 200 μl whole blood sample or 200 μl ethanol standard add 3 ml n-propanol followed by 250 μl sodium tungstate and 250 μl sulphuric acid, mixing between each addition. Leave to stand for 5 min and centrifuge for 2 min. First prime the column by injecting 5 μl water as a blank and then inject 5 μl of the standard extract followed by 5 μl of the blood extract.

Cooper used Poropak Q at 170°C with a flame ionisation detector. Satisfactory results can also be obtained with Carbowax 400 at 85°C with hydrogen and nitrogen flows at 50 ml/min and air at 500 ml/min. The order of elution on Poropak Q is water, methanol, ethanol, n-propanol and on Carbowax 400, methanol, ethanol, n-propanol and water. Read peak

Drugs and Poisons 317

heights of the ethanol and propanol in the standard and compare with those obtained for the test solution.

Calculation. Blood ethanol (mg/l) =

$$\frac{\text{Peak height } n\text{-propanol in standard}}{\text{Peak height ethanol in standard}} \times$$

$$\frac{\text{Peak height ethanol in unknown}}{\text{Peak height } n\text{-propanol in unknown}} \times 800$$

INTERPRETATION

Ingested ethanol is rapidly distributed throughout the body water reaching equilibrium with the brain and liver within a few minutes and with muscle within an hour. Ethanol is excreted unchanged with water in urine, expired air and perspiration, the hourly rates being about 0.24, 0.50, and 0.12 per cent of the total alcohol content of the body respectively. Over 90 per cent of the alcohol is removed by tissue oxidation giving a total average rate of disappearance of 100 mg kg^{-1} h^{-1}. The average hourly rate of fall of blood alcohol concentration is about 200 mg/l in normals but may be 500 mg/l in habitual drinkers and much less if serious liver damage is present. There are minor differences in the ethanol concentration of venous and capillary blood and between whole blood and plasma. For legal purposes it is usual to allow for these variables and the analytical error of the method by deducting 60 mg/l up to 1 000 mg/l and 6 per cent of all figures beyond this.

The current maximal legal blood alcohol concentration for drivers of vehicles in the United Kingdom is 800 mg/l. Above 1 g/l varying degrees of intoxication are apparent but there is considerable variation in the correlation of blood levels and clinical effects. In particular, regular heavy drinkers show tolerance of concentrations which produce severe intoxication in the non-drinker. On average, definite confusion is apparent above 2 g/l leading to stupor at 3 g/l and coma at 4 g/l and beyond. The concentration in urine is about a third higher than the blood. This arises from the different water content and the fact that the urine is being collected over a period when blood levels are falling quickly. The legal limit for urinary ethanol concentration for vehicle drivers is 1.07 g/l.

Considerable care is needed in the interpretation of ethanol concentrations in post-mortem material, particularly if much autolysis has occurred. Ethanol may be formed by microbiological activity and may be destroyed by enzyme activity. The same may be true for unpreserved blood kept at 37° under non-sterile conditions.

For a useful review of methods for ethanol determination and many aspects of ethanol intoxication see Harger (1961), Ritchie (1970), Cravey *et al.* (1974), Mason and Dubowski (1974).

318　　　　　　　　　　　　　　　　　　*Practical Clinical Biochemistry*

HYPNOTICS OTHER THAN BARBITURATES

A group of drugs has been introduced for their hypnotic action in an effort to avoid the undesirable effects of barbiturates. They are often taken in self-poisoning and several have been responsible for deaths (Table 7,1). They may create dependence like the barbiturates. The group includes substances of very different composition and in many cases identification of the agent involved may be more helpful than quantitative determination in the clinical management of the patient. Drugs included in this group are carbromal, chloral hydrate and its derivatives, ethchlorvynol, ethinamate, glutethimide, methaqualone, methyprylone, and the benzodiazepines, nitrazepam and flurazepam. The latter have been discussed previously (p. 303).

Carbromal

This substituted urea is almost entirely prescribed in combination with pentobarbitone as Carbrital. Its structure is shown on the left and its metabolic product, 2-hydroxy-2-ethylbutyric acid on the right. The

$$Br - \underset{\underset{C_2H_5}{|}}{\overset{\overset{C_2H_5}{|}}{C}} - CO \cdot NH \cdot CO \cdot NH_2 \rightarrow HO - \underset{\underset{C_2H_5}{|}}{\overset{\overset{C_2H_5}{|}}{C}} - COOH$$

bromine is released as the bromide ion (see p. 309). Very little carbromal is detectable in blood or urine but gastric aspirate can be subjected to a simple screening test.

Screening Test for Carbromal in Gastric Aspirate

Prepare an ether extract of acidified gastric aspirate as outlined in Table 7,3 up to the stage of the first water wash. Evaporate to dryness after filtering. Dissolve the residue in 2 drops of sodium hydroxide solution, 50 g/l, transfer to a white porcelain dish or tile and dry with gentle heating. Cool, add 2 drops of fluorescein solution, 10 g/l, 4 drops glacial acetic acid and 4 drops of strong hydrogen peroxide solution ("100 volumes"). Evaporate to dryness on a boiling water bath. Carbromal gives a red residue.

If this test is positive, blood should be examined for the presence of pentobarbitone and bromide. The usual therapeutic dose is 250 mg carbromal with 100 mg pentobarbitone. The ingestion of 10 g carbromal may prove fatal.

Drugs and Poisons 319

Chloral Hydrate

This is a long established hypnotic with a burning taste. Its formula and metabolic fate is shown below:

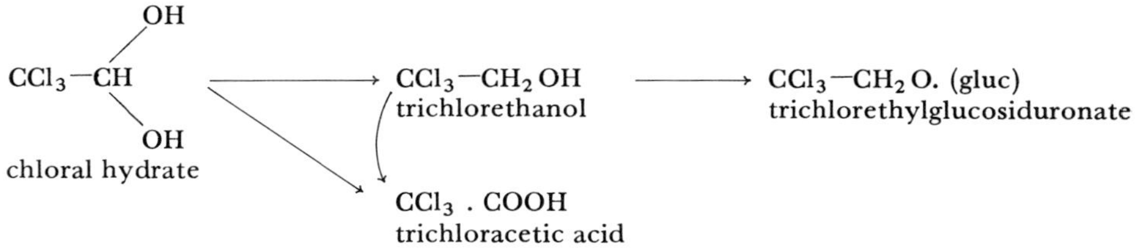

$$CCl_3-CH \begin{matrix} OH \\ \\ OH \end{matrix} \longrightarrow CCl_3-CH_2OH \longrightarrow CCl_3-CH_2O. \text{ (gluc)}$$

chloral hydrate   trichlorethanol   trichlorethylglucosiduronate

$$CCl_3 . COOH$$
trichloracetic acid

Trichlorethanol is probably the active substance. Various liquid preparations of chloral hydrate are available but are now less widely used than more convenient proprietary products. These include Noctec (chloral hydrate capsules): the phosphate ester of trichlorethanol, triclofos (Tricloryl) which is rapidly hydrolysed to the alcohol; the complex of chloral and phenazone, dichloralphenazone (Paedo-Sed, Welldorm) which is rapidly dissociated in the stomach yielding chloral.

The different substances and other trichlorinated compounds are detected by Fujiwara's test.

Fujiwara's Test for Trichloro-compounds

For blood or gastric aspirate make an ether extract from the acidified fluid as in Tables 7,3 and 7,4. Evaporate and redissolve in 1 ml water. For urine take 1 ml. To either add 1 ml sodium hydroxide solution, 100 g/l, and 1 ml pyridine. Heat in a boiling water bath for 2 min. A positive test is shown by a pink or red colour in the pyridine layer.

The test is given by several chlorinated hydrocarbons used as anaesthetics or cleaning fluids. They include chloroform, trichlorethylene and trichloroethane.

The usual dose of chloral or its equivalent is 1 to 2 g. Fatal poisoning has occurred with as little as 10 g but there is a wide variation and recovery from 30 g is recorded.

Ethchlorvynol

This substance, available also as Serenesil, has the structure shown. It is not often involved in deaths from poisoning (Table 7,1) but can be detected by a simple screening test.

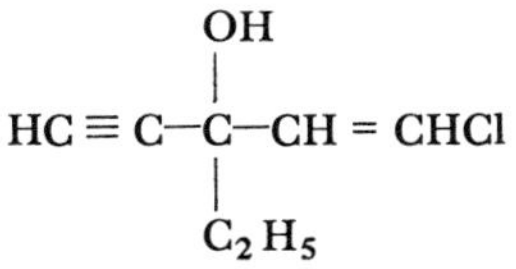

$$HC \equiv C - \underset{\underset{C_2H_5}{|}}{\overset{\overset{OH}{|}}{C}} - CH = CHCl$$

Practical Clinical Biochemistry

Simple Screening Test for Ethchlorvynol in Blood, Urine or Gastric Aspirate

Prepare an ether extract as outlined in Table 7,3 up to the first water wash. Dry with a little anhydrous sodium sulphate and mix 2 ml with 0.4 ml of a freshly prepared solution of phloroglucinol in ethanol (100 mg/ml). Add 3.6 ml concentrated hydrochloric acid and heat in a boiling water bath for 30 min. A positive test is shown by the rapid development of a greenish colour which slowly becomes orange. The intensity is proportional to the amount of ethchlorvynol.

The usual dose is 0.5 to 1 g and the lethal dose about 15 g. Quantitative determination by spectroscopy (Wallace *et al.,* 1974b) and GLC (Evenson and Poquette, 1974) is possible.

Glutethimide

Glutethimide, also available as Doriden, is an important cause of poisoning in this group (see Table 7,1). The structural similarity to the barbiturates and some anticonvulsant drugs suggests that it will also ionise in alkaline solution to give a characteristic absorption in the ultraviolet.

Glutethimide (α-ethyl-α-phenyl glutarimide)

Determination of Serum Glutethimide. Method of Dauphinais and McComb (1965)

Glutethimide is readily extracted into chloroform. The extract is washed with alkali and acid and then evaporated to dryness. UV-absorbing material besides glutethimide still present is removed by partition between ethanol/water and hexane, the non-glutethimide component passing into the hexane. The extinction of the ethanol solution is read at 235 nm for the blank, and is read again after making alkaline. Glutethimide is thereby hydrolysed over 30 min, with reduction of the extinction. Several readings are made during this time to enable the extinction at zero time to be calculated. The difference between this and the extinction in neutral solution is used in the calculation. This action of alkali is used to prevent interference by glutethimide in the determination of barbiturates (p. 293).

Reagents. 1. Chloroform, spectroscopic grade.

2. Sodium hydroxide, 450 mmol/l, 18 g/l.

3. Hydrochloric acid, 600 mmol/l. Dilute 25 ml concentrated acid to 500 ml with water.

4. Ethanol, analytical reagent grade.

Drugs and Poisons 321

5. *n*-Hexane, spectroscopic grade.

6. Ethanol/water, blank solution. Mix 5 ml water with 20 ml ethanol.

7. Potassium hydroxide solution, 10 mol/l. Dissolve 56 g in about 80 ml water and make to 100 ml when cool.

8. Glutethimide standard, 50 mg/l. Dissolve 10 mg purified crystalline glutethimide in chloroform and dilute to 200 ml. A solution in chloroform is as stable as in ethanol and is more suitable.

Technique. To 2 ml serum contained in a 150 ml separating funnel add 25 ml chloroform from a measuring cylinder. For the standard take 2 ml water, 2 ml standard, and 23 ml chloroform. Stopper and shake for 3 min with intermittent removal of the stopper to release the pressure. Filter the lower chloroform layer through a Whatman No. 541 paper into a second separating funnel. Add 5 ml sodium hydroxide to the filtered extract and shake again for 3 min. Repeat filtration into a third separating funnel, add 5 ml hydrochloric acid and shake again for 3 min. Transfer 15 ml of the chloroform solution to a 150 x 15 mm ground glass-stoppered tube and evaporate to dryness on a rotary evaporator at $50°C$ or on a water bath at $80°C$ using a stream of air. Remove from the bath immediately the chloroform has evaporated to avoid any destruction of glutethimide. To each tube add 2 ml ethanol, 5 ml hexane and 0.5 ml water, mix thoroughly and allow layers to separate. Remove the top hexane layer and discard.

Set up 3 silica cuvettes as follows: test, 1 ml ethanol-water extract of serum; standard, 1 ml ethanol-water extract of standard; blank, 1 ml ethanol-water blank solution. To each add a further 2 ml ethanol and 1 ml water, mix thoroughly and read test and standard against the blank at 235 nm to give the readings in neutral solution. Add 0.1 ml potassium hydroxide to the blank cuvette, cap with parafilm and mix thoroughly. Use this to zero the spectrophotometer at 235 nm. Add 0.1 ml potassium hydroxide to the standard cuvette, start a stop watch, cap and mix. Read at 1 min intervals for 5 min. Repeat this procedure with the test cuvette. Plot the readings against time and extrapolate back for readings of test and standard at zero time.

Calculation. Serum glutethimide (mg/l)

$$= \frac{\text{Reading of unknown at zero time} - \text{Reading of neutral solution of unknown}}{\text{Reading of standard at zero time} - \text{Reading of neutral solution of standard}} \times 50$$

INTERPRETATION

Glutethimide poisoning resembles barbiturate poisoning but shock, myocardial damage and metabolic acidosis may be more severe. At glutethimide levels of 10 mg/l, drowsiness is apparent. In patients who have not developed tolerance, figures above 30 mg/l are associated with severe poisoning with the possibility of a fatal outcome. Higher levels with recovery are seen in patients who have become habituated to the drug with

322   *Practical Clinical Biochemistry*

the development of tolerance. The usual therapeutic dose is 0.5 g and recovery is uncertain in the dose range of 5 to 10 g. It is probable that several metabolites of the drug, present in the plasma, are also involved in the depression of the CNS. The situation is demonstrable by gas chromatography but its interpretation is uncertain (Gold *et al.*, 1974; Hansen and Fisher, 1974).

Methaqualone

Methaqualone (Melsedin, Revanol) is almost entirely prescribed in combination with diphenhydramine as Mandrax. The development of dependence is not uncommon and addiction is well recognised so that

methaqualone

preparations are now controlled under the Misuse of Drugs Act. It is an important member of the non-barbiturate hypnotics in causing death by poisoning (Table 7,1).

The drug is rapidly absorbed and is metabolised to a series of hydroxylated derivatives (Bonnichsen *et al.*, 1974). Several of these are present in blood and some are extracted with methaqualone itself in the basic fraction when chloroform is used as the solvent. This leads to a discrepancy between GLC and spectroscopic methods of determining methaqualone in the extract as the metabolites have a similar spectrum to that of methaqualone. The disagreement may be such that the spectroscopic method overestimates the methaqualone concentration by several fold (Bailey and Jatlow, 1973). Some hydroxylated metabolites are phenols and this may account for earlier observations that the drug is also extracted in small amounts in the neutral and weak acid fractions (Lawson and Brown, 1967; Curry, 1969a). These polar metabolites are not extracted by *n*-hexane and this method, given below, gives a good correlation with GLC techniques. Methods for the latter have been described using 3 per cent OV-17 (Bailey and Jatlow, 1973) and 3 per cent OV-1 (Evenson and Lensmeyer, 1974).

Determination in Serum (Bailey and Jatlow, 1973)

Methaqualone is extracted into hexane and re-extracted into acid before determination by spectroscopy.

Reagents. 1. Sodium hydroxide solution, 1 mol/l, 40 g/l.
2. Sodium hydroxide solution, 450 mmol/l, 18 g/l.
3. *n*-Hexane, analytical grade, redistilled.

Drugs and Poisons

4. Hydrochloric acid, 1 mol/l.

5. Methaqualone standards in serum, 20 and 40 mg/l.

Technique. Place 1 ml serum in a ground glass-stoppered tube and adjust to pH 12 approximately using sodium hydroxide, 1 mol/l. Add 5 ml *n*-hexane, stopper, and shake 3 min. After separation of the hexane, remove this and filter it through Whatman No. 1 paper into a second tube. Repeat the extraction and filtration step with a second 5 ml hexane. Shake the combined extracts with 3 ml sodium hydroxide, 450 mmol/l, for 2 min. Separate and remove the alkaline layer. Add 3 ml hydrochloric acid, shake 3 min, and separate. Centrifuge, if necessary, to clarify. Transfer the acid layer to a 1 cm path silica cuvette and scan from 200 to 350 nm. Methaqualone gives a peak at 234 nm with a second peak near 210 nm and a weak peak at 269 nm. Measure the extinction at 234 nm for the samples and for standards and water blanks put through the same procedure, reading against the water blank.

Calculation.

$$\text{Serum methaqualone (mg/l)} = \frac{\text{Reading of Unknown}}{\text{Reading of Standard}}$$

$$\times \text{ concentration of standard.}$$

Notes. 1. The recovery of the drug in the extraction is only 50 to 55 per cent. Chloroform gives 55 to 60 per cent. Hence the use of serum standards is important.

2. The calibration curve is linear from 0 to 40 mg/l.

3. The coefficient of variation over a 12 day period is reported as 6.6 per cent.

INTERPRETATION

The effects of methaqualone overdosage are deep unconsciousness, convulsions, signs of pyramidal involvement, acute myocardial damage and sometimes acute pulmonary oedema. Therapeutic concentrations in plasma are in the range 2 to 3 mg/l. Much higher values are seen in patients who have acquired tolerance to the drug by frequent intake. In the absence of such tolerance there is usually loss of consciousness at levels above 8 mg/l and figures up to 22 mg/l are reported. Rather higher figures are found if chloroform extraction is used. Then values over 30 mg/l indicate potentially serious toxic effects and figures up to 60 mg/l may be seen.

The normal dose is 200 to 400 mg and serious poisoning occurs after 5 g is taken. Only about 2 per cent of the drug is excreted in the urine unchanged so serum determinations are preferable.

The ingestion of Mandrax involves diphenhydramine intake of one tenth that of methaqualone. This does not seem to have any additional serious effects.

324 *Practical Clinical Biochemistry*

LEAD

Lead is a good example of an environmental hazard. The metal itself is used in various ways in sheet, foil or pipe forms. Alloys with antimony and/or tin are used for bearings, printing type, accumulator plates, solder, bullets and shot. White lead (PbO) and lead carbonate are used in pottery glazing and red lead (Pb_3O_4) is a protective primer for steel. The use of white lead in paints is now much less frequent than previously. The organic compound, lead tetraethyl, is an "anti-knock" agent added to high octane petroleum. It is converted into finely particulate inorganic forms of lead during combustion and discharged into the atmosphere.

Lead may enter the body directly as lead shot but is usually either ingested or inhaled. Ingestion includes lead from water pipes, gnawing of lead paints in children and contamination of the hands and later of the food in workers handling lead in any form. Inhalation of lead fumes occurs in the general public from atmospheric pollution but to a potentially much greater degree in industrial workers involved in the manufacture of batteries, rubber, linoleum, paint, vitreous enamel or glazed pottery. Particular hazards arise in paint burning, shipbreaking and casting.

Although acute lead poisoning can occur following sudden excessive exposure, most cases involve chronic lead poisoning. The absorption of lead is slow, but prolonged exposure can result in toxic effects. Lead accumulates in the body, particularly in the bones from which it is only slowly released. Mild symptoms of lead poisoning include tiredness, lassitude, anorexia, constipation, abdominal discomfort, irritability, anaemia and sleep disturbances. These are common and non-specific complaints, so objective confirmation of lead toxicity is needed in the form of laboratory tests. In more severe lead poisoning there is severe intermittent abdominal colicky pain with reduction of muscle power, muscle tenderness and paraesthesiae as features of a peripheral neuropathy. There may also be serious disturbances in cerebral function particularly in children with the possibility of a fatal outcome or permanent brain damage. In some cases a "lead line" may be seen in the gums due to deposition of lead sulphide. The degree of toxicity again requires investigation by laboratory tests.

The methods for the investigation of lead poisoning or lead exposure involve determination of the metal itself or the detection of its toxic effects. Lead exists in the blood almost entirely in combination with the red cells and whole blood should be taken for analysis. Lead in the plasma, the metabolically active fraction, is partly excreted in the urine so that the rate of urinary lead excretion may be a useful determination. Lead interferes with haem synthesis (Chap. 27, Vol. 1). Several aspects of this interference are used in the early detection of lead toxicity (Editorial, 1970). There is an increased excretion in urine of coproporphyrin III in lead workers. Greater output and a rise in coproporphyrin I excretion is seen in lead poisoning. The urinary excretion of δ-aminolaevulinic acid

Drugs and Poisons 325

(δ-ALA) is also increased and may be a rather more sensitive indicator of early toxicity. The most sensitive is the measurement of the enzyme δ-ALA dehydratase (E.C. No. 4.2.1.24) whose activity is reduced in lead toxicity. This may have a place in monitoring the urban population rather than the lead worker.

Methods for the determination of lead in biological materials are currently of three main types. Firstly, the colorimetric method using dithizone is a well-established reference method applicable without complex instrumentation and is given below. Secondly the modified polarographic technique known as anodic stripping can be employed on appropriate digests of biological samples (Searle *et al.*, 1973). Thirdly the use of atomic absorption spectrophotometry allows the determination to be carried out directly on small samples of blood. For good results the sample must be heated in a controlled fashion so that the organic matter is burned before the lead is volatilised. This normally requires special equipment and a double beam instrument is usually necessary to allow for non-specific interfering substances. The technique is appropriate for highly specialised laboratories. (See for example, Evenson and Prendergast, 1974).

The treatment of lead toxicity involves avoiding further exposure and the removal of lead from the body, mainly from the skeleton. Any condition causing bone catabolism may result in increased release of lead with toxic effects. Lead is bound to chelating agents, particularly BAL, the calcium disodium salt of EDTA, or penicillamine. The treatment may be given in repeated courses to remove lead becoming available as a consequence of constant remodelling of bone. The ability to remove lead from the labile part of the skeleton by such chelating agents may be used for diagnostic purposes.

The Colorimetric Determination of Lead. Method of King*

Lead forms a red coloured complex with diphenylthiocarbazone, dithizone. Interference from other metals, such as copper and iron, is eliminated by extraction of the lead-dithizone complex from alkaline solution (pH > 11) in the presence of cyanide. The unreacted dithizone is removed with ammonium hydroxide-cyanide solution and the red complex remaining in the chloroform layer is determined spectrophotometrically. The whole procedure, except for spectrophotometry, is performed in one digestion tube, thereby eliminating the use of separating funnels and the usual transfer steps. The method given here resembles that proposed by Rice *et al.* (1965) which is a development of that of Bessman and Layne (1955). The present procedure uses more carefully controlled heating conditions.

Equipment. *Digestion Rack.* (Fig. 7,2). This is constructed from electrical quality asbestos board as end plates joined with appropriate

* Personal communication. E. King, National Occupational Hygiene Service, Manchester.

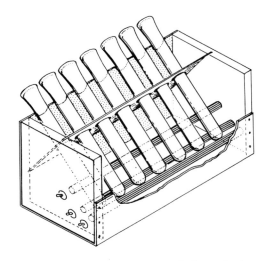

Fig. 7,2. Digestion rack for lead determinations. (After King).

aluminium alloy or equivalent. Each tube is supported on bottom electrical element after passing through the hole in the baffle plate. The upper end of the tube is located in a groove cut in the back plate. The heaters are 300 W electric bar elements, 30 cm long, with porcelain ends, positioned so that the bottom element supports the tube with other elements 3 mm from the tube and higher up it. The elements are operated by individual switches so that the amount of heat applied can be controlled according to the stage of digestion.

Digestion-extraction tubes. These are Pyrex glass about 100 ml capacity,– 200 × 28 mm, with ground sockets and stoppers. Before use, the bottom of the internal surface should be etched with carborundum to prevent superheating. Clean by adding 10 ml concentrated sulphuric acid and heating until the whole of the internal surface is being refluxed with acid. Cool, wash out with tap water, fill with concentrated nitric acid (commercial grade), stopper and store. Immediately before use return the nitric acid to stock, wash tubes with tap water and three times with distilled water.

Reagents. Reagents 1 to 6 can be obtained from British Drug Houses as lead-free reagents for foodstuff analysis.

All water should be made lead-free by distillation or deionisation. This can be checked by extracting with dithizone at pH 9.5 in the presence of cyanide. All reagents except the distilled water should be stored in Pyrex containers. Polythene, in particular, should not come into contact with the citrate-cyanide reagents since it releases metals to them.

1. Concentrated sulphuric acid, lead-free.
2. Concentrated nitric acid, 69-72 per cent, lead-free.
3. Perchloric acid, 60 per cent, lead-free.

Drugs and Poisons 327

4. Concentrated ammonia solution sp. gr. 0.88, lead-free.

5. Potassium cyanide, lead-free. Prepare a 100 g/l solution in water.

6. Ammonium citrate solution, approximately 460 g/l. Solid ammonium citrate may contain chelating material and should not be used routinely unless checked for its absence. King prefers to prepare an approximately 500 g/l solution of ammonium citrate by neutralising citric acid with concentrated ammonia. Dissolve 210 g citric acid monohydrate in 250 ml water, carefully add concentrated ammonia solution, approximately 150 ml, until the pH is 9.5 and make up to 500 ml with water. In either case extract repeatedly with dilute dithizone solution until this remains green, wash with chloroform, filter and store. Traces of ammonia will discolour dithizone and as the organic layer is removed it should be transferred to a test tube and bubbled with air to remove excess ammonia.

7. Citrate buffer. Make 150 ml ammonium citrate to 400 ml with concentrated ammonia solution.

8. Cyanide buffer. Make 30 ml potassium cyanide, 3 ml ammonium citrate, and 10 ml ammonia solutions up to 1 litre with water.

9. Cyanide wash reagent. Make 10 ml potassium cyanide and 10 ml concentrated ammonia to 1 litre with water.

10. Chloroform, analytical reagent grade. Occasional batches contain oxidising agents which destroy dithizone as shown by a purple rather than green colour in dilute solution. Redistil if necessary as follows. Dissolve 0.5 g dithizone in 2 litres chloroform and distil in all glass apparatus discarding the first 100 ml and collecting approximately 1 800 ml.

11. Dithizone solution. Prepare a *stock* solution in chloroform as follows. Dissolve about 20 mg dithizone in 30 to 40 ml chloroform and extract this with about 10 ml ammonia solution (50 ml/l). Reprecipitate the dithizone by adding hydrochloric acid, 1 mol/l, to the ammonia extract and extract again into chloroform. Repeat the sequence and after the second extraction into chloroform store in the refrigerator under hydrochloric acid, 100 mmol/l, to which a few crystals of sodium sulphite have been added. Dilute 1 ml stock solution with chloroform and titrate against lead solution. Calculate dilution of stock required to give the *dilute* solution of which 10 ml equals 10 μg lead.

12. Stock standard lead solution, 5 mmol/l. Dissolve 189.7 mg lead acetate trihydrate, $(CH_3 CO.O)_2 Pb.3H_2 O$, in water containing 1 ml glacial acetic acid and dilute to 100 ml with water. This solution is stable at room temperature if stored in a tightly stoppered plastic container.

13. Working standard lead solution containing 25 μmol/l. Dilute 1 ml stock solution to 200 ml with water.

Technique. Whole blood collected in a plastic syringe and transferred to a heparinised container must be used. Urine samples should be collected in well-washed containers containing 1 to 2 g EDTA (free acid) for 24 h samples or 100 to 200 mg EDTA for random samples. To about 3 g blood (weighed) or 20 ml urine in the digestion tube add 1 ml sulphuric acid and 5 ml of a perchloric acid-nitric acid mixture (2 vols: 5 vols). Set up at the same time 3 blank tubes containing acid only and recovery tubes containing 1 and 3 µg lead as required. Place in the digestion rack and heat. For urine use the top bar initially followed as the volume reduces by the second bar and finally by the two lower bars. For blood use only the middle bar until the reaction subsides when the two lower bars are used. Continue heating until the sulphuric acid refluxes up the tube for the greater part of its length. Do not overheat since the method depends upon a low sulphuric acid loss. Allow to cool, add 10 ml water and 5 ml citrate buffer. Check pH with indicator paper to ensure alkalinity for the dithizone extraction, and to avoid possible later liberation of hydrogen cyanide. Add 5 ml cyanide buffer and 10 ml dilute dithizone solution and shake vigorously for exactly 20 s. Allow to settle, remove aqueous layer with suction pipette. Add 10 ml cyanide wash, shake vigorously, allow to settle and remove aqueous layer. Repeat to give 4 washes in all. After removal of the aqueous layer add one 7 cm Whatman No. 41 filter paper to absorb residual water, shake and allow to settle. Decant through a folded 5 cm Whatman No. 41 filter paper into a cuvette of 20 mm path length and read against chloroform at 515 nm. Read the blanks and recovery standards. Subtract blank reading from that of test and standards.

Calculation

$$\text{Blood lead } (\mu\text{mol/l}) = \frac{\text{Reading of test}-\text{Reading of blank}}{\text{Reading of standard}-\text{Reading of blank}} \times 25 \times \frac{1\ 000}{3}$$

$$\text{Urinary lead } (\mu\text{mol/l}) = \frac{\text{Reading of test}-\text{Reading of blank}}{\text{Reading of standard}-\text{Reading of blank}} \times 25 \times \frac{1\ 000}{20}$$

To convert to µg/l from µmol/l multiply by 207.

Notes. 1. In the absence of a digestion rack use the technique of Rice *et al.*, (1965). Prepare freshly a digestion reagent by mixing 25 vols concentrated nitric acid with 10 vols concentrated sulphuric acid and add 5 ml to urine and blood samples, standards and blanks contained in digestion-extraction tubes. Heat over a micro burner under a fume hood until thin white fumes appear. Remove the burner and allow each tube to cool to *room temperature*. At this stage blood is dark brown, urine samples are yellow and the blank and standards are essentially colourless. Add 0.6 ml perchloric acid to each cool tube and cover with an inverted 50 ml beaker. Reheat each tube and continue heating while the solution goes through the following stages; yellow, colourless, yellow again with frothing until finally colourless and clear. Blood digests may remain very faintly yellow. At times the solution goes colourless on addition of the perchloric acid, it must still be heated through the yellow stage to ensure complete digestion. With these different amounts of digestion reagents and less standardised heating conditions additional care must be taken with the neutralisation before the addition of cyanide and more ammonia solution may be required.

Drugs and Poisons

2. The method is based on complexing all interfering metals other than bismuth with cyanide. In practice bismuth is not found in either blood or urine samples. Bismuth contamination from polythene can be recognised by the brown, instead of pure pink, colour of the final dithizonate.

3. Occasionally a urine sample will show excess zinc, as a purple colour. If observed add more cyanide buffer at the appropriate stage.

4. Under the conditions given an extinction of 0.06 is obtained with 5 nmol (1 μg) of lead. Gross deviations from this value should be investigated.

5. Since the method depends upon quantitative removal of unused dithizone, wash conditions are critical. Underwashing gives incorrectly high "blank" levels due to excess dithizone, and overwashing removes the lead dithizonate.

6. While the samples may be stored when acid after digestion, once they are made alkaline the operation must be completed without delay to avoid loss of lead onto the glassware.

7. As with all dithizone techniques sunlight should be avoided.

8. Blank values under the conditions given should approximate to 1.5 nmol (0.3 μg) lead.

INTERPRETATION

People exposed to lead inevitably absorb some but may be symptom free. The diagnosis of lead poisoning is based on clinical findings supported by laboratory evidence of excessive absorption and perhaps by a history of unusual exposure to lead. A suggested set of ranges of blood lead, and the urinary excretion of lead, coproporphyrins and δ-ALA are given in Table 7,14. These figures refer to samples taken *concurrently* with exposure to lead and the onset of symptoms, if any. Column A refers to a population in whom there has been no occupational or known abnormal exposure. Column B refers to occupational or abnormal exposure which is

TABLE 7,14

Biochemical Findings in Lead Exposure

Test	A Normal	B Acceptable	C Excessive	D Dangerous
Blood lead (μmol/l)	<1.93	1.93-3.87	3.87-5.80	>5.80
Blood lead (μg/l)	<400	400-800	800-1 200	>1 200
Urinary lead (μmol/l)	<0.39	0.39-0.73	0.73-1.21	>1.21
Urinary lead (μg/l)	<80	80-150	150-250	>250
Urinary coproporphyrin (μg/l)	<150	150-500	500-1 500	>1 500
Urinary δ-ALA (mg/l)	<6	6-20	20-40	>40

For details see text.
Based on Statement, 1968.

330   *Practical Clinical Biochemistry*

occupationally acceptable and unlikely to produce symptoms specifically attributable to lead. Column C applies to excessive occupational or other exposure which may be associated with mild or moderate symptoms. Continued exposure is likely to lead to toxic episodes and long term consequences. Column D concerns dangerous absorption of lead often associated with symptoms of toxicity and the probability of chronic poisoning.

The urinary lead determinations are best performed on 24 h collections but this is often difficult in industry. Random samples are then examined, preferably on several occasions. Dilute samples (sp. gr. less than 1.010) should be rejected. Where doubt exists as to lead accumulation in the skeleton, a 24 h collection of urine can be made during the administration of 3 doses of calcium, disodium EDTA, 25 mg/kg, at 8 hourly intervals. If more than 500 μg lead is excreted this is suggestive of lead toxicity.

Many patients in category C or D are anaemic and a blood haemoglobin determination is helpful. The effect of lead on the red cell detected as punctate basophilia is probably less reliable than the biochemical tests. However, anaemia may occur from many unrelated causes. Where marked it is likely to reduce the blood lead concentration below that expected for a particular degree of lead exposure.

LITHIUM

Lithium carbonate, introduced in 1949 for the treatment of mania or hypomania, is now used more frequently with an increasing awareness of its toxic side effects if serum lithium concentrations increase above the therapeutic range. Even when optimal serum levels have been maintained, therapy may lead to hypothyroidism with reduction in serum T_4 or protein-bound iodine concentrations and an increase in thyroid stimulating hormone (Linstedt *et al.*, 1973). A diffuse goitre may develop. This suppressive action of lithium salts has been used in treating hyper-thyroidism (Temple *et al.*, 1972).

Determination of Serum Lithium Using Flame Photometry

Flame photometry is the method of choice as with other alkali metals. Emission techniques have a sensitivity at least as great as that for sodium and potassium under optimal conditions, but the low concentrations present make for difficulties with the relatively low temperature flames of older equipment. The flame temperature of an air-natural gas flame can be increased to give better sensitivity if the samples are diluted with 20 per cent acetone (Denswill *et al.*, 1972), but even then only one fifth of the full scale deflection is achieved at therapeutic concentrations using the EEL 100, 150, or 227 Flame Photometers. The Coleman Model 51 instrument using a total consumption burner and an oxygen-propane flame gives

Drugs and Poisons 331

greater sensitivity as does an air-acetylene flame with photomultiplier detector (Robertson *et al.*, 1973). Adequate sensitivity is obtained using a sample diluted 100-fold. See also Brown and Legg (1970) and Woollen and Wells (1973).

The newer internal standard emission flame photometers such as the EEL 450, IL 343 or Beckman KLiNa models include the facility to measure lithium using potassium as internal standard. The IL 343 instrument uses a 50-fold dilution of the sample with a solution containing 1.5 mmol/l of potassium.

The emission from lithium at therapeutic concentrations is modified by the much higher concentrations of sodium and potassium. Appropriate concentrations of these ions are therefore included in the standard solutions.

Several workers have compared flame emission and absorption techniques. Using an earlier version of the IL flame photometer, the IL 143. Levy and Katz (1970) found under their conditions that the emission method was more sensitive and convenient but less precise. Pybus and Bowers (1970) found good agreement between the two methods. They used water as the diluent for serum and were unable to demonstrate any protein interference if standards and blanks contained similar sodium and potassium concentrations.

Method of Pybus and Bowers (1970) Using Atomic Absorption Spectroscopy

This is described as used with the EEL 140 instrument, an air-acetylene flame, a scale expander and external recorder.

Reagents. 1. Stock lithium standard, 20 mmol/l. Transfer 369.4 mg dried lithium carbonate to a 500 ml volumetric flask and add 10 ml hydrochloric acid, 100 mmol/l. Shake to dissolve and make to the mark with water.

2. Stock blank solution containing sodium 280 mmol/l and potassium, 100 mmol/l. Dissolve in water 8.1816 g sodium chloride and 0.3728 g potassium chloride, previously dried to constant weight, and make to 500 ml with water.

3. Prepare a set of working standards as below:

Serum lithium (mmol/l)	0	0.5	1.0	1.5	2.0	2.5
Stock lithium standard (ml)	0	0.5	1.0	1.5	2.0	2.5

To each add 10 ml stock blank solution and make to 200 ml with water.

Technique. Switch on the lithium lamp, light the flame, and set the monochromator to the resonance wavelength of 670 nm. While aspirating the most concentrated standard adjust the flame position and gas flows to give maximal absorption. Dilute 0.5 ml serum samples with 4.5 ml water. Spray the working blank solution and adjust to zero extinction. Then spray

332   *Practical Clinical Biochemistry*

the standards followed by the diluted sera interspersed with the working blank after every three or four samples. Repeat the set of standards at the end.

Use the blank readings to assess any drift in the instrument readings. Correct the recorded readings of the unknowns and standards for base-line drift, prepare a calibration curve and read the concentrations of samples from this.

INTERPRETATION

Normal serum contains 3 nmol/l of lithium. Serum concentrations during therapy depend on the time elapsing since the last dose and the preparations used. Some workers collect the specimen before the morning dose, others use a fixed time (12 to 18 h) after the last dose. Of the lithium carbonate preparations available, Priadel and Phasal are slow-release formulations minimising fluctuations during the 24 h after each dose.

For the optimal effect, the serum lithium concentration at least 10 h after the last dose should be between 2.0 and 2.5 mmol/l. According to Marks *et al.* (1973) maintained levels of less than 2.0 mmol/l rarely give trouble, but values above 3.0 mmol/l are potentially life-threatening. Concentrations above 4.5 mmol/l are almost invariably fatal unless arising acutely as a result of a suicidal attempt. The highest figure recorded for such cases is 8.2 mmol/l. The concentration is reduced by stopping administration of the drug while maintaining adequate salt and water intake. The risk of high concentrations developing is greater if patients are retaining sodium.

For a discussion of the value of monitoring serum lithium concentrations during treatment see Fry and Marks (1971) and for a review of lithium therapy, Marks *et al.* (1973).

MERCURY

Mercury is a highly volatile metal which can pollute the atmosphere producing toxic effects. The metal is an industrial hazard when used on a large scale such as in the manufacture of electrical switchgear. In the laboratory, mercury which has been accidentally spilled and incompletely recovered can also produce unacceptably high concentrations in the atmosphere.

Methyl mercury derivatives are used in organic chemical syntheses or as fungicides and are very toxic. Outbreaks of poisoning have occurred following ingestion of grain treated with mercurial fungicides and intended for planting. Of the inorganic salts, calomel (mercurous chloride) was formerly used as a component of teething powders. Such preparations given to infants carried the risk of producing pink disease.

Drugs and Poisons 333

Although such techniques as atomic absorption spectroscopy (Linstedt, 1970) and neutron activation analysis (Howie and Smith, 1967) have been developed in recent years, the colorimetric determination of urinary mercury using dithizone is still useful. Organic matter is destroyed under mild conditions by treating with hot acid permanganate. Prolonged heating with concentrated acids is avoided. Mercury is extracted from the acid solution into an organic phase containing dithizone. A two-fold change occurs. The formation of the pink-coloured mercury dithizonate with maximal absorption at 485 to 490 nm is the most sensitive and specific means of quantitation. The decrease in green dithizone colour at 620 nm is less specific as urinary constituents may occasionally occur which oxidise dithizone. In order to correct for unchanged dithizone present, Clarkson and Kench (1956) read at two wavelengths and used the equation:

Corrected reading at 490 nm = Actual reading at 490 nm − 0.23 × reading at 600 nm

Tompsett and Smith (1959) read at 620 nm before and after treatment with thiosulphate to destroy the dithizonate. The difference is proportional to the amount of mercury present. Milton and Hoskins (1946) destroyed excess dithizone with ammonia leaving the metal complex unchanged and reading at 480 nm. The purity of the dithizone used is critical as impurities prevent complete removal of excess dithizone.

Goldberg and Clarke (1970) reviewing available dithizone methods recommended that of Wall and Rhodes (1956) with modifications given below.

Magos and Cernik (1969) determined mercury in vapour form using ultraviolet absorption, following liberation of the metal from urine and other biological samples using a simple chemical method. Stannous chloride at high pH frees mercury from sulphydryl bonds and converts it to the metal. Initially cysteine is added to prevent any loss of mercury from the solution until it is transferred to a closed system. The reaction is then triggered by adding excess sodium hydroxide and entraining the mercury in a stream of gas which passes into the absorption cell in a photometer. The overall time for the determination is said to be less than 2 min (see also Sayers, 1970). Gage and Warren (1970) also applied this technique for mercury in organic form.

Determination of Mercury in Urine. Method of Goldberg and Clarke (1970)

Organic matter is destroyed by means of potassium permanganate the excess of which is removed by hydroxylamine. The mercury is then extracted with dithizone and estimated colorimetrically at 485 nm.

Reagents. 1. Sulphuric acid. Add 1 volume of concentrated acid to 2 volumes of water.

2. Solid potassium permanganate.

334   *Practical Clinical Biochemistry*

3. Hydroxylamine hydrochloride, 500 g/l. Dissolve 50 g in water and make up to 100 ml.

4. Dithizone solution. Prepare from high grade dithizone in crystalline form; Eastman Kodak, catalogue number 3092, is satisfactory. Otherwise to purify, dissolve in chloroform, extract with dilute ammonia solution, 50 ml (sp. gr. 0.88)/l in water, precipitate with weak hydrochloric acid from the ammonia extract, take up in chloroform, evaporate and dry in the incubator. Dissolve about 1 mg in 10 ml chloroform and add approximately 250 ml carbon tetrachloride to give an extinction of 0.20 to 0.25 when read against carbon tetrachloride in a 10 mm cuvette. Prepare freshly each day, stopper and keep in the dark when not in use.

5. Stock mercury standard solution, 5 mmol/l. Dissolve 136 mg mercuric chloride, dried in a desiccator, in 100 ml water.

6. Working mercury standard solution, 50 μmol/l (10 mg Hg/l). Dilute 1 ml stock standard to 100 ml with water.

All chemicals should be of analytical grade as free from heavy metals as possible. All glassware should be soaked in nitric acid, 500 ml concentrated acid/l in water, thoroughly rinsed with water and then filled with a dilute solution of dithizone. Any showing a change of colour with dithizone should be rejected.

Technique. To 50 ml urine in a 250 ml conical flask add 3 g potassium permanganate and 10 ml sulphuric acid, stand for 10 min to allow frothing to subside, then cover the neck of the flask with a watch glass and transfer to a hot plate set to keep the contents of the flask at a temperature of $50 \pm 2°$ C. Simmer in this way for 30 min then carefully add 0.5 ml portions of hydroxylamine until the solution is decolourised. Add a further 0.5 ml and cool. Transfer quantitatively to a separating funnel, add 10 ml dithizone solution and shake vigorously for 30 s. Allow the layers to separate and run off the lower organic layer into a centrifuge tube. Subsequent treatment depends upon the amount of mercury present. If the green colour of the dithizone appears unaltered the sample contains less than 25 nmol (5 μg). Add a little anhydrous sodium sulphate, shake, and centrifuge at 2 000 rpm for two minutes. Read the extinction at 485 and 620 nm, against carbon tetrachloride solution. If the green colour of the dithizone solution is completely removed or at least markedly decreased add a further 10 ml dithizone solution and repeat the extraction. Three extractions suffice for 75 to 100 nmol (15 to 20 μg). Mix the combined extracts thoroughly with anhydrous sodium sulphate and centrifuge before reading. If the amount of mercury present is greater than this take a smaller sample originally or measure the volume after destroying the organic matter and adding hydroxylamine and take an aliquot for extraction with dithizone.

With each batch of tests take 50 ml water instead of urine for a reagent blank, and 0.5 and 1.0 ml of the working standard diluted to 50 ml with water and proceed as before.

Drugs and Poisons 335

Calculation

$$\text{Urinary mercury (nmol/l)} = \frac{\text{Reading of unknown} - \text{reading of blank}}{\text{Reading of standard} - \text{reading of blank}}$$

$\times$ number of extractions $\times$ ml standard $\times$ 1 000

(The readings are those made at 485 nm).

Urinary mercury (μg/l) = 0.2 $\times$ nmol/l.

Notes. 1. The increase in extinction at 485 nm and decrease at 620 nm are proportional to the amount of mercury present only if extraction is continued until the green colour persists. The precision is worse at 620 nm, however, due to the high extinctions.

2. Mercury dithizonate is much more stable than dithizone. If the extracts in stoppered tubes are stored in the dark for 2.5 h, the reading at 485 nm is unaltered but that at 620 falls by 15 per cent. Similar extracts exposed to light for this time show decreases in extinction at 485 and 620 nm of 8 and 24 per cent respectively.

3. The decrease in extinction at 620 nm is not specific for mercury: other metals can cause distortion of the absorption curves or decrease in extinction at 620 nm without a corresponding increase at 485 nm.

4. The reading at 620 nm serves as an indication of the presence in the urine of substances capable of oxidising dithizone and causing a decrease in extinction at both 485 and 620 nm. Goldberg and Clarke (1970) found recovery of mercury added to such urines to range from 101 to 65 per cent based on readings at 485 nm. It was thought this might be due to metabolites of drugs such as aspirin, codeine, and paracetamol, but this was not confirmed. Should such a reduction in the reading at 620 nm occur, collect a further specimen of urine after withdrawing all drugs.

INTERPRETATION

Using this method Goldberg and Clarke found no detectable mercury or oxidation of dithizone in 24 healthy laboratory staff. The limit of detection was 2.5 nmol (0.5 μg). Urines from 50 hospital patients not suspected of exposure to mercury gave negative results; in eight the first specimen showed oxidation of dithizone. One industrial worker who was symptom-free showed levels falling from 750 to 275 nmol/24 h (149 to 54 μg/24 h). Much higher values, up to 13 μmol/24 h (2.6 mg/24 h) have been reported by Magos and Cernik (1969) for industrial exposure. The decrease probably reflects increasing awareness of the toxicity of mercury. The withdrawal of teething powders containing calomel has also reduced the incidence of acrodynia (pink disease) in infants in whom levels as high as 10 μmol/l (2 mg/l) were formerly recorded.

Published results for normal subjects using other dithizone methods vary appreciably : Monier Williams (1949), 2.5 to 5 nmol/24 h (0.5 to

336   *Practical Clinical Biochemistry*

1 µg/24 h); Simonsen (1953), none detected; Tompsett and Smith (1959),- up to 25 nmol/24 h (5 µg/24 h); Nobel and Nobel (1958), up to 150 nmol/l (30 µg/l); Nobel and Leifert (1961), up to 150 nmol/24 h (30 µg/24 h). Warkany and Hubbard (1951) in a study of infants with pink disease detected none in 71, 5 to 250 nmol/l (1 to 50 µg/l) in 14, and 250 to 500 nmol/l (50 to 100 µg/l) in 2 of their control population. Buckell *et al.* (1946) in 14 controls found 5 between zero and 60 nmol/24 h (12 µg/24 h), 4 between 100 and 150 nmol/24 h (20 to 30 µg/24 h), 3 between 200 and 250 nmol/24 h (40 to 50 µg/24 h) and 2 had concentrations of 325 and 450 nmol/24 h (65 and 90 µg/24 h). In our laboratory we also found an upper limit of 400 nmol/l (80 µg/l) in persons not known to have been exposed to mercury, with the great majority below 150 nmol/l (30 µg/l).

Howie and Smith (1967) using neutron activation found in their 46 normal controls a range of 0.5 to 665 nmol/l urine (0.1 to 133 µg/l) with a median of 65 nmol/l (13 µg/l) and a mean of 115 nmol/l (23 µg/l). The distribution curve was markedly skewed with about two-thirds of results below 100 nmol/l (20 µg/l) and very few above 250 nmol/l (50 µg/l). Skewed distribution has been obtained by others as shown above. Although Howie and Smith suggest that their patients may not be typical of the country as a whole they had no known mercury exposure other than to dental fillings. The preparation of dental amalgam was shown by them to be a slight hazard and they found increased mercury content in the hair and nails of dental assistants. A further factor which may distort the distribution curves is the considerable day to day variation in urinary mercury excretion (Warkany and Hubbard, 1951).

PARAQUAT

This quaternary ammonium base, used as a herbicide, has been implicated in accidental and deliberate poisoning (Table 7,1). It is related to another weedkiller, diquat.

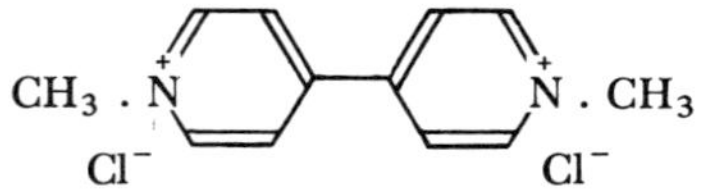

$$CH_3 . \overset{+}{N} \bigcirc\bigcirc \overset{+}{N} . CH_3 \qquad Cl^- \qquad Cl^-$$

Paraquat 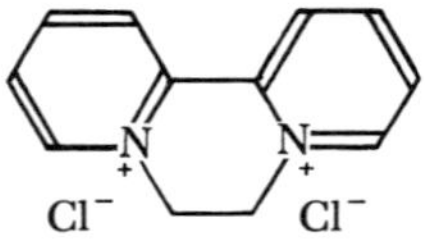   Diquat

On the basis of animal work they were originally considered to have only moderate toxicity, but they are much more toxic in man. After a single oral dose, acute ulcerative damage occurs in those parts of the skin and mucous membranes in contact with the poison. More serious effects on the liver, kidney and heart occur 2 or 3 days later. Still later, signs of pulmonary

Drugs and Poisons

TABLE 7,15
Paraquat Preparations

Liquids	
Containing 200 g/l:	Dextrone X, Esgram, Gramoxone
Containing 100 g/l:	
+ diquat	Priglone, Spray-seed
+ diuron	Dexuron, Gramuron, Tota-Col
+ monlinuron	Gramonol
+ simazine	Terraklene
Solids	
Containing 25 g/kg	
+ diquat	Duantl, Weedol, Weedrite
+ diquat, simazine	Pathclear

dysfunction appear with dyspnoea and pulmonary oedema leading to a progressive fatal pulmonary fibrosis.

Paraquat is available in liquid and solid formulations (Table 7,15) sometimes in conjunction with other herbicides. The liquid preparations are more concentrated and hence more dangerous. A dose of 3 g is likely to be lethal and this is contained in only 15 ml of the most potent preparations. Accidental poisoning has occurred as a result of storing liquids containing paraquat in unlabelled or mislabelled domestic bottles.

The paraquat ion can be detected in urine by the blue colour following reduction in alkaline solution. The reaction is the basis for quantitative determination in plasma or urine.

Qualitative Test for Paraquat in Urine.

A blue colour is produced by reduction with alkaline dithionite.

Reagents. 1. Sodium hydroxide solution, 1 mol/l.

2. Sodium dithionite, solid. Dissolve 100 mg in 10 ml sodium hydroxide immediately before use.

Technique. Add 1 ml dithionite reagent to 1 ml urine. A strong blue colour indicates the presence of paraquat, diquat or both. The natural colour of the urine produces a greenish colour with lower concentrations. Then the sensitivity may be improved by shaking with alumina and decanting before testing with dithionite.

Note. Berry and Grove (1971a) preferred to increase the urine volume used to 5 ml claiming that 1 mg/l could be detected in clear urine and 1.5 mg/l in cloudy specimens.

Determination of Paraquat in Urine or Blood

After deproteinisation, paraquat is adsorbed onto a cation exchange column and, after washing the column, eluted and determined colori-

338 *Practical Clinical Biochemistry*

metrically (Calderbank and Yuen, 1965). The method below is based on that of Berry and Grove (1971a) and an ICI Monograph (1974).

Reagents. 1. Trichloracetic acid solution, 50 g/l.

2. Trichloracetic acid solution, 250 g/l.

3. Hydrochloric acid, 2 mol/l.

4. Ammonium chloride solution, 25 g/l.

5. Ammonium chloride solution, saturated (approx. 270 g/l).

6. Alkaline dithionite solution, freshly prepared as described above.

7. Paraquat stock standard solution. Dissolve 69.1 mg paraquat dichloride ("methyl viologen") in reagent 5 to make 500 ml. This contains 100 mg/l expressed as a paraquat ion. Store in the refrigerator and avoid exposure to sunlight.

8. Working standard solution. Dilute 5 ml stock standard to 50 ml with reagent 5 to give a concentration of 10 mg/l. Store as before.

9. Dowex AG 50W -X8 (50 to 100, or 100 to 200 mesh) cation exchange resin in H^+ form.

Technique. *Preparation of sample.* For *urine* collect a timed sample and preserve by adding a little thymol or by freezing. After measuring the total volume, take 100 ml, add 25 ml reagent 2 and mix. Centrifuge at 1 500 g for 15 min, pour off the supernatant fluid and resuspend the precipitate in 50 ml reagent 1. Centrifuge at 700 g for 5 min, pour off the supernatant fluid and mix with the first one.

For *blood*, pipette 2 ml into a centrifuge tube, add 8 ml reagent 1 and centrifuge at 500 g for 15 min. Decant the supernatant fluid and resuspend the precipitate in 10 ml reagent 1. Centrifuge at 500 g for 5 min and combine with the first one.

Ion exchange separation. Prepare a resin column using 3 g of the Dowex resin in a long glass column. Wash with 50 ml water. Pass the deproteinised extract through the column at a rate less than 5 ml/min. Wash at a flow rate not greater than 3 ml/min with the following fluids successively: 25 ml water, 50 ml hydrochloric acid, 25 ml water, 25 ml reagent 4, 25 ml water. When the last wash has drained to just above the column surface, add 30 ml reagent 5, reduce the flow rate to not more than 1 ml/min, collect the first 25 ml of eluate and mix.

Colorimetric determination. To 10 ml eluate add 2 ml sodium dithionite reagent. Set up a blank and appropriate standard using 10 ml reagent 5 or standard in place of the eluate. After 3 to 5 min read at 600 nm using 1 cm cells for urine and 4 cm cells for blood.

Prepare a calibration curve for urine as follows:

Paraquat concentration (mg/l)	0	20	40	60	80	100
Paraquat working standard (ml)	0	2	4	6	8	10
Reagent 5 (ml)	10	8	6	4	2	0

To each add 2 ml sodium dithionite reagent

Drugs and Poisons 339

For blood cover the range 0 to 25 mg/l by taking 0, 0.5, 1.0, 2.0, 2.5 ml working standard, make to 10 ml with reagent 5 and proceed as before.

Calculation. Urinary paraquat (mg/l)

$$= \frac{\text{Reading of unknown}}{\text{Reading of standard}} \times \text{concentration of standard} \times \frac{25}{100}$$

$$\text{Blood paraquat (mg/l)} = \frac{\text{Reading of unknown}}{\text{Reading of standard}}$$

$$\times \text{concentration of standard} \times \frac{25}{2}$$

Note. A similar extraction procedure can be used for tissues or faeces (ICI Monograph, 1974).

INTERPRETATION

The urinary excretion of paraquat is maximal in the first day or so after ingestion before any of the toxic effects other than local ones are apparent. If the diagnosis is made at this stage there is no specific therapy. Gastric aspiration, adsorption of paraquat in the gut onto Fuller's Earth, purgation, and forced diuresis by intravenous fluid administration until paraquat disappears from the urine form the basis of treatment. The appropriate tests are carried out to assess hepatic, renal and pulmonary function.

If the urine test is negative during the first 48 h then absorption is so little that systemic toxic effects are very unlikely. The amount of paraquat excreted over the first 48 h gives some indication of the amount absorbed and hence the prognosis. In animals about 90 per cent of the absorbed dose is excreted in this time. The same is true for human poisoning cases undergoing forced diuresis. It is important that urine passed after ingestion of paraquat is not discarded if a proper assessment of urinary excretion is to be made. Recovery has occurred with excretion in the first 24 h of up to 200 mg. The blood concentrations may be much lower than in the urine. Kerr *et al.* (1968) found an initial serum concentration of 850 μg/l falling to undetectable levels in 15 h during forced diuresis in a patient who recovered.

PHENOTHIAZINES

The phenothiazines are derived from the parent substance, phenothiazine, $R_1 = R_2 = H$ in Table 7,16, an anthelmintic used in veterinary work. A related substance is the azaphenothiazine, prothipendyl (Tolnate)

prothipendyl

$$CH_2 . CH_2 . CH_2 . N(CH_3)_2$$

TABLE 7,16

Phenothiazines

General formula

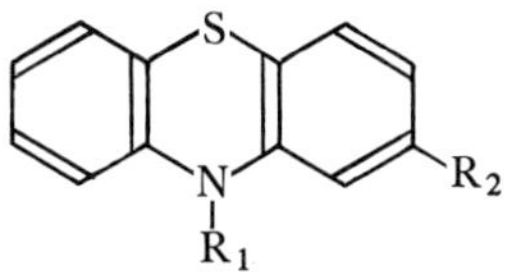

Name	R_1	R_2
Promazine (Sparine)	$-CH_2 . CH_2 . CH_2 . N(CH_3)_2$	H
Chlorpromazine (Amargyl, Chloractil, Largactil)	$-CH_2 . CH_2 . CH_2 . N(CH_3)_2$	Cl
Promethazine (Avomine, Phenergan)	$-CH_2 . CH(CH_3) . N(CH_3)_2$	H
Dimethothiazine (Banistyl)	$-CH_2 . CH(CH_3) . N(CH_3)_2$	$SO_2 . N(CH_3)_2$
Ethopropazine (Lysivane)	$-CH_2 . CH(CH_3) . N(C_2H_5)_2$	H
Trimeprazine (Vallergan)	$-CH_2 . CH(CH_3) . CH_2 . N(CH_3)_2$	H
Methotrimeprazine (Veractil)	$-CH_2 . CH(CH_3) . CH_2 . N(CH_3)_2$	OCH_3
Prochlorperazine (Stemetil, Vertigon)	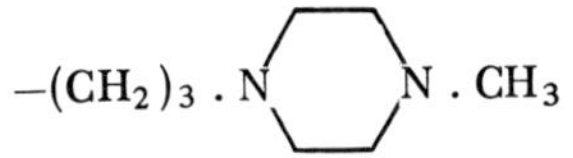 $-(CH_2)_3 . N\langle\text{piperazine}\rangle N . CH_3$	Cl
Trifluoperazine (Stelazine)	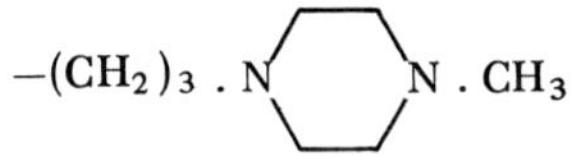 $-(CH_2)_3 . N\langle\text{piperazine}\rangle N . CH_3$	CF_3
Thiethylperazine (Torecan)	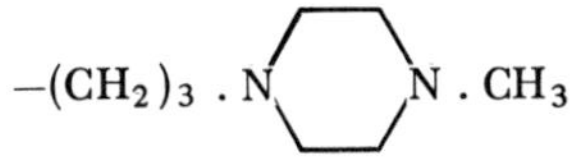 $-(CH_2)_3 . N\langle\text{piperazine}\rangle N . CH_3$	SC_2H_5

Perphenazine (Fentazin)	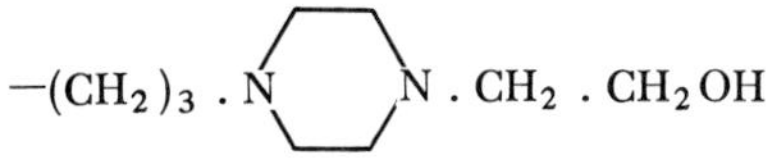 $-(CH_2)_3$. N〈 〉N . CH_2 . CH_2 OH	Cl
Fluphenazine (Modecate, Moditen)	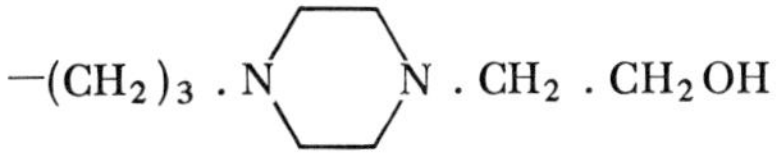 $-(CH_2)_3$. N〈 〉N . CH_2 . CH_2 OH	CF_3
Thiopropazate (Dartalan)	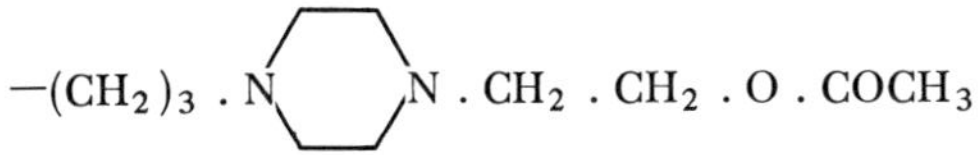 $-(CH_2)_3$. N〈 〉N . CH_2 . CH_2 . O . COCH_3	Cl
Methdilazine (Dilosyn)	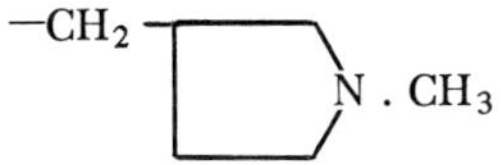 $-CH_2$ 〈 〉N . CH_3	H
Thioridazine (Melleril)	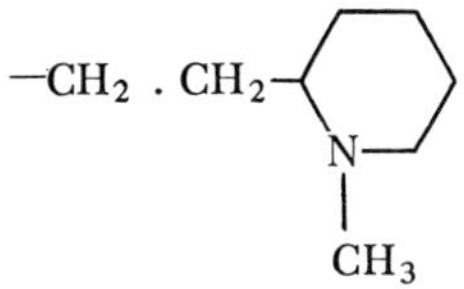 $-CH_2$. CH_2 〈 〉N—CH_3	SCH_3
Pericyazine (Neulactil)	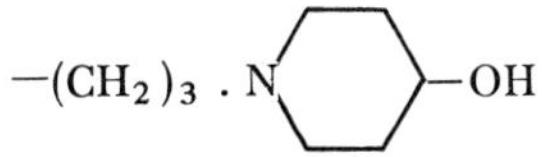 $-(CH_2)_3$. N〈 〉—OH	CN

Mixed Preparations

Steladex	:	trifluoperazine + dexamphetamine
Motival	:	fluphenazine + nortriptyline (tricyclic antidepressant)
Amylozine	:	trifluoperazine + amylobarbitone
Protamyl	:	promethazine + amylobarbitone
Sonergan	:	promethazine + butobarbitone

342   *Practical Clinical Biochemistry*

Many derivatives are used in current practice. A number of them are potent tranquillisers used for psychotic patients. Some are antihistamines, for example promethazine, dimethothiazine and trimeprazine. Many are anti-emetics, and a few are especially used for this or for motion sickness, namely promethazine, prochlorperazine, thiethylperazine, and prothipendyl. The parasympatholytic activity of ethopropazine (Lysivane) is useful for the treatment of Parkinsonism.

They are all tertiary amines and are extracted with other basic drugs. Most of them when freshly excreted in the urine as a mixture of metabolites, give colour reactions with the FPN reagent of Forrest and Forrest (1960). See also Forrest *et al.* (1961) and Clarke (1969, 1975) and Table 7,17.

Many phenothiazines are given in high doses for psychotic disorders. The possibility of monitoring therapeutic levels has been investigated. Also these substances are sometimes taken with suicidal intent and help in identifying such cases may be sought.

Phenothiazines are rapidly absorbed from the intestine and are rapidly taken up by the liver and converted into a variety of metabolites. Chlorpromazine has been extensively studied. The main changes are oxidation of the $=S$ atom to $=SO$ or even $=SO_2$, some oxidation of the nuclear $=N$ to $=NO$, hydroxylation at position 7, dealkylation of the side chain, and formation of conjugates (mainly glucosiduronates). The changes occur singly or in combination. At least 75 metabolites have been recognised (Turano *et al.*, 1973). Many are present in both urine and plasma and most are therapeutically inert. The pattern of metabolites in the urine varies between individuals. The colour reactions with the FPN reagent may vary somewhat between different metabolites and thus the colours quoted in Table 7,17 should be taken as a general guide only.

This rapid metabolism results in rather low levels of chlorpromazine itself in the plasma and urine. It is the plasma concentration, however, which is correlated with the therapeutic response and there are individual variations in dose needed to achieve a satisfactory concentration and clinical effect (Curry, 1971). The methods required for such study are beyond the scope of this book but involve preparation of a partially purified extract of basic drugs from the plasma followed by GLC. The sensitivity for this halogenated drug is increased by using an electron capture detector. The therapeutic range for peak concentrations after a dose of chlorpromazine in patients on long term therapy is 25 to 300 μg/l. The metabolism of other phenothiazines has been less extensively investigated but appears to follow a broadly similar pattern. Not all are halogenated and the electron-capture detector is not applicable to all phenothiazines.

In acute poisoning the plasma concentration of active drugs is still very low. There is no specific therapy for such overdoses and measurement of plasma levels has little place in monitoring recovery. Investigation of the excretion of urinary metabolites may however be helpful.

Drugs and Poisons · 343

Screening Tests for Phenothiazines in Urine

A variety of colour tests are available for freshly-voided urine (Table 7,17). They may be affected by the amount and relative proportions of the many metabolites although extraction procedures may separate metabolites and the unchanged drug. The colour reactions in the Table are those given by the parent phenothiazines in concentrations corresponding to those achieved in the urine after normal therapeutic doses. The reactions are not unique to phenothiazines and some are given also by benzodiazepines (Table 7,12) and the tricyclic antidepressants (Table 7,21).

A. FPN reagent (Forrest and Forrest, 1960)

1. Ferric chloride solution, 50 g/l in water.
2. Perchloric acid. Make 200 ml of the 72 per cent acid to 1 litre with water.
3. Nitric acid solution. Make 500 ml concentrated acid to 1 litre with water.

These reagents are stable indefinitely. For the FPN reagent mix reagents 1, 2, and 3 in the proportion 1/9/10 respectively, and use fresh.

B. Thioridazine reagent (Forrest et al., 1960a)

Mix 2 ml reagent 1 above with 98 ml sulphuric acid (300 ml concentrated acid diluted to 1 litre).

C. Forrest reagent (Forrest et al., 1960b)

For details of composition see p. 355.

Technique. Add 1 ml of the appropriate reagent (A, B or C) to 1 ml urine and note the colour developed immediately.

D. Phosphoric acid—ceric sulphate reagent (Meunier et al., 1970)

In a flask place 3.162 g ceric ammonium sulphate and 50 ml water. Shake until dispersed and then add 450 ml orthophosphoric acid, sp. gr. 1.71. Shake well until solution is complete.

E. Sulphuric acid-formol reagent (Meunier et al., 1970)

1. Concentrated sulphuric acid.
2. Formaldehyde solution, "35 per cent"; formalin.

F. Phosphoric acid reagent (Meunier et al., 1970)

Phosphoric acid, sp. gr. 1.71.

TABLE 7,17

Colour Reactions of Phenothiazines

	FPN reagent[1]	Thioridazine reagent[2]	Forrest reagent[3]	Ce/H$_3$PO$_4$ reagent[4]	H$_2$SO$_4$ reagent[4]	Formaldehyde reagent[4]	H$_3$PO$_4$ reagent[4]
Promazine	orange-pink	orange-pink	orange	pink-orange	orange	deep red	pink
Chlorpromazine	pink-purple	purple	pink-orange	faint pink	pink-red	deep purple	pink-purple
Promethazine	pink	faint pink	pink-orange	faint pink	salmon pink	deep purple	pale pink
Dimethothiazine	pale pink	—	green-yellow	pink	orange	deep red	salmon pink
Ethopropazine	rose pink	pale pink	orange-pink	pink	pink-red	deep red	salmon pink
Trimeprazine	pale pink	pale pink	—	pink	salmon pink	pink	pale pink
Methotrimeprazine	violet-purple	violet	—	purple	—	—	purple
Trifluoperazine	orange	—	—	—	purple	blue	—
Thiethylperazine	transient blue	faint blue	—	faint pink	—	orange pink	blue
Fluphenazine	—	—	—	—	pale yellow	—	—
Thiopropazate	violet-pink	violet	—	faint pink	pink	deeper pink	pink
Methdilazine	faint pink	faint pink	—	faint pink	pale pink	pink	faint pink
Thioridazine	blue	deep blue	green	blue	deep blue	deep purple	deep blue

1 = Forrest and Forrest, 1960.

2 = Forrest *et al.*, 1960a.

3 = Forrest *et al.*, 1960b.

4 = Meunier *et al.*, 1970.

Drugs and Poisons 345

Technique. For D, E and F prepare an extract of urine (or gastric contents if available) in dichloroethane as follows. In a 250 ml separating funnel place 100 ml urine, 25 ml sodium hydroxide, 400 g/l, and 100 ml dichloroethane. Shake for 2 min and allow the phases to separate. If an emulsion forms, transfer to a centrifuge bottle and spin for 5 min. Remove the organic phase and shake it with 20 ml water. Aspirate the upper water phase and any interface emulsion. Transfer the organic phase to a clean flask and shake with 5 g anhydrous sodium sulphate. Filter off the solid and divide the extract into 4 parts. Evaporate two to dryness.

For the ceric-phosphoric acid reaction add 3 ml of this reagent to one of the liquid dichloroethane extracts. Shake vigorously for 15 s and allow the layers to separate. Note any colour in the lower acid layer. The reagent also gives colours with some tricyclic antidepressants (p. 354).

For the sulphuric-formol reaction add 3 ml sulphuric acid to one of the dried extracts and shake until dissolved. Note any colour developed and then add 1 ml formaldehyde solution. Observe any colour change. These reactions are also given by the benzodiazepines (p. 308) and the tricyclic antidepressants (p. 354).

For the phosphoric acid test add 2 ml reagent to the other dried extract and shake until dissolved. Note any colour change.

Spectrophotometry of Phenothiazines

Phenothiazines as basic drugs are extracted from alkaline solution into organic solvents.

Technique. Prepare an extract in dichloroethane as described in the last section. Transfer to a cuvette of 1 cm path length and scan in a double beam spectrophotometer against dichloroethane in the reference beam over the range 230 to 330 nm. Most phenothiazines give two peaks at approximately 260 and 310 nm. Details are given in Table 7,18.

TABLE 7,18

Absorption Maxima (nm) of Phenothiazines in Dichloroethane

Promazine	255,	310	
Chlorpromazine	260,	310	
Promethazine	258,	307	
Dimethothiazine	240,	268,	310
Ethopropazine	257,	310	
Methotrimeprazine	258,	310	
Prochlorperazine	237,	260	
Thiethylperazine	269		
Fluphenazine	270		
Thiopropazate	261		
Methdilazine	258,	307	
Thioridazine	270		

346   *Practical Clinical Biochemistry*

INTERPRETATION

Negative tests are a good indication that phenothiazines have not been taken. Weakly positive tests with ferric salts are given by a few other drugs and by urobilinogen in excessive quantities. Benzodiazepines do not interfere but some tricyclic antidepressants do (p. 354). The other colour tests are sometimes more sensitive but are less specific as benzodiazepines (p. 308) and tricyclic antidepressants (p. 354) also react. Clearly positive tests with both ferric reagents strongly suggest phenothiazine ingestion. The colour intensity and hue vary for different phenothiazines. Thioridazine is the only one giving consistent blue colours but some confusion can arise with the tricyclic antidepressants (p. 354).

In patients receiving long term phenothiazine treatment, strong colour reactions appear and even after stopping therapy, excretion of urinary metabolites may continue for several weeks. With acute ingestion the excretion drops more quickly. Effects on the central nervous system of a particular dose are very different for a single isolated dose and one during long-term treatment probably because of the different concentrations of unchanged drug and the induction of metabolising enzymes by repeated drug administration. The total excretion of drug and metabolites may, however, be similar.

SULPHONAMIDES

With the recognition of the antibacterial action of sulphanilamide ($R_1 = R_2 = H$, Table 7,19) a wide range of substituted sulphanilamides referred to collectively as the sulphonamides have been introduced. Many are still in use (Table 7,19). They are derived by replacement of one H atom in the $-SO_2NH_2$ group with a basic group. Sulphacetamide is an exception. If the aromatic $-NH_2$ group of sulphathiazole is substituted, the products are poorly absorbed from the small intestine and are slowly hydrolysed in the large intestine exerting their effects there. These preparations, mainly used for treating intestinal infection, are coded I in Table 7,19. The related substance, sulphasalazine is used in treating ulcerative colitis. Many sulphonamides are acetylated during metabolism with increase in their solubility. This is important in avoiding their crystallisation in the urinary tract. Some sulphonamides are bound to serum proteins and following rapid absorption are slowly excreted so that therapeutic levels are maintained in the circulation for many hours. These slowly cleared drugs are coded S in Table 7,19. A number are less well-bound to proteins and are more rapidly excreted achieving higher concentrations in the urine. They are useful for urinary tract infections and are coded R in Table 7,19. Some are intermediate, being moderately slowly excreted and are coded as M. Most sulphonamides are relatively insoluble in water but a few are sufficiently soluble for local application as in eye drops. These are coded L in Table 7,19.

Drugs and Poisons   347

Determination in Blood. Method of Bratton and Marshall (1939). Micro-modification

After precipitating the proteins with trichloracetic acid the sulphonamide present in the filtrate is diazotised and then coupled with N-(1-naphthyl)-ethylenediamine dihydrochloride after destroying excess nitrite with sulphamic acid. The resulting colour is read at 540 nm.

Reagents. 1. Trichloracetic acid solution, 200 g/l.

2. Sodium nitrite solution, 1 g/l. Prepare freshly at frequent intervals.

3. Ammonium sulphamate solution, 5 g/l.

4. N-(1-Naphthyl)-ethylenediamine dihydrochloride, 500 mg/l aqueous solution. Keep in a dark coloured bottle. A 1 g/l solution in ethanol (950 ml/l) has been used and is said to be less likely to give rise to turbidity.

5. Hydrochloric acid, 4 mol/l.

6. Stock standard solution of the sulphonamide, 100 mg/l. Dissolve 100 mg in water and make up to 1 litre. While it is most satisfactory to use the actual sulphonamide which is being determined, a solution of any one of them can be used and the necessary correction made for the difference in molecular weight. Sulphanilamide has been frequently used but the molecular weights of sulphapyridine, sulphadiazine and sulphathiazole are near to each other and to other commonly used ones, so that one of these is perhaps more suitable.

7. Standard solution for use, 2.5 mg/l. Add 40 ml trichloracetic acid to 5 ml stock standard and make up to 200 ml with water.

Technique. Pipette 3 ml water into a test tube and add 100 μl capillary or venous blood. Mix and add 0.9 ml trichloracetic acid, mix well and stand for a few min. Filter through a 7 cm No. 1 Whatman filter paper, or centrifuge. Pipette 2 ml filtrate, standard solution or water for test, standard and blank respectively into test tubes and add 0.2 ml ammonium sulphamate, mix and after 2 min add 1 ml coupling agent. Allow to stand 10 min and read against the blank at 540 nm or using a yellow-green filter.

Calculation.

$$\text{Blood sulphonamide (mg/l)} = \frac{\text{Reading of unknown}}{\text{Reading of standard}} \times \frac{4}{0.1} \times 2.5$$

$$= \frac{\text{Reading of unknown}}{\text{Reading of standard}} \times 100$$

Notes. 1. A standard curve should be prepared to check that Beer's Law is obeyed. Make up a series of standards by adding 1.25, 2.5, 5.0, 7.5 and 10 ml stock standard to 40 ml trichloracetic acid and make to 200 ml. These correspond to 25, 50, 100, 150 and 200 mg sulphonamide/l blood.

2. The method given above estimates the free drug. A certain amount is present as the acetyl derivative. However, only the free sulphonamide is active so that it alone needs to be determined. Total sulphonamide can be estimated by heating some of the filtrate with hydrochloric acid after

TABLE 7,19

Sulphonamides in Current Use

$$R_2N{-}\langle\text{benzene}\rangle{-}SO_2NHR_1$$

Type	Name	R_1	R_2
I	Calcium sulphaloxate (Enteramide)	$-CONHCH_2OH$	(benzene ring with $COOH$ and $-CO-$, $-H$)
I	Phthalylsulphathiazole (Thalazole)	(thiazole ring)	$-H$, $CO \cdot CH_2CH_2COOH$
I	Succinylsulphathiazole (Sulfasuxidine)	(thiazole ring)	H_2
S	Sulfametopyrazine (Dalysep, Kelfizine)	(pyrazine ring, CH_3O)	H_2
L,R	Sulphacetamide (Albucid, Ocusol, Vasosulf)	$-COCH_3$	H_2
R	Sulphadiazine	(pyrimidine ring)	H_2
S	Sulphadimethoxine (Madrinon)	(pyrimidine ring, OCH_3, OCH_3)	H_2
R	Sulphadimidine (Sulphamethazine)	(pyrimidine ring, CH_3, CH_3)	H_2
R,L	Sulphafurazole (Gantrisin)	(isoxazole ring, CH_3, CH_3)	H_2

R	Sulphamerazine		H_2
R	Sulphamethizole (Methisul, Urolucosil)		H_2
M	Sulphamethoxazole (Gantanol)		H_2
S	Sulphamethoxydiazine (Durenate)		H_2
S	Sulphamethoxypyridazine (Lederkyn, Medicel)		H_2
M	Sulphaphenazole (Orisulf)		H_2
R	Sulphapyridine (M & B 693)		H_2
I	Sulphasalazine (Salazopyrin)		
R	Sulphathiazole (Triazamide)		H_2

Mixed Preparations

Albamycin	—Sulphamethizole and novobiocin
Bactrim, Septrin	—Sulphamethoxazole and trimethoprim
Cremotresamide	—Sulphadiazine, sulphamerazine, sulphadimidine
Sulphatriad	—Sulphadiazine, sulphamerazine, sulphathiazole.

350   *Practical Clinical Biochemistry*

precipitating the proteins, before carrying out the diazotisation. Heat 2 ml
of such filtrate with 0.2 ml of 4 mol/l hydrochloric acid in boiling water for
one hour. Cool and make up to 2 ml with water. Proceed as before.

3. Urea solution, 5 g/l may be used instead of ammonium sulphamate
for removing excess nitrite.

4. For values above 200 mg/l use 50 μl blood and for low values 200 μl.

5. The method is applicable to other fluids, for example, cerebrospinal
fluid in cases of meningitis or cerebral abscess. The concentration in this
fluid is usually 50-70 per cent of the blood level for the sulphonamides
labelled R in Table 7,19. For those labelled S, their binding to plasma
proteins reduces the figure to 30 per cent. High levels are achieved by direct
injection into the theca.

For urine a preliminary dilution of 10 to 50-fold is usually required.

6. For those sulphonamides labelled I in Table 7,19 the method is only
applicable after acid hydrolysis to release the free amino group. This is not
important if blood concentrations are measured, as absorption only occurs
following hydrolysis in the gut. It would be relevant if a faecal homogenate
was to be analysed.

INTERPRETATION

Sulphonamide determinations are now required much less frequently
than formerly, mainly due to the use of other antibiotics. The therapeutic
concentration varies with the drug used and the manufacturer's literature
should be consulted for details of the optimal range. For the rapidly
excreted sulphonamides (R, Table 7,19) the concentration varies appreciably with time after the last dose but plasma levels are much less variable
for the slowly cleared (S) type.

Whole blood is convenient if capillary blood is used. The plasma
concentration is greater than in the cells and can be over 25 per cent higher
than for whole blood.

TRICYCLIC ANTIDEPRESSANTS

This group of drugs is widely prescribed in the more severe forms of
depression. The several members may be subdivided into different groups
but share the common chemical feature of having two benzene rings joined
by a seven-membered ring (Table 7,20). The latter is a cycloheptene in the
dibenzocycloheptenes, but contains one or two N atoms in the
dibenzazepines and dibenzdiazepines respectively. Others contain an O or S
atom in the seven-membered ring. A basic side chain is attached to the
central ring in all cases and these drugs are found amongst the basic group
in the usual extraction procedures.

Drugs and Poisons 351

The group as a whole is rapidly absorbed and the drugs enter the tissues leaving only a small quantity in the circulation. They are readily metabolised in the liver and the conjugated metabolites are rapidly cleared by the kidney. An important step in metabolism is demethylation. Thus imipramine is converted to desipramine and amitriptyline to nortriptyline. The urine contains mainly metabolites. Most of a dose is usually cleared from the body within 24 h.

The rate of metabolism shows wide individual variation so that the plasma concentration may vary widely from one patient to another on a constant dose. Thus Braithwaite and Widdop (1971) found a 15-fold range for amitriptyline and a 12-fold range for nortriptyline under such conditions. In view of this, methods have been developed for monitoring plasma levels to achieve better therapeutic control. It is claimed (Kragh-Sørensen *et al.,* 1973) that for nortriptyline the optimal concentration in plasma is 175 μg/l with less satisfactory effects at higher or lower figures. The prescription of these substances to depressed patients is associated with the risk of deliberate self-poisoning. The ingestion of more than 1 g is likely to have serious effects. The clinical features are specially centred on the nervous and cardiovascular systems. There may be hallucinations, hyper-reflexia, convulsions and varying degrees of unconsciousness but rarely profound coma. Depression of respiration, dilation of pupils, dryness of the mouth and urinary retention are seen. The cardiovascular effects include tachycardia, hypotension and a tendency to develop severe arrhythmias leading to cardiac arrest. These features become apparent within an hour or two after ingestion and severe symptoms rarely persist for longer than 18 to 24 h. Intensive supportive therapy may be needed during this time and the rapid detection of the metabolites in the urine may aid in the detection of the cause of poisoning and the need for such care.

Quantitation in plasma for monitoring therapy has usually involved gas-liquid chromatography (Braithwaite and Windop, 1971; Kragh-Sørensen *et al.,* 1973). Simple colour tests applied to urine are more appropriate for the rapid detection in overdose cases.

Screening Tests for Tricyclic Antidepressants in Urine or Gastric Contents

Several colour reactions have been employed. They are not specific for this group of drugs as some are given by phenothiazines (p. 344) and benzodiazepines (p. 308). The results of the various tests are collected together in Table 7,21.

A. FPN reagent (see p.343)

352   *Practical Clinical Biochemistry*

TABLE 7,20

Tricyclic Antidepressants

Dibenzazepines

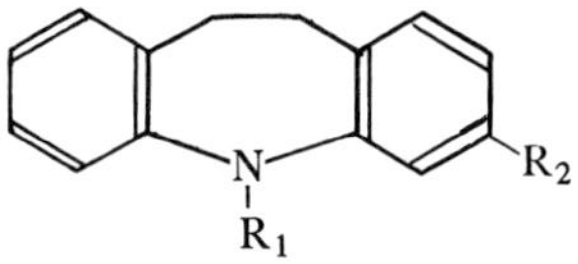

(structure of dibenzazepine nucleus with substituents R_2 on the ring and N–R_1)

	R_1	R_2
Clomipramine (Anafranil)	$-CH_2 . CH_2 . CH_2 N(CH_3)_2$	Cl
Desipramine (Pertofran)	$-CH_2 . CH_2 . CH_2 NHCH_3$	H
Imipramine (Berkomine, Dimipressin, Ethipram, Norpramine, Praminal, Tofranil)	$-CH_2 . CH_2 . CH_2 N(CH_3)_2$	H
Opipramol (Insidon)	$-CH_2 . CH_2 . CH_2 . N$ 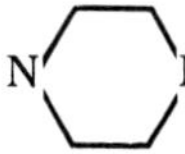 (piperazine ring) $N . CH_2 . CH_2 OH$ (also extra double bond in 7-membered ring)	H
Trimipramine (Surmontil)	$-CH_2 . CH(CH_3) . CH_2 N(CH_3)_2$	H

Dibenzocycloheptenes

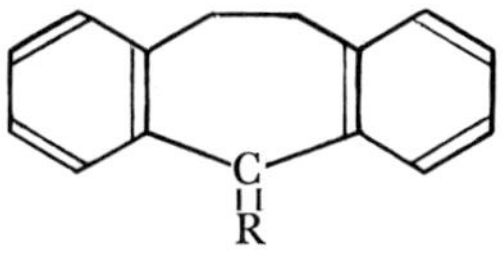

(structure of dibenzocycloheptene nucleus with =C–R substituent)

$$R$$

Amitriptyline (Laroxyl, Lentizol, Saroten, Tryptizol) $\quad =CH . CH_2 . CH_2 N(CH_3)_2$

Nortriptyline (Allegron, Aventyl, Motival) $\quad =CH . CH_2 . CH_2 NHCH_3$

Protriptyline (Concordin) $\quad <^{CH_2 . CH_2 . CH_2 NHCH_3}_{H}$

Compare the *antihistamine*,

cyproheptadine (Periactin)

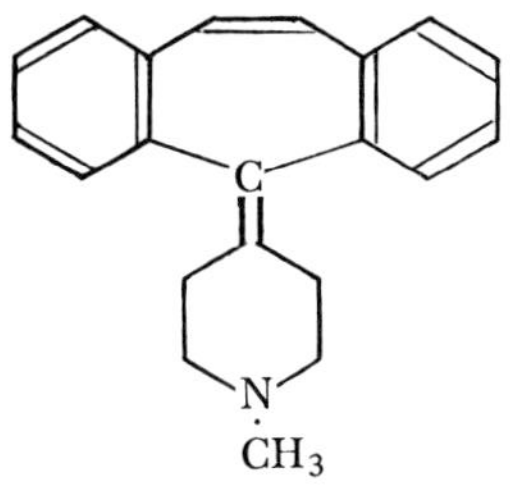

Dibenzdiazepine

Dibenzepin (Noveril)

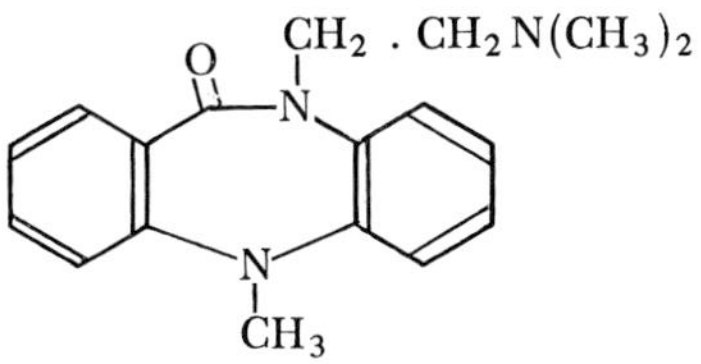

Dibenzthiepin and Dibenzoxepin

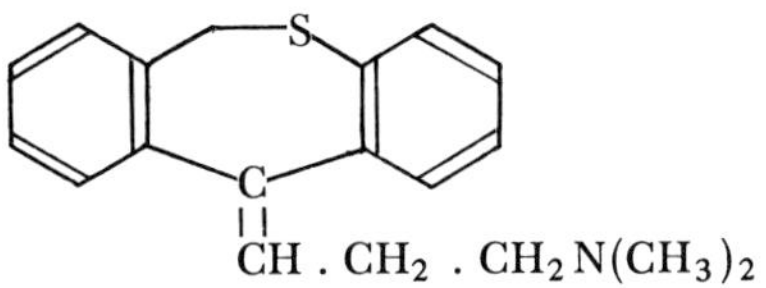

Dothiepin (Prothiaden)

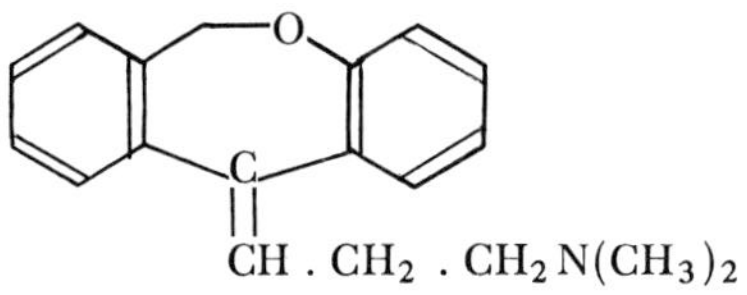

Doxepin (Sinequan)

TABLE 7,21

Colour Reactions of Tricyclic Antidepressants

	FPN reagent	Forrest reagent	Ceric–H$_3$PO$_4$ colour	Ceric–H$_3$PO$_4$ fluoresc.	H$_2$SO$_4$ + colour	Formalin → colour	Fluorescence initial	Fluorescence diluted	H$_3$PO$_4$ colour	Lead dioxide colour (fluorescence)
Clomipramine	blue	green	deep blue	–	–	–	–	–	–	deep blue
Desipramine	deep blue	blue	deep blue	–	–	–	–	–	–	deep blue
Imipramine	blue	blue	deep blue	–	–	–	–	–	–	deep blue
Trimipramine	blue	blue	deep blue	–	–	–	–	–	–	deep blue
Amitriptyline	–	–	–	–	deep orange	brown	green-yellow	yellow	–	brown (green-yellow)
Nortriptyline	–	–	–	faint green	deep orange	deep orange	yellow	pale blue	–	light brown (yellow)
Protriptyline	–	–	faint purple	green	pale yellow	pale yellow	blue	blue	–	light brown (yellow-green)
Cyproheptadine	–	–	–	–	pale yellow	pale yellow	blue	blue	–	light brown (green)
Dothiepin	–	–	–	–	dark brown	green	–	–	–	light brown (green)
Doxepin	–	–	grey-blue	–	deep orange	brown	yellow	green-yellow	–	light brown (–)

Drugs and Poisons 355

B. **Forrest reagent** (Forrest *et al.*, 1960b)

1. Potassium dichromate solution, 2 g/l.
2. Sulphuric acid, 300 ml/l. Add 30 ml concentrated acid carefully to 70 ml water.
3. Perchloric acid solution. Add 20 ml "72 per cent" perchloric acid to 80 ml water.
4. Nitric acid, 500 ml/l. Mix equal parts of concentrated acid and water. Mix equal volumes of reagents 1 to 4. The mixture is stable indefinitely.

Technique. To 1 ml urine add 1 ml reagent and note any colour produced. For a known positive reaction grind one 25 mg imipramine tablet with water and make up to 100 ml.

C. **Ceric sulphate—phosphoric acid reagent** (Meunier *et al.*, 1970)

For preparation see p. 343.

Technique. Prepare a dichloroethane extract as on p. 345. To 25 ml of the liquid extract add 3 ml reagent. Shake vigorously for 15 s and allow to separate. Note any colour in the lower acid layer. After 5 min examine under a UV lamp at 365 nm for any fluorescence. If phenothiazines are present they may also give colours. In this case the interference is less if 6 ml ether is added to the dichloroethane extract followed by 10 ml reagent.

D. **Sulphuric acid—formaldehyde reagent** (Meunier *et al.*, 1970)

For preparation see p. 343.

Technique. Prepare a dichloroethane extract and evaporate 25 ml to dryness as on p. 345. To the residue add 3 ml sulphuric acid and shake to dissolve. Observe any colour developed, then add 1 ml formaldehyde and note the colour. Examine the fluorescence with a UV lamp at 365 nm. Then carefully add, with shaking, 10 ml water and reobserve the fluorescence.

E. **Phosphoric acid—lead dioxide reagent** (Meunier *et al.*, 1970)

1. Phosphoric acid, sp. gr. 1.71.
2. Lead dioxide, solid.

Technique. Prepare a dichloroethane extract and evaporate 25 ml to dryness as on p. 345. To the residue add 2 ml phosphoric acid and note any colour change. Add a small quantity of lead dioxide and record the colour. The reaction is also given by phenothiazines (p. 344) and is only useful in their absence. Finally examine the fluorescence using a 365 nm source.

F. **Ultraviolet Absorption Spectra of Tricyclic Antidepressants**

Prepare an extract of urine or gastric contents in dichloroethane as on

TABLE 7,22

Absorption Maxima (nm) of Tricyclic Antidepressants in Dichloroethane

Clomipramine	228,	258,	276 (shoulder)
Desipramine	228,	258,	275 (shoulder)
Imipramine	228,	258,	275 (shoulder)
Trimipramine	228,	258,	275 (shoulder)
Amitriptyline	233		
Nortriptyline	243		
Protriptyline	234,	294	
Cyproheptadine	232,	247 (shoulder),	285
Dothiepin	242,	262 (shoulder),	303
Doxepin	233,	255 (shoulder),	297

p. 345. Transfer to a 10 mm cuvette and scan the spectrum from 200 to 400 nm in a double beam UV spectrophotometer against dichloroethane in the reference beam.

The absorption peaks are listed in Table 7,22. Several compounds show a shoulder on the longer wavelength side of a peak.

INTERPRETATION

The colour reactions are those given by therapeutic doses. Those reactions carried out on dichloroethane extracts avoid interference by polar, phenolic or acidic metabolites. The dibenzazepines have identical colour reactions and spectra. The blue colours may lead to confusion with thioridazine (Table 7,17), particularly if only the FPN reagent has been used. Thioridazine gives a weaker colour with the Forrest reagent and gives a blue colour with phosphoric acid alone. The dibenzazepines do not give any colour with the thioridazine reagent (Table 7,21) unlike thioridazine. The fluorescent products in the sulphuric-formol reaction are helpful for the dibenzocycloheptenes and doxepin. Fluorescence is not seen with the phenothiazines but is found with the benzodiazepine, oxazepam (p. 308). The fluorescence in the phosphoric acid—lead dioxide reaction is more characteristic than the colour developed. The dibenzocycloheptenes and dothiepin give yellow or green fluorescent products and these may be confused with some of the benzodiazepines which also fluoresce under these conditions (p. 308).

URINE SCREENING PROCEDURES FOR DRUGS OF ABUSE

The common drugs of abuse, which are those controlled by the Misuse of Drugs Act, are classified as:

1. Narcotics and analgesics, both alkaloids and synthetic drugs—e.g. heroin, morphine, codeine, methadone, pethidine, dextropropoxyphene.

Drugs and Poisons 357

2. Sympathomimetic amines—e.g. amphetamine, methylamphetamine.
3. Hypnotics and sedatives—e.g. barbiturates, glutethimide, methaqualone, phenothiazines.
4. Hallucinogens—e.g. cannabis, lysergide, mescaline.

Patients who are addicted to such drugs often take members of these different types simultaneously. It is therefore necessary when investigating suspects to choose methods which allow screening for a wide variety of drugs. Such methods are available for the first three groups but there are difficulties with the hallucinogens. Although techniques involving GLC, mass spectrometry and immunological reactions are being developed, most work has relied on the resolving power of TLC using silica gel. For early methods see Mulé (1964, 1969, 1971), Dole *et al.* (1966), Parker and Hine (1967), Davidow *et al.* (1968), Ono *et al.* (1969), Berry and Grove (1971b).

The best fluid for analysis is urine. An extract is made and applied to the TLC plate which is then developed in one or more solvent mixtures. Multiple detecting sprays or other visualisation procedures allow recognition of many substances by their R_F values and reactions. Published methods vary considerably. The following methods have been selected from more recent publications.

Extraction Procedures

The required drugs include acidic, neutral and basic substances. Earlier methods involved extractions into organic solvents at several different pH values but more recently simpler, efficient techniques have been devised.

Single Extraction using an Organic Solvent (Stoner and Parker, 1974)

Extraction at pH 6 removes neutral and acidic drugs. Basic drugs are converted to soluble salts with bromcresol purple, thus permitting simultaneous extraction.

Reagents 1. Bromcresol purple buffer, pH 6.0. Dissolve 1.7 g Na_2HPO_4, 12.0 g KH_2PO_4 and 0.4 g bromcresol purple sodium salt in about 500 ml water and dilute to 1 litre. Check the pH.
2. Extracting solvent. Mix 75 ml chloroform and 25 ml 2-propanol.

Technique. Add 15 ml urine to 2.0 ml buffer in a 50 ml stoppered centrifuge tube. Check that the pH is 5.7 to 6.3, adjusting if required. Add 25 ml solvent and shake mechanically for 5 min. Centrifuge for 10 min at 400 g, aspirate and discard the upper aqueous layer. Evaporate to dryness in a water bath at 70°C. A water vacuum pump connected to a tube projecting into the upper part of the centrifuge tube aids the process. Dissolve the dried residue by washing down the sides of the tube with 100 μl methanol, and transfer an aliquot to the TLC plate.

Use of a Resin Column (Weissman *et al.*, 1971)

The non-ionic resin, Amberlite XAD-2 has been used by several workers.

358   *Practical Clinical Biochemistry*

This absorbs drugs from aqueous solution, but releases them to methanol.

Reagents. 1. Amberlite XAD-2 resin, 20-50 mesh (Mallinckrodt Chemical Co.). Wash by stirring with 5 volumes methanol for 2 h. Allow to settle and decant. Repeat the process twice more. Rinse the resin 3 times with 10 volumes water and store at $4°C$ under methanol: water, 300 ml/l.

2. Methanol, anhydrous.

Technique. Place a small plug of glass wool in the bottom of a glass column 1×16 cm. Pour the resin suspension into the column to produce a 6 cm height of resin. Wash with 20 ml water. Carefully centrifuge the urine to remove all particulate matter, transfer 5 ml to the column and allow to enter the column fully. Wash with 60 ml water and after draining apply suction to the bottom of the column to remove as much water as possible. Add 10 ml methanol and collect the eluate.

Evaporate the solvent in a water bath at $45°C$ under a nitrogen stream. When evaporation is almost complete, rinse the walls with 1 ml methanol and take to dryness. Dissolve the residue in $30 \mu l$ methanol and transfer an aliquot to the TLC plate.

Use of Charcoal (Meola and Vanko, 1974)

Drugs are adsorbed onto charcoal from which they can be eluted with small volumes of solvent. Differential elution simplifies the TLC pattern.

Reagents. 1. Charcoal, "Norit A", neutral, pharmaceutical grade.

2. Carbonate buffer, pH 11.0. Dissolve $21 g$ Na_2CO_3 and $420 mg$ $NaHCO_3$ in about 700 ml water. Adjust to pH 11.0 ± 0.1 if necessary and dilute to 1 litre. Store in the refrigerator.

3. Charcoal slurry. Mix 500 mg charcoal and 200 ml buffer using a magnetic stirrer. After settling for 10 min aspirate as much buffer as possible. Before use, resuspend the charcoal.

4. Diethyl ether, pure.

5. Chloroform, 2-propanol mixture. Add 20 ml 2-propanol to 80 ml chloroform.

Technique. Into a 16×150 mm screw-capped tube place 10 ml urine, 5 ml buffer and 0.5 ml charcoal slurry. Mix by repeated inversion and allow to settle for 5 min. Centrifuge for 5 min, then aspirate as much of the fluid as possible. To elute barbiturates, glutethimide and cocaine add 2 ml ether and shake vigorously by hand. After the charcoal has settled decant the ether into a clean 10×75 mm tube. Re-extract the charcoal with 0.5 ml ether and add to the first extract. Evaporate at room temperature in a stream of nitrogen. Dissolve the residue in 2 drops methanol for chromatography.

Extract the amphetamines, narcotic alkaloids and other drugs by adding 2 ml chloroform-propanol to the charcoal and shaking vigorously. Filter through a 5.5 cm Whatman No. 1 paper, moistened with clean solvent, into a 5 ml beaker. Re-extract the charcoal with 0.5 ml chloroform-propanol and filter through the same paper. To a 10×75 mm clean tube add 1 drop

Drugs and Poisons 359

hydrochloric acid, 100 mmol/l, followed by the solvent from the beaker, rinsing this with a few drops of clean solvent. Evaporate to dryness at room temperature in a stream of nitrogen. Dissolve the residue in 2 drops methanol for chromatography.

Thin Layer Chromatography

Silica gel layers have been almost entirely used, either prepared in the laboratory or as commercially manufactured prepared plates. The degree of separation achieved varies with the manufacturer of the gel or plate, making the use of standards, preferably in urine, essential for identification.

A variety of developing solvents has been employed. Some are intended for a particular group of drugs and are useful for selective detecting agents or extracts containing part of the whole range of drugs of abuse. Others are intended for separation of all drugs on a single plate followed by a series of detection procedures. Cochin and Daly (1963) give details of four systems for separating antihistamines, benzodiazepines, phenothiazines and tricyclic antidepressants namely: glacial acetic acid/butanol/butyl ether (10/40/80); ammonium hydroxide/benzene/dioxan (5/60/35); glacial acetic acid/ ethanol/water (30/50/20); *n*-butanol/methanol (40/60). The same authors separated barbiturates and other hypnotics using three other systems: glacial acetic acid/benzene (10/90); ammonium hydroxide/benzene/dioxan (5/75/20); acetone/chloroform (10/90). Mulé (1964) used two systems for the narcotic analgesics: ammonium hydroxide/benzene/dioxan/ethanol (5/50/40/5); glacial acetic acid/ethanol/water (30/60/10).

For the extraction procedures described earlier, Weissman *et al.* (1971) used ammonium hydroxide/ethyl acetate/methanol (5/85/10) for separation of all drugs on one plate, while Stoner and Parker, and Meola and Vanko prefer to use two plates. Stoner and Parker (1974) use acetone chloroform (10/90) to separate barbiturates and the same system as Weissman *et al.*, for basic drugs. For their first extract Meola and Vanko (1974) also use acetone/chloroform (10/90) followed by ammonium hydroxide/acetone/chloroform (2/10/90) for the lower half of the plate. For their second extract they use ammonium hydroxide/*n*-butanol/ chloroform (3/10/190) followed by the mixture of Weissman *et al.* for the lower three quarters of the plate.

For a particular choice of silica gel plate, several systems from the above list should be tried to assess which gives the most critical separation.

Detection Procedures

These vary with different authors as does the composition of supposedly identical spraying agents.

The usual sprays are:

1. Ninhydrin, followed by heating and exposure to ultraviolet light to detect amphetamines, phenothiazines and tricyclic antidepressants. This

360 *Practical Clinical Biochemistry*

can be followed by buffered bromocresol green when the colours of amphetamine and methadone change characteristically.

2. Dilute sulphuric acid followed by inspection in UV light, 365 nm, for the intense blue fluorescence of quinine and metabolites.

3. Diphenylcarbazone in aqueous acetone followed by mercuric sulphate detects barbiturates and glutethimide as purple spots which fade on heating when phenothiazines are revealed.

4. Iodoplatinate reagent prepared from potassium iodide and chloroplatinic acid is a general reagent for bases. Characteristic colours are given by the alkaloids, synthetic narcotics, methaqualone, methylamphetamine etc.

5. Dragendorff's reagent, bismuth subnitrate and potassium iodide in acetic acid, may be employed after the last reagent to produce characteristic changes in colours to aid identification.

6. Tollens reagent, ammoniacal silver nitrate, is used after the iodoplatinate spray to intensify certain spots, particularly those due to morphine and pentazocine.

In many cases these sprays can be used sequentially. For details of composition, order and colour changes see the various references already quoted. Neesby (1973) suggests also the use of diazotised p-nitroaniline for narcotics and Meola and Vanko (1974) also employ fluorescamine for amphetamines.

Notes. 1. Urines need not be stored under special conditions before testing. Even after 14 days at room temperature without preservation, satisfactory results are obtained (Frings and Queen, 1972).

2. Urines containing known amounts of different drugs of abuse can be prepared in the laboratory (Frings and Queen, 1972) and are also available commercially (Lederle Diagnostics Ltd.).

3. Prepacked kits for the extraction, chromatography and detection of drugs of abuse are available commercially from the Gelman Instrument Company, Ann Arbor, Michigan.

REFERENCES

Baer, D. M. (1965). *Amer. J. clin. Path.*, **44**, 114.
Bailey, D. N. and Jatlow, P. I. (1973). *Clin. Chem.*, **19**, 615.
Barbour, R. F., Pilkington, F. and Sargent, W. (1963). *Brit. med. J.*, **2**, 397.
Berry, D. J. and Grove, J. (1971a). *Clin. chim. Acta*, **34**, 5.
Berry, D. J. and Grove, J. (1971b). *J. Chromatog.*, **61**, 111.
Bessman, S. P. and Layne, E. C., Jr. (1955). *J. lab. clin. Med.*, **45**, 159.
Bochner, F., Hooper, W. D., Tyrer, J. H. and Eadie, M. J. (1972). *J. Neurol. Neurosurg. Psychiat.*, **35**, 873.
Bonnichsen, R., Mårde, Y. and Ryhage, R. (1974). *Clin. Chem.*, **20**, 230.
Braithwaite, R. A. and Widdup, B. (1971). *Clin. chim. Acta*, **35**, 461.
Bratton, A. C. and Marshall, E. K. (1939). *J. biol. Chem.*, **128**, 537.
British Medical Association Special Committee (1958). Recognition of Intoxication, revised edition.

Drugs and Poisons

361

Brodie, B. B. and Axelrod, J. (1948). *J. Pharmacol. exp. Therap.*, **94**, 22.
Brodie, B. B., Udenfriend, S. and Coburn, A. F. (1944) *J. Pharmacol. exp. Therap.*, **80**, 114.
Broughton, P. M. G. (1956). *Biochem. J.*, **63**, 207.
Broughton, P. M. G., Higgins, G. and O'Brien, J. R. P. (1956). *Lancet*, **1**, 180.
Brown, P. B. and Legg, E. F. (1970). *Ann. clin. Biochem.*, **7**, 13.
Brown, S. S. (1971). *Ann. clin. Biochem.*, **8**, 98.
Buckell, M., Hunter, D., Milton, R. and Perry, K. M. A. (1946). *Brit. J. industr. Med.*, **3**, 55.
Calderbank, A. and Yuen, S. H. (1965). *Analyst*, **90**, 99.
Cavett, J. W. (1938). *J. lab. clin. Med.*, **23**, 543.
Chefetz, L., Daly, R. E., Schriftman, H. and Lomner, J. J. (1971). *J. pharm. Sci.*, **60**, 463.
Christiansen, J. and Dam, M. (1973). *Acta Neurol. Scand.*, **49**, 543.
Clarke, E. G. C. (editor). (1969). *Isolation and Identification of Drugs*, Pharmaceutical Press, London.
Clarke, E. G. C. (editor). (1975). *Isolation and Identification of Drugs*, Volume 2, Pharmaceutical Press, London.
Clarkson, T. W. and Kench, J. E. (1956). *Biochem. J.*, **62**, 361.
Cochin, J. and Daly, J. W. (1963). *J. Pharmacol. exp. Therap.*, **139**, 154, 160.
Connell, P. M. (1958). *Amphetamine Psychosis*, Maudesley Monographs, No. 5, Chapman and Hall, London.
Conway, E. J. (1957). *Microdiffusion Analysis and Volumetric Error*, 4th Edition, p. 249, Crosby Lockwood.
Cooper, J. D. H. (1971). *Clin. chim. Acta*, **33**, 483.
Cravey, R. H. and Jain, N. C. (1974). *J. chromatog. Sci.*, **12**, 209.
Curry, A. S. (1961). In *Toxicology, Mechanisms and Analytical Methods*, (Stolman, A. and Stewart, C. P., eds.), vol. 2, p. 153, Academic Press, London and New York.
Curry, A. S. (1963). *Brit. med. J.*, **2**, 1040.
Curry, A. S. (1964). *Brit. med. J.*, **1**, 354.
Curry, A. S. (1969a). *Poison Detection in Human Organs*, 2nd edn., Thomas, Springfield, Illinois.
Curry, A. S. (1969b, 1975). In *Isolation and Identification of Drugs*, (Clarke, E. G. C., ed.), Pharmaceutical Press, London, pp. 43, 922.
Curry, S. H. (1971). *Proc. Roy. Soc. Med.*, **64**, 285.
Dauphinais, R. M. O. and McComb, R. (1965). *Amer. J. clin. Path.*, **44**, 440.
Davidow, B., Petri, N. L. and Quame, B. (1968). *Amer. J. clin. Path.*, **50**, 714.
Denswill, E. H. and Ditmers, J. P. (1972). *Clin. chim. Acta*, **40**, 129.
Dill, W. A., Clincot, L., Chang, T. and Glazko, A. J. (1971). *Clin. Chem.*, **17**, 1200.
Dole, V. P., Kim, W. K. and Eglitis, I. (1966). *J. Amer. med. Ass.*, **198**, 349.
Douglas, A. P., Hamlyn, A. N. and James, O. (1976). *Lancet*, **1**, 111.
Editorial. Early Detection of Lead Toxicity. (1970). *Lancet*, **1**, 705.
Evenson, M. A. and Lensmeyer, G. L. (1974). *Clin. Chem.*, **20**, 249.
Evenson, M. A. and Poquette, M. A. (1974). *Clin. Chem.*, **20**, 212.
Evenson, M.A. and Prendergast, D. D. (1974). *Clin. Chem.*, **20**, 163.
Fincham, R. W., Schottelius, D. D. and Sahs, A. L. (1974). *Arch. Neurol.*, **30**, 259.
Forrest, I. S. and Forrest, F. M. (1960). *Clin. Chem.*, **6**, 11.
Forrest, I. S., Forrest, F. M. and Mason, A. S. (1960). *Amer. J. Psychiat.*, **116**, 928 (a); 1021 (b).
Forrest, F. M., Forrest, I. S. and Mason, A. S. (1961). *Amer. J. Psychiat*, **118**, 300.
Fox, R. H. (1969, 1975). In *Isolation and Identification of Drugs*, (Clarke, E. G. C., ed.), Pharmaceutical Press, London, pp. 31, 921.
Frings, C. S. and Queen, C. A. (1972). *Clin. Chem.*, **18**, 1440, 1442.
Fry, D. E. and Marks, V. (1971). *Lancet*, **2**, 886.
Gage, J. C. and Warren, J. M. (1970). *Ann. occup. Hyg.*, **13**, 115.

362   *Practical Clinical Biochemistry*

Garvey, K. and Bowden, C. H. (1966). *Proc. Ass. clin. Biochem.*, **4**, 20.

Gibson, P. F. (1972). *Lancet*, **2**, 607.

Glynn, J. P. and Kendal, S. E. (1975). *Lancet*, **1**, 1147.

Golbey, M. J. (1971). *Ann. clin. Biochem.*, **8**, 117.

Gold, M., Tassoni, E., Etzl, M. and Mathew, G. (1974). *Clin. Chem.*, **20**, 195.

Goldberg, D. M. and Clarke, A. D. (1970). *J. clin. Path.*, **23**, 178.

Greaves, M. S. (1974). *Clin. Chem.*, **20**, 141.

Grove, J. (1971). *J. Chromatog.*, **59**, 289.

Hansen, A. R. and Fischer, L. J. (1974). *Clin. Chem.*, **20**, 236.

Harger, R. N. (1961). In *Toxicology, Mechanisms and Analytical Methods*, (Stolman, A. and Stewart, C. P. eds.), vol. 2, p. 86, Academic Press, London and New York.

Higgins, G. and Leach, H. (1975). In *Isolation and Identification of Drugs*, (Clarke, E. G. C., ed.), vol. 2, p. 873, The Pharmaceutical Press, London.

Howie, R. A. and Smith, H. (1967). *J. forensic Sci. Soc.*, **7**, 90.

I.C.I. Monograph. (1974). *The Treatment of Paraquat Poisoning*, Industrial Hygiene Laboratories.

Jackson, J. V. (1960). In *Chromatographic and Electrophoretic Techniques*, (Smith, I., ed.), vol. 1, p. 494, Heinemann Medical Books, London.

Jamieson, A. and Frew, M. W. (1973). *Ann. clin. Biochem.*, **10**, 37.

Keller, W. J. (1947). *Amer. J. clin. Path.*, **17**, 415.

Kerr, F., Patel, A. R., Scott, P. D. R. and Tompsett, S. L. (1968). *Brit. med. J.*, **3**, 291.

Kragh-Sørensen, P., Åsberg, M. and Eggert-Hansen, C. (1973). *Lancet*, **1**, 113.

Lawson, A. A. and Brown, S. S. (1967). *Scot. med. J.*, **12**, 63.

Leach, H. (1969, 1975). In *Isolation and Identification of Drugs*, (Clarke, E. G. C., ed.), Pharmaceutical Press, London, pp. 59, 925.

Leech, H. and Jones, O. P. (1971). *Ann. clin. Biochem.*, **8**, 73.

Lehmann, J. and Karamustafaoglu, V. (1962). *Scand. J. clin. lab. Invest.*, **14**, 554.

Levvy, G. P. (1940). *Biochem. J.*, **34**, 73.

Levy, A. L. and Katz, E. M. (1970). *Clin. Chem.*, **16**, 840.

Lindstedt, G. (1970). *Analyst*, **95**, 264.

Lindstedt, G., Lundberg, P. A., Tofft, M., Akesson, H. O. and Ohman, R. (1973). *Clin. chim. Acta*, **48**, 127.

Lubran, M. A. (1961). *Clin. chim. Acta*, **6**, 594.

Lundquist, F. (1959). In *Methods of Biochemical Analysis*, (Glick, D., ed.), **7**, 217.

Magos, L. and Cernik, A. A. (1969). *Brit. J. industr. Med.*, **26**, 144.

Marks, V., Lindup, W. E. and Baylis, E. M. (1973). *Adv. Clin. Chem.*, **16**, 47.

Martindale. (1972). *The Extra Pharmacopoeia*, 26th edn., (Blacow, N. W., ed.). Pharmaceutical Press, London.

Mason, M. F. and Dubowski, K. M. (1974). *Clin. Chem.*, **20**, 126.

Mawer, G. E., Mullen, P. W., Rodgers, M., Robins, A. J. and Lucas, S. B. (1974). *Brit. J. clin. Pharmacol.*, **1**, 163.

Meade, B. W., Widdop, B., Blackmore, D. J., Brown, S. S., Curry, A. S., Goulding, R., Higgins, G., Matthew, H. J. S. and Rinsler, M. G. (1972). *Ann. clin. Biochem.*, **9**, 35.

Meola, J. M. and Vanko, M. (1974). *Clin. Chem.*, **20**, 184.

Meunier, J., Lemontey, Y. and Lafargue, P. (1970). *Ann. Biol. clin.*, **28**, 431.

Milton, R. F. and Hoskins, J. L. (1947). *Analyst*, **72**, 6.

Monier-Williams, G. W. (1949). *Trace Elements in Foods*, Chapman and Hall, London, p. 453.

Mulé, S. J. (1964). *Anal. Chem.*, **36**, 1907.

Mulé, S. J. (1969). *J. Chromatog.*, **39**, 302.

Mulé, S. J. (1971). *J. Chromatog.*, **55**, 255.

Mullen, P. W. (1974). *Clin. Chem.*, **20**, 1478.

Neesby, T. (1973). *Clin. Chem.*, **19**, 356.

Nobel, S. and Leifheit, H. C. (1961). *Stand. Meth. Clin. Chem.*, **3**, 176.

Drugs and Poisons

Nobel, S. and Nobel, D. (1958). *Clin. Chem.*, 4, 150.

Ono, M., Englke, B. F. and Fulton, C. (1969). *Bull. Narcotics*, 21, 31.

Parker, K. D. and Hine, C. H. (1967). *Bull. Narcotics*, 19, 51.

Payne, J. P., Foster, D. V., Hill, D. W. and Wood, D. G. L. (1967). *Brit. med. J.*, 3, 819.

Prescott, L. F. (1971). *J. Pharm. Pharmacol.*, 23, 807.

Prescott, L. F. and Matthew, H. (1974). *Lancet*, 1, 998.

Prescott, L. F., Swainson, C. P., Forrest, A. R. W., Newton, R. W., Wright, N. and Matthew, H. (1974). *Lancet*, 1, 588.

Prescott, L. F., Wright, N., Roscoe, P. and Brown, S. S. (1971). *Lancet*, 1, 519.

Proudfoot, A. T. and Wright, N. (1970). *Brit. med. J.*, 4, 557.

Pybus, J. and Bowers, C. N. (1970). *Clin. Chem.*, 16, 139.

Report of the Joint Sub-Committee of the Standing Medical Advisory Committee, Hospital Treatment of Acute Poisoning (1968). HM 68 (92). HMSO. London.

Rice, E. W., Fletcher, D. C. and Stumpff, A. (1965). *Stand. Meth. Clin. Chem.*, 5, 121.

Richens, A. (1974). *Proc. Roy. Soc. Med.*, 67, 1227.

Ritchie, J. M. (1970). In *The Pharmacological Basis of Therapeutics*, 4th edn. (Goodman, L. S. and Gilman, A., eds.), Macmillan, New York.

Robertson, R., Fritze, K. and Crof, P. (1973). *Clin. chim. Acta*, 45, 23.

Routh, J. I., Shore, N. A., Arrendonde, E. G. and Paul, W. D. (1967). *Clin. Chem.*, 13, 734.

Routh, J. I., Shore, N. A., Arrendonde, E. G. and Paul, W. D. (1968). *Clin. Chem.*, 14, 882.

Sayers, M. H. P. (1970). *J. clin. Path.*, 23, 741.

Searle, B., Chan, W. and Davidow, B. (1973). *Clin. Chem.*, 19, 76.

Simonsen, D. G. (1953). *Amer, J. clin. Path.*, 23, 789.

Simpson, E. and Stewart, M. J. (1973). *Ann. clin. Biochem.*, 10, 171.

Smith, M. J. H. and Talbot, J. M. (1950. *Biochem. J.*, 46, v.

Special Issue on Toxicology. (1971). *Ann. clin. Biochem.*, 8, 73.

Special Issue: Toxicology and Drug Assay. (1974). *Clin. Chem.*, 20, 111.

Statement. Diagnosis of Inorganic Lead Poisoning. (1968). *Brit. med. J.*, 4, 501.

Stevenson, G. W. (1961). *Anal. Chem.*, 33, 1374.

Stewart, M. J. and Simpson, E. (1973). *Ann. clin. Biochem.*, 10, 173.

Stewart, M. J. and Willis, R. G. (1975). *Ann. clin. Biochem.*, 12, 4.

Stolman, A. and Stewart, C. P. (editors). (1960, 1961). *Toxicology, Mechanisms and Analytical Methods*, vols. 1 and 2, Academic Press, London and New York.

Stoner, R. E. and Parker, C. (1974). *Clin. Chem.*, 20, 309.

Sunshine, I. (1963). *Amer. J. clin. Path.*, 40, 576.

Sunshine, I. (1969). *Handbook of Analytical Toxicology*, Chemical Rubber Co., Cleveland.

Sunshine, I. and Nenad, R. (1953). *Anal. Chem.*, 25, 653.

Svensmark, O. and Kristensen, P. (1963). *J. lab. clin. Med.*, 61, 501.

Temple, R., Borman, M., Carlsson, H. E., Robbins, J. and Wolff, J. (1972). *J. clin. Invest.*, 51, 2746.

Tompsett, S. L. and Smith, D. C. (1959). *J. clin. Path.*, 12, 219.

Toseland, P. A., Grove, J. and Berry, D. J. (1972). *Clin. chim. Acta*, 35, 321.

Trinder, P. (1954). *Biochem. J.*, 57, 301.

Turano, P., Turner, W. J. and Menden, A. A. (1973). *J. Chromatog.*, 75, 277.

Valentour, J. C., Monforte, J. R., Lorenzo, B. and Sunshine, I. (1975). *Clin. Chem.*, 21, 1976.

Vessell, E. S. and Passananti, G. T. (1971). *Clin. Chem.*, 17, 851.

Walker, W. H. C. and Wood, J. K. (1965). *J. clin. Path.*, 18, 482.

Wall, H. and Rhodes, C. (1966). *Clin. Chem.*, 12, 837.

Wallace, J. E. (1966). *J. Forensic Sci.*, 11, 522.

Wallace, J. E. (1969). *Clin. Chem.*, 15, 323.

Wallace, J. E., Briggs, J. and Dahl, H. V. (1965). *Anal. Chem.*, 37, 410.

364 *Practical Clinical Biochemistry*

Wallace, J. E., Farquhar, J. K., Hamilton, H. E. and Everhart, B. A. (1974a). *Clin. Chem.*, **20**, 515.

Wallace, J. E., Hamilton, H. E., Riloff, J. A. and Blum, K. (1974b). *Clin. Chem.*, **20**, 159.

Warkany, J. and Hubbard, D. M. (1951). *Amer. J. Dis. Childh.*, **81**, 335.

Watson, D. and Dillion, G. (1973). *Ann. clin. Biochem.*, **10**, 31.

Watson, E. and Kalman, S. M. (1972). *Clin. chim. Acta*, **38**, 33.

Weissman, N., Lowe, M. L., Beattie, J. M. and Demetriou, J. A. (1971). *Clin. Chem.*, **17**, 875.

Willoughby, C. E. and Wilkins, E. S. (1938). *J. biol. Chem.*, **124**, 639.

Woollen, J. W. and Wells, M. G. (1973). *Ann. clin. Biochem.*, **10**, 85.

Wright, J. T. (1954). *J. clin. Path.*, **7**, 61.

APPENDICES

Standards for Volumetric Analysis

The following chemicals of a very high degree of purity are used as primary standards. They are anhydrous and may be dried by heat without changing their composition. Hopkin and Williams Ltd. provide these reagents as "Purified for Volumetric Standardisation". The following amounts (g) made up to one litre give a concentration of 100 mmol/l.

Benzoic acid	12.212
Potassium dichromate	29.419
Potassium iodate	21.400
Sodium carbonate	10.599
Sodium chloride	5.844
Sulphamic acid	9.709

Secondary standards are liable to gain or lose moisture in accordance with the humidity of the atmosphere and the care with which they are stored. The following amounts (g) made up to one litre give a concentration of 100 mmol/l.

Antimony potassium tartrate	32.492
Ferrous ammonium sulphate, hexahydrate	39.214
Oxalic acid, dihydrate	12.607
Potassium hydrogen phthalate	20.423
Silver nitrate	16.987
Sodium tetraborate, decahydrate	38.138

BDH and HW supply ampoules of concentrated volumetric solutions which when diluted with distilled water give a standard solution with concentration accurate to within ± 0.1 per cent. They cover all the commonly used volumetric reagents.

Indicators

The following well-tried indicators are available from several manufacturers either in solid form or as prepared solutions.

	pH range	Colour change
Phenol red (acid range)	0.0- 2.0	pink to yellow
Cresol red (acid range)	0.2- 1.8	red to yellow
m-Cresol purple (acid range)	0.6- 2.4	red to yellow
Thymol blue (acid range)	1.2- 2.8	red to yellow
Bromophenol blue*	2.8- 4.6	yellow to blue
Methyl orange*	2.8- 4.6	red to yellow
Methyl orange, screened	3.0- 4.6	violet to green
Congo red*	3.0- 5.0	blue to red
Bromocresol green*	3.8- 5.4	yellow to blue
Methyl red*	4.2- 6.3	red to yellow
Chlorophenol red*	4.8- 6.8	yellow to red
Litmus*	5.0- 8.0	red to blue

Bromocresol purple*	5.2- 6.8	yellow to purple
Bromothymol blue*	6.0- 7.6	yellow to blue
Neutral red	6.8- 8.0	yellow to red
Phenol red	6.8- 8.4	yellow to red
Cresol red	7.2- 8.8	yellow to red
m-Cresol purple	7.6- 9.2	yellow to purple
Thymol blue	8.0- 9.6	yellow to blue
Phenolphthalein*	8.3-10.0	colourless to purple-red
Thymolphthalein	9.3-10.5	colourless to blue
Alizarin yellow GG	10.0-12.0	colourless to yellow
Tropaeolin O	11.1-12.7	yellow to orange

The following mixed indicators are supplied by BDH.

"4460"	4.4- 6.0	red to green
"4.5"	3.5- 6.0	orange red to blue
"6676"	6.6- 7.6	orange to violet
"7785"	7.7- 8.5	green to purple
"9011"	9.0-11.0	yellow to violet-grey
"1113"	11.0-13.0	yellow to red-purple

Several wider range mixed indicators are useful for approximate determination of pH. They are available from BDH and HW.

BDH "4080"	4.0- 8.0	red-yellow-bluish green
BDH "678"	5.0-10.0	orange-green-grey-violet
BDH "1014"	10.0-14.0	green-pink-orange
BDH "Full Range"	1.0-14.0	red to violet (spectral colours)
BDH "Universal Indicator"	4.0-11.0	red to violet (spectral colours)
HW "BTL Universal Indicator"	1.0-12.0	red to purple (spectral colours)

A number of indicators, indicated by * in the list above are also supplied in paper form. Sets of narrow range indicator papers are supplied by BDH and HW to cover the following ranges of pH: 1 to 4, 4 to 6, 6 to 8, 8 to 10, 10 to 12, 12 to 14; 1.0 to 3.5, 3.6 to 5.1, 5.2 to 6.7, 6.8 to 8.3, 8.4 to 10.0. Universal indicator papers are also available.

Buffer Mixtures

The following mixtures are suitable for general purposes. In each case details are given for making 1 litre of solution. $\Delta pH/^{\circ}C$ refers to the rate of change of pH with temperature. The ionic strength (I) is in mmol/l as is the osmolarity.

1. KCl-HCl (Clark and Lubs) at 20° C

pK = 1.33 $\quad \Delta pH/^{\circ}C \approx 0 \quad$ I = 147 to 57 (pH 1 to 2.2)
Osmolarity = 294 to 114

Appendices 367

Volume (ml) 200 mmol/l hydrochloric acid to be added to 250 ml of 200 mmol/l potassium chloride followed by dilution to 1 litre with water.

pH	ml	pH	ml	pH	ml
1.0	485	1.6	131.5	2.2	35.5
1.2	322.5	1.8	84		
1.4	207.5	2.0	53		

2. *Glycine-HCl (Sørensen) at 18° C*

pK = 2.35 ΔpH/° C $\approx$ 0   I = 100 to 189 (pH 1.2 to 3.6) Osmolarity = 200 to 289

Volume (ml) of glycine-sodium chloride mixture, 100 mmol/l of each, to be diluted to 1 litre with 100 mmol/l hydrochloric acid.

pH	ml	pH	ml	pH	ml
1.2	150	2.2	583	3.2	856
1.4	287	2.4	645	3.4	903
1.6	382	2.6	702	3.6	945
1.8	457	2.8	756		
2.0	523	3.0	808		

3. *Phthalate-HCl (Clark and Lubs) at 20°C*

pK_1 = 2.95 Δ pH/° C = 0.001   I = 50 (constant) Osmolarity = 147 to 103

Volume (ml) of 200 mmol/l hydrochloric acid to be added to 250 ml of 200 mmol/l potassium hydrogen phthalate followed by dilution to 1 litre with water.

pH	ml	pH	ml	pH	ml
2.2	233.5	2.8	132	3.4	49.8
2.4	198	3.0	101.5	3.6	30.0
2.6	165	3.2	74.0	3.8	13.2

4. *Acetate-acetic acid (Walpole) at 23° C*

pK = 4.76 ΔpH/° C = -0.004 I = 7 to 90 (pH 3.6 to 5.6) Osmolarity = 107 to 190

Volume (ml) of A: 200 mmol/l acetic acid and volume (ml) of B: 200 mmol/l sodium acetate to be diluted to 1 litre with water.

pH	A	B	pH	A	B	pH	A	B
3.6	463	37	4.4	305	195	5.2	105	395
3.8	440	60	4.6	255	245	5.4	88	412
4.0	410	90	4.8	200	300	5.6	48	452
4.2	368	132	5.0	148	352			

368 — Practical Clinical Biochemistry

5. Phthalate-NaOH (Clark and Lubs) at 20° C

$pK_2 = 5.41$ $\Delta pH/°C = 0.001$ $I = 51$ to 144 (pH 4.0 to 6.2)
Osmolarity = 100 to 147

Volume (ml) of 200 mmol/l sodium hydroxide to be added to 250 ml of 200 mmol/l potassium hydrogen phthalate followed by dilution to 1 litre with water.

pH	ml	pH	ml	pH	ml
4.0	2.0	4.8	87.5	5.6	198.5
4.2	18.3	5.0	128.3	5.8	215.5
4.4	36.8	5.2	148.8	6.0	227.0
4.6	60.0	5.4	176.3	6.2	235.0

6. Tris-maleate-NaOH (Gomori) at 23° C

pK's = 6.24, 8.08   I uncertain   Osmolarity = 107 to 187

Volume (ml) of 200 mmol/l sodium hydroxide to be added to 250 ml of tris [hydroxymethyl] aminomethane—maleic acid, 200 mmol/l of each, followed by dilution to 1 litre with water.

pH	ml	pH	ml	pH	ml
5.2	35	6.4	185	7.6	290
5.4	54	6.6	213	7.8	318
5.6	78	6.8	225	8.0	345
5.8	103	7.0	240	8.2	375
6.0	130	7.2	255	8.4	405
6.2	158	7.4	270	8.6	433

7. Phosphate (Sørensen) at 18° C

$pK_2 = 7.20$ $\Delta pH/°C = -0.003$ $I = 77$ to 191 (pH 5.8 to 7.9)
Osmolarity = 139 to 195

Volume (ml) of 1/15 mol/l monopotassium phosphate to be diluted to 1 litre with 1/15 mol/l disodium phosphate.

pH	ml	pH	ml	pH	ml
5.80	920	6.85	475	7.40	192
5.90	901	6.90	446	7.45	175
6.00	878	6.95	418	7.50	159
6.10	847	7.00	389	7.55	143
6.20	814	7.05	361	7.60	130
6.30	776	7.10	334	7.65	118
6.40	733	7.15	308	7.70	106
6.50	682	7.20	280	7.75	95
6.60	625	7.25	256	7.80	85
6.70	565	7.30	232	7.90	68
6.80	504	7.35	211		

Appendices 369

8. Barbitone-HCl (Michaelis) at 23° C

pK = 7.98 ΔpK/°C = −0.008   I = 52 to 99 (pH 6.8 to 9.6)
Osmolarity = 152 to 199
Volume (ml) of 100 mmol/l sodium barbitone to be diluted to 1 litre with 100 mmol/l hydrochloric acid.

pH	ml	pH	ml	pH	ml
6.8	522	7.8	662	8.8	908
7.0	536	8.0	716	9.0	936
7.2	554	8.2	769	9.2	952
7.4	581	8.4	823	9.4	974
7.6	615	8.6	871	9.6	985

9. Tris-HCl (Gomori) at 23° C

pK = 0.08 ΔpH/°C = −0.020   I = 44 to 5 (pH 7.2 to 9.0)
Osmolarity = 94 to 55
Volume (ml) of 200 mmol/l hydrochloric acid to be added to 250 ml of 200 mmol/l tris[hydroxymethyl] aminomethane and diluted to 1 litre with water.

pH	ml	pH	ml	pH	ml
7.2	221	8.0	134	8.8	41
7.4	207	8.2	110	9.0	25
7.6	192	8.4	83		
7.8	163	8.6	61		

10. Borate-KCl-NaOH (Clark and Lubs) at 20° C

pK = 9.24 ΔpH/°C = −0.006   I = 97 to 56 (pH 7.8 to 10)
Osmolarity = 153 to 194
Volume (ml) of 200 mmol/l sodium hydroxide to be added to 250 ml of boric acid−potassium chloride mixture, 200 mmol/l of each, and diluted to 1 litre with water.

pH	ml	pH	ml	pH	ml
7.8	13.3	8.6	60.0	9.4	160.0
8.0	20.0	8.8	82.0	9.6	184.3
8.2	29.5	9.0	107.0	9.8	204.0
8.4	42.8	9.2	133.5	10.0	219.5

11. Glycine-NaOH (Sørensen) at 18° C

pK_2 = 9.78 ΔpH/°C = −0.025   I = 193 to 100 (pH 8.4 to 13.0)
Osmolarity = 293 to 208

370 *Practical Clinical Biochemistry*

Volume (ml) of glycine-sodium chloride mixture, 100 mmol/l of each, to be diluted to 1 litre with 100 mmol/l sodium hydroxide.

pH	ml	pH	ml	pH	ml
8.4	965	10.0	630	11.6	488
8.6	948	10.2	590	11.8	478
8.8	921	10.4	561	12.0	462
9.0	885	10.6	537	12.2	436
9.2	842	10.8	522	12.4	400
9.4	790	11.0	510	12.6	334
9.6	732	11.2	503	12.8	242
9.8	677	11.4	497	13.0	75

12. Na_2CO_3-$NaHCO_3$ (Delory and King) at $23°C$

$pK_2 = 10.33$ $\Delta pH/°C = -0.008$ $I = 58$ to 135 (pH 9.2 to 10.6) Osmolarity = 104 to 143

Volume (ml) of A: 200 mmol/l sodium carbonate and B: 200 mmol/l sodium bicarbonate to be diluted to 1 litre with water.

pH	A	B	pH	A	B	pH	A	B
9.2	20	230	9.8	110	140	10.4	193	58
9.4	48	203	10.0	138	113	10.6	213	38
9.6	80	170	10.2	165	85			

13. Wide range buffer, citrate-phosphate-borate-barbitone (Britton and Welford) at $25°C$

pK's = 2.15, 3.13, 4.76, 7.20, 7.98, 9.24, 12.38. $\Delta pH/°C = 0$ at pH 2.6 to -0.020 at pH 12 I = uncertain   Osmolarity = 149 to 171.

Dissolve 6.004 g citric acid monohydrate, 3.888 g potassium dihydrogen phosphate, 1.767 g boric acid, and 5.263 g sodium barbitone (all 28.57 mmol/l) in water and make to 1 litre. Volume (ml) of 200 mmol/l sodium hydroxide to be added to 1 litre of the above solution.

pH	ml	pH	ml	pH	ml	pH	ml
2.6	20	5.0	271	7.4	558	9.8	793
2.8	43	5.2	295	7.6	586	10.0	808
3.0	64	5.4	318	7.8	617	10.2	820
3.2	83	5.6	342	8.0	637	10.4	829
3.4	101	5.8	365	8.2	656	10.6	839
3.6	118	6.0	389	8.4	675	10.8	849
3.8	137	6.2	412	8.6	693	11.0	860
4.0	155	6.4	435	8.8	710	11.2	877
4.2	176	6.6	460	9.0	727	11.4	897
4.4	199	6.8	483	9.2	740	11.6	920
4.6	224	7.0	506	9.4	759	11.8	950
4.8	248	7.2	529	9.6	776	12.0	996

Appendices 371

14. *Zwitterionic biological buffers (Good) at 20° C*

The buffers listed above have restrictions when used in the usual physiological pH range. Component ions may combine with reactants or products or may interfere with their determination. The following compounds which possess both acidic and basic groups ("zwitterions") cover the physiological range of pH, react very little with enzymes or substrates, do not enter cells and interfere to only a slight degree with spectrophotometric measurements. They are available from HW. They are dissolved in water at the required concentration and the pH is adjusted to that desired by addition of acid or base.

Substance	pKa	pH range	pH/$^{\circ}$C
2-(N-Morpholino)ethanesulphonic acid, MES	6.15	5.8- 6.5	−0.011
N-(2-Acetamido)iminodiacetic acid, ADA	6.62	6.2- 7.2	−0.011
Piperazine-NN′-bis (2-ethanesulphonic acid), PIPES	6.80	6.4- 7.2	−0.0085
N-(2-Acetamido)-2-aminoethanesulphonic acid, ACES	6.88	6.4- 7.4	−0.020
NN-(Bis-2-hydroxyethyl)-2-aminoethanesulphonic acid, BES	7.15	6.6- 7.6	−0.016
3-(N-Morpholino)propanesulphonic acid, MOPS	7.20	6.5- 7.9	−0.011
N-((Trishydroxymethyl) methyl)-2-aminoethane-sulphonic acid, TES	7.50	7.0- 8.0	−0.020
N-2-Hydroxyethylpiperazine-N′-2-ethanesulphonic acid, HEPES	7.55	7.0- 8.0	−0.014
N-2-Hydroxyethylpiperazine-N′-3-propanesulphonic acid, EPPS	8.00	7.6- 8.6	−0.011
N-((Trishydroxymethyl)methyl)glycine, TRICINE	8.15	7.6- 8.8	−0.021
NN-(Bis-2-hydroxyethyl)glycine, BICINE	8.35	7.8- 8.8	−0.018
2-(Cyclohexylamino)ethanesulphonic acid, CHES	9.55	9.0- 10.1	−0.011
3-(Cyclohexylamino)propanesulphonic acid, CAPS	10.40	9.7-11.1	−0.021

Properties of Common Laboratory Reagents

Acids	Density[a] (kg/kg)	Sp. gr.	Concentration (mol/l)	Volume for[b] diluting (ml)
Acetic, "glacial"	>0.99	1.048-1.051	17.4	115
Hydrochloric, "concentrated"	0.36	1.18	11.7	172
Nitric, "concentrated"	0.69-0.71	1.412-1.417	15.5-16.0	129-125
Orthophosphoric, "88%"	0.88	1.75	15.7	127
"10%"	0.095-0.105	1.051-1.057	1.02-1.13	—
Perchloric, "72%"	0.72	1.70	12.2	164
"60%"	0.60	1.54	9.2	218
Sulphuric, "concentrated"	0.98	1.84	18.4	109
Bases				
Ammonia solution,				
"concentrated"	0.35	0.880	18.1	111
"26%"	0.26	0.908	13.9	144
Other				
Hydrogen peroxide, "100 volumes"	0.28-0.29[c]	1.11	8.9	224
"20 volumes"	0.06[c]	1.02	1.8	—
"10 volumes"	0.03[c]	1.01	0.9	—

a = or "per cent w/w ÷ 100".
b = volume of reagent to be diluted to 1 litre with water to give a solution of concentration, 2 mol/l.
c = kg/l.

Appendices   373

Properties of Common Solvents

Name	BP (°C)	Density (kg/l)
Diethyl ether	35	0.71
Dichloromethane	40	1.31
Carbon disulphide	46	1.27
Acetone	56	0.79
1,1-Dichloroethane	57	1.17
Chloroform	61	1.48
Methanol	65	0.79
n-Hexane	69	0.65
Ethyl acetate	77	0.90
Carbon tetrachloride	77	1.58
Ethanol	78	0.79
Benzene	80	0.88
Cyclohexane	81	0.78
Propan-2-ol (*iso*-propanol)	82	0.79
2-Methylpropan-2-ol (*tert*-butanol)	82	0.78
1,2-Dichloroethane	84	1.25
Trichloroethylene	87	1.48
Propan-1-ol (*n*-propanol)	97	0.80
Butan-2-ol (*sec*-butanol)	100	0.80
Water	100	1.00
Formic acid	101	1.21
1,4-Dioxane	101	1.03
2-Methylpropan-1-ol (*iso*-butanol)	108	0.80
Toluene	111	0.86
3-Methylbutan-2-ol	112	0.81
Pyridine	115	0.98
Pentan-3-ol	115	0.82
Butan-1-ol (*n*-butanol)	118	0.81
Acetic acid	118	1.05
Pentan-2-ol	119	0.81
2-Methoxyethanol (methyl cellosolve)	125	0.96
2-Methylbutan-1-ol	129	0.82
3-Methylbutan-1-ol	131	0.81
2-Ethoxyethanol (ethyl cellosolve)	136	0.93
Pentan-1-ol (*n*-amyl alcohol)	138	0.81
p-Xylene	138	0.86
m-Xylene	139	0.86
Acetic anhydride	140	1.09
2-Methylbutan-2-ol	142	0.81
o-Xylene	144	0.88
2-Methoxyethyl acetate (methyl cellosolve acetate)	145	1.00
Amyl acetate	149	0.88
Dimethylformamide	153	0.94
2-Ethoxyethyl acetate (cellosolve acetate)	156	0.97
Ethanolamine	170	1.01
Aniline	184	1.02
Dimethylsulphoxide	189	1.10
Ethylene glycol	197	1.11
Formamide	211	1.13
Nitrobenzene	211	1.21

P.C.B.(II)—13

374 *Practical Clinical Biochemistry*

Desirable Weights According to Height and Age

The following figures adapted from the Statistical Bulletin, Metropolitan Life Insurance Company, *40,* November to December, 1959, apply to people with the greatest life expectancy.

Heights and weights are measured in indoor clothing without shoes. For clothing weight allow 3.6 kg (8 lb) for men and 1.8 kg (4 lb) for women.

The figures refer to age 25 and over. For women in the age range 18 to 25 subtract 0.45 kg (1 lb) for every year under 25.

Height (cm)	Small frame	Weight (kg) Medium frame	Large frame
	Men		
154	50.5–54	53 –58	56.5–63
156	51.5–55	54 –59.5	58 –64.5
158	52.5–56	55 –60.5	59 –66
160	53.5–57.5	56 –61.5	60 –67
162	54.5–58.5	57.5–63	61 –68.5
164	55.5–59.5	58.5–64	62 –70
166	57 –61	59.5–65.5	63 –71.5
168	58.5–62.5	61 –67	64.5–73
170	59.5–64	62.5–68.5	66.5–75
172	61 –65.5	64 –70.5	68 –76.5
174	62.5–67	65.5–72	69.5–78.5
176	64 –68.5	67 –73.5	71 –80
178	65.5–70	68 –75.5	72.5–81.5
180	67 –71.5	69.5–77	74 –83.5
182	68.5–73	71 –78.5	76 –85
184	69.5–74.5	72.5–80.5	77.5–87
186	71 –76	74 –82	79 –88.5
188	72.5–77.5	76 –83.5	80.5–90
190	74 –79	77.5–85.5	82 –92
	Women		
142	41.5–44.5	43.5–48.5	47 –54
144	42.5–45.5	44 –49.5	48 –55
146	43 –46.5	45 –50.5	48.5–56
148	44 –47.5	46 –51.5	50 –57
150	45 –48.5	47 –52.5	51 –58
152	46 –49.5	48.5–54	52 –59
154	47 –51	49.5–55	53 –60
156	48 –52	50.5–56	54 –61.5
158	49.5–53	51.5–57.5	55.5–63
160	50.5–54	52.5–59	56.5–64.5
162	51.5–55.5	54 –60.5	58 –66
164	52.5–57	55.5–62	59.5–67
166	54 –58.5	57 –63.5	61 –68.5
168	55.5–60	58.5–65	62.5–70
170	57 –61.5	59.5–66.5	64 –71.5
172	58.5–63	61 –68	65.5–73.5
174	60 –64.5	62.5–69.5	66.5–75
176	61.5–66	64 –71	68 –77
178	63 –67	65.5–72.5	69.5–78.5

Appendices 375

	Height			Weight (lb)	
ft	in	in	Small frame	Medium frame	Large frame
Men					
5	1	61	112—120	118—129	126—141
5	2	62	115—123	121—133	129—144
5	3	63	118—126	124—136	132—148
5	4	64	121—129	127—139	135—152
5	5	65	124—133	130—143	138—156
5	6	66	128—137	134—147	142—161
5·	7	67	132—141	138—152	147—166
5	8	68	136—145	142—156	151—170
5	9	69	140—150	146—160	155—174
5	10	70	144—154	150—165	159—179
5	11	71	148—158	154—170	164—184
6	0	72	152—162	158—175	168—189
6	1	73	156—167	162—180	173—194
6	2	74	160—171	167—185	178—199
6	3	75	164—175	172—190	182—204
Women					
4	8	56	92— 98	96—107	104—119
4	9	57	94—101	98—110	106—122
4	10	58	96—104	101—113	109—125
4	11	59	99—107	104—116	112—128
5	0	60	102—110	107—119	115—131
5	1	61	105—113	110—122	118—134
5	2	62	108—116	113—126	121—138
5	3	63	111—119	116—130	125—142
5	4	64	114—123	120—135	129—146
5	5	65	118—127	124—139	133—150
5	6	66	122—131	128—143	137—154
5	7	67	126—135	132—147	141—158
5	8	68	130—140	136—151	145—163
5	9	69	134—144	140—155	149—168
5	10	70	138—148	144—159	153—173

Atomic Weights

Selected from the Table of Atomic Weights, 1967 (IUPAC) with revisions of 1971, which is based on the assigned mass of exactly 12 for ^{12}C. Some of the figures have been rounded off.

Element	Symbol	Atomic number	Atomic weight	Element	Symbol	Atomic number	Atomic weight
Aluminium	Al	13	26.98	Molybdenum	Mo	42	95.94
Antimony	Sb	51	121.75	Neon	Ne	10	20.18
Argon	Ar	18	39.95	Nickel	Ni	28	58.71
Arsenic	As	33	74.92	Nitrogen	N	7	14.01
Barium	Ba	56	137.34	Osmium	Os	76	190.2
Beryllium	Be	4	9.012	Oxygen	O	8	16.00
Bismuth	Bi	83	208.98	Palladium	Pd	46	106.4
Boron	B	5	10.81	Phosphorus	P	15	30.97
Bromine	Br	35	79.90	Platinum	Pt	78	195.09
Cadmium	Cd	48	112.40	Potassium	K	19	39.10
Caesium	Cs	55	132.91	Radium	Ra	88	226.03
Calcium	Ca	20	40.08	Radon	Rn	86	222
Carbon	C	6	12.01	Rubidium	Rb	37	85.47
Cerium	Ce	58	140.12	Scandium	Sc	21	44.96
Chlorine	Cl	17	35.45	Selenium	Se	34	78.96
Chromium	Cr	24	52.00	Silicon	Si	14	28.09
Cobalt	Co	27	58.93	Silver	Ag	47	107.87
Copper	Cu	29	63.55	Sodium	Na	11	22.99
Fluorine	F	9	19.00	Strontium	Sr	38	87.62
Gallium	Ga	31	69.72	Sulphur	S	16	32.06
Gold	Au	79	196.97	Tantalum	Ta	73	180.95
Helium	He	2	4.003	Technetium	Tc	43	98.91
Hydrogen	H	1	1.008	Tellurium	Te	52	127.60
Iodine	I	53	126.90	Thallium	Tl	81	204.37
Iridium	Ir	77	192.22	Thorium	Th	90	232.04
Iron	Fe	26	55.85	Tin	Sn	50	118.69
Krypton	Kr	36	83.80	Titanium	Ti	22	47.90
Lanthanum	La	57	138.92	Tungsten	W	74	183.85
Lead	Pb	82	207.2	Uranium	U	92	238.03
Lithium	Li	3	6.941	Vanadium	V	23	50.94
Magnesium	Mg	12	24.31	Xenon	Xe	54	131.30
Manganese	Mn	25	54.94	Zinc	Zn	30	65.38
Mercury	Hg	80	200.59	Zirconium	Zr	40	91.22

BIBLIOGRAPHY

The following short list of books, which is not meant to be comprehensive, has been found useful by the authors.

Advances in Clinical Chemistry, volume 1, 1958 to volume 16, 1975 (various editors). Academic Press, London and New York.

Baron, D. N. *A Short Textbook of Chemical Pathology*, 3rd Edition, 1973. English Universities Press, London.

Cantarow, A. and Trumper, M. *Clinical Biochemistry*, (Latner, A. L., ed.), 7th Edition, 1975. W. B. Saunders Co., London, Philadelphia, Toronto.

Clinics in Endocrinology and Metabolism, volume 1, 1971 to volume 4, 1975 (various editors). W. B. Saunders Co., London, Philadelphia, Toronto.

Gray, C. H. *Clinical Chemical Pathology*, 7th Edition, 1974, Arnold, London.

Hall, R., Anderson, J. and Smart, G. A. *Fundamentals of Clinical Endocrinology*, 2nd Edition, 1974, Pitman Medical, London.

Harrison, G. A. *Chemical Methods in Clinical Medicine*, 4th Edition, 1957, Churchill, London.

Henry, R. J., Cannon, D. C. and Winkelman, J. W. *Clinical Chemistry, Principles and Technics*, 2nd Edition, 1974, Harper and Row, New York, San Francisco, London.

Methods of Biochemical Analysis, (Glick, D., ed.), volume 1, 1953 to volume 22, 1974; supplemental volume, Biogenic Amines, 1971; Interscience Publishers Inc., New York.

Peters, J. P. and Van Slyke, D. D. *Quantitative Clinical Chemistry*, 1st Edition, volume 1, Interpretations; volume 2, Methods, 1932: 2nd Edition, volume 1, part I, 1946.

Recent Advances in Clinical Pathology, (Dyke, S. C., ed.), 1st Edition, 1947 to Series 6, 1973, Churchill Livingstone, Edinburgh and London.

Recent Advances in Medicine, 1st Edition, 1924 to 16th Edition, 1973, (various editors), Churchill Livingstone, Edinburgh and London.

Scientific Tables, 7th Edition, 1970, Documenta Geigy, Basle.

Smith I. *Chromatographic and Electrophoretic Techniques, Clinical and Biochemical Applications*, 2 volumes, 2nd Edition, 1960, Heinemann, London.

Standard Methods of Clinical Chemistry, volume 1, 1953 to volume 7, 1972 (various editors), Academic Press, London and New York.

Symposium on Advanced Medicine, 1st, 1965 to 11th, 1975, (various editors), Pitman Medical, London.

Thompson, R. H. S. and Wootton, I. D. P. *Biochemical Disorders in Human Disease*, 3rd Edition, 1970, Churchill, London.

Tietz, N. W. *Fundamentals of Clinical Chemistry*, 2nd Edition, 1975, W. B. Saunders Co., London, Philadelphia and Toronto.

Vogel, A. I. *Textbook of Quantitative Analysis*, 3rd Edition, 1961, Longmans Green, London.

Whitby, L. G., Percy-Robb, I. W. and Smith, A. F. *Lecture Notes on Clinical Chemistry*, 1975, Blackwell Scientific Publications, Oxford, London, Edinburgh and Melbourne.

White, A., Handler, P. and Smith, E. L. *Principles of Biochemistry*, 5th Edition, 1973, McGraw-Hill Kogakusha Ltd., Tokyo, New York etc.

Williams, R. H. (ed.) *Textbook of Endocrinology*, 5th Edition, 1974, W. B. Saunders Co., Philadelphia, London and Toronto.

Wootton, I. D. P. *Micromethods in Medical Biochemistry*, 5th Edition, 1974, Churchill Livingstone, Edinburgh and London.

Zilva, J. F. and Pannall, P. R. *Clinical Chemistry in Diagnosis and Treatment*, 2nd Edition, 1975, Lloyd Luke, London.

INDEX

INDEX

Abortion, threatened
  determination of progesterone and
       pregnanediol in, 172
    of HCG in, 174
    of HPL in, 173
Absorption spectra,
  amphetamines and related substances,
    273
  aspirin, 277
  barbiturates, 289, 293, 294
  benzodiazepines, 309
  methaqualone, 323
  phenothiazines, 345
  tricyclic antidepressants, 356
Acetanilide, 278
Acetazolamide, inhibition of T_4
    formation in the thyroid, 39
Acetylcoenzyme A, 224
Acetylsalicylic acid, see Aspirin
Acidosis, metabolic
  in aspirin poisoning, 276
  in glutethimide poisoning, 321
Acrodynia, see Pink disease
Acromegaly, TRH stimulation test in, 25
ACTH, adrenocorticotrophic hormone
Addison's disease, 102
  ACTH stimulation test in, 103
  biochemical changes in, 103-104
  investigation of, 103-104
Adenylate kinase in thyroid disease, 36
Adrenal androgens, control of secretion
    of, 83
Adrenal cortex
  steroid hormones of, 45, 82
    metabolism of, 84
  stimulation of, 88
  suppression of, 89
  tumours of, 95-102
Adrenal medulla, 193
  hormones of, 193
  tumours of, 193
Adrenaline, 193 *et seq.*
  determination in urine, 200, 201
    in tissue extracts, 203
  formation and metabolism of, 193-194
  oxidation of, 195
Adrenochrome, 195
Adrenocortical dysfunction, 90-104

hyperfunction, 90-102
  in CAH, 91-94
  in Cushing's syndrome, 95-102
hypofunction, 102-104
Adrenocorticotrophic hormone (ACTH),
  82
  overproduction of, 90
  plasma, in Addison's disease, 103-104
    in ectopic ACTH syndrome, 102
  reducing plasma TBG, 39
  stimulation tests, 88
    in Addison's disease, 103
    in Cushing's syndrome, 99
  suppression of, using dexamethasone,
    89
Adrenogenital syndrome, 84
Adrenolutine, 195
Adroyd, reducing plasma TBG, 47
Aetiocholanolone, 46, 70, 84
  formula of, 51, 52
  increased urine excretion in CAH, 93
  metabolite of corticosteroids, 51
  originating from testis, 61
  Zimmermann colour equivalent of, 56
δ-ALA, δ-aminolaevulinic acid
Alanine aminotransferase (ALT), as
    indicator of liver damage, 283
Albamycin, 349
Albucid, 348
Alcohols, deaths from poisoning by, 264
Aldosterone, 46, 63
  chief mineralocorticoid, 82
  control of secretion of, 83
  formula, 49, 50
  in Addison's disease, 103
  increased secretion of, 91
Alkaline phosphatase isoenzymes from
    the placenta, 176
Alkaloids, 264, 269, 270, 274, 275, 279,
    291, 303, 356 *et seq.*
Alkalosis, metabolic, in aldosteronism, 91
  in Cushing's syndrome, 95, 102
  respiratory, in aspirin poisoning, 276
Allegron, 353
Allen correction formula, 57, 79, 159,
    161
Allopregnane, 47
Allopregnanediol, 48, 49, 52

Index

Allopregnanolone, 49, 52
Allo-series of steroids, 47
Allotetrahydro E and F, 70
ALT, alanine aminotransferase
Amargyl, 340
Amenorrhoea, primary
in CAH, 93
in hirsutism, 147
in simple virilism, 95
infertility in, 148
secondary in Cushing's syndrome, 95
infertility in, 149
investigation of, 149-150
Amethopterin, antagonist of folate
reductase, 236
Amino acid oxidase, 229
γ-Aminobutyric acid, deficiency in
infants, 235
Aminoglutethimide, inhibiting T_4
formation in the thyroid, 39
δ-Aminolaevulinic acid (δ-ALA)
dehydratase activity, reduced in lead
poisoning, 325
urinary, increased in lead poisoning,
325
Aminophylline, effect on excretion of
catecholamines, 200
Aminopterine, antagonist of folate
reductase, 236
p-Aminosalicylic acid (PAS), inhibition of
T_4 formation in the thyroid, 39
Amitriptyline, 263, 268, 351, 353
absorption maximum of, 356
colour reactions for, 354
GLC for, 303
Amniocentesis, 112
Amniotic fluid
bilirubin determination in, 112,
176-179
bilirubin/protein ratio in, 179
composition of, 111-112
fetal cells in, 112, 118
α-fetoprotein in, 112, 188
formation of, 111
phospholipids, determination in,
183-185
in respiratory distress syndrome,
182, 185
pregnanetriol in, in CAH, 188
volume of, 111, 185
determination of, 186
Amphetamine(s) 264, 270-274
absorption spectra of, 273
combined with other drugs, 275, 279
determination of by GLC, 273

drugs of abuse, 270, 274, 357
excretion of, 274
screening test for, in urine, 272
spectroscopic identification of, 272
Ampicillin, interfering in determination
of catecholamines, 200
Amylobarbitone (Amytal), 262, 275,
279, 290, 291, 341
extinction coefficient of, 296
R_f value by TLC, 300
Amylozine, 291, 341
Anabolic steroids, reducing plasma TBG,
39
Anadin, 275
Anaemia, see also Megaloblastic and
Pernicious anaemia
low serum tocopherol in, in infants,
223
Anaesthesia, induction of, by
barbiturates, 288
plasma cortisol increased by, 77
Anafranil, 352
Analgesics, 267, 275-283, 356
deaths from poisoning by, 263
drugs of abuse, 356
reducing plasma TBG, 39
Analgin, 275, 279
Anapolon, reducing plasma TBG, 39
Androgens, 46
effect at puberty, 142
formation of, 84
reducing plasma TBG, 39
reducing plasma transcortin, 77
Androstane, 45
5α-Androstane, 47
5β-Androstane, 47
effects on plasma transcortin, 77
5α-Androstane-3α, 17α-diol, 70
plasma, at puberty, 142
5β-Androstane-3α, 17α-diol, 70
5α-Androstane-3α, 11β, 17-triol, 71
5β-Androstane-3α, 11β, 17-triol, 71
Δ4-Androstenediol, 135
Δ5-Androstenediol, 49, 135
plasma, at puberty, 142
during the menstrual cycle, 137
in polycystic ovary syndrome, 147
in simple hirsutism, 146
index of androgen production, 63
menopausal and post-menopausal, 146
Androsterone, 46, 52, 61, 70, 84
Zimmermann colour equivalent of, 56
Aneurin, see Thiamine, 223 et seq.
Angiotensin 1 and II, 83
Angiotensinogen, 83

Index

383

Anorchia, 144
Anorectic amines, 270-271
Anovular cycles, 115, 142, 145, 148, 151
Antazoline, 264
Anterior pituitary
   secretion of ACTH by, 82
      of FSH and LH by, 105
      of TSH by, 1
   stimulated by TRH, 24
Anthelmintic, 339
Antibiotics, effect on determination of
   17-OGS, 61
Anticonvulsant drugs, 267, 268, 283-288
   barbiturates as, 284, 288
   deaths from poisoning by, 264
   displacing T_4 from binding to TBG, 39
   GLC for, 302
   inhibiting T_4 formation in the thyroid,
     39
   interaction between, 285
   monitoring of, 288
Antidepressants see also Tricyclic
     antidepressants
   deaths from poisoning by, 263
Antidol, 279
Antiemetics, phenothiazines as, 342
Antihistamines, 342
   deaths from poisoning by, 264
Antoin, 275
Apisate, 271
Appetite-suppressant drugs, 270
Ascorbic acid, 249-257
   determination in leucocytes, 256
     in plasma, 253, 254
     in urine, 250
     in buffy layer, 256
   properties of, 249
   saturation tests, 252
Aspartate aminotransferase (AST), used in
   testing for liver damage, 283
Aspirin, 263, 267, 275-278
   combinations with other drugs, 275,
     291
   determination in postmortem blood,
     277
     in serum, 277
   displacing T_4 from binding to TBG, 39
   effect on 17-OGS excretion, 71
   interference in oestrogen
     determination, 169
   poisoning, symptoms in, 276
     treatment of, 276
Atensine, 304
Ativan, 304

Atomic absorption spectroscopy
   determination of lead by, 325
   determination of lithium by, 331
Atomic weights, Table of, 376
AutoAnalyzer methods,
   for catecholamines (reference only),
     196
   for oestrogens, 163, 166
   for thyroxine, semiautomated, 12
Autoimmune thyroid disease
   (Hashimoto's disease), 41
Aventyl, 353
Avomine, 340
Azaphenothiazine, 339
Azospermia, 152

Bactrim, 349
BAL (British Anti-Lewisite), 325
Bananas, increased excretion of
     catecholamines after eating, 199
Banistyl, 340
Barbitone, 262, 290
   extinction coefficients of, 296
   R_f value by TLC, 300
Barbiturates, 283, 288-302
   absorption spectra of, 293, 294
   classification of, 290-291
   determination in blood, 292 et seq.
     by complexing with mercury, 289,
       292
     by GLC, 301
     by UV spectrophotometry, 289,
       293-297
   drugs interfering with, 293, 294, 297
   deaths from poisoning by, 262
   determination in urine and gastric
     aspirate, 295
   drugs of abuse, 288, 357
   effect on cortisol metabolism, 71
     on determination of 17-OS, 61
     on folate metabolism, 237
   extinction coefficients of, 296
   identification of types of, 295, 298
   mixed preparations containing, 291
   overdose, blood values in, 298
   TLC of, 298-300
Basal metabolism, 25-36
   definition of, 26
   effect of age on, 27-28
     body size on, 26
     fever on, 35
     previous diet on, 35
     sex on, 27
   interpretation, 35

384   *Index*

Basal metabolism—*cont.*
  in thyroid disease, 35
  measurement of, 28-35
    by closed circuit method using
      Benedict-Roth apparatus, 30
    by open circuit method, 30
    on out-patients, 33
    standards for, 27
Base deficit, in aspirin poisoning, 276
Basic drugs, GLC of, 303
Beclamide, 284
Bemegride, interference in barbiturate
  determination, 297
Benuride, 284
Benzedrex, 270
Benzodiazepines, 303-309
  absorption maxima of, 309
  clinical effects of overdose of, 304
  colour reactions for, 306, 308
  fluorimetric reaction for, 306
  GLC for (reference only), 309
  metabolism of, 304
  screening test for in urine, 305-308
  spectroscopic identification of, 308
Berkomine, 352
Bilirubin, determination in amniotic
  fluid, 176-182
Biloptin, interference in the
  determination of T_4, 14, 38
Bismuthate, sodium, as oxidising agent
  for C_{21} steroids, 65
Blind loop syndrome, 243
Blood, determination of substances in,
  see individual substances.
Borohydride as reducing agent
  in 17-oxogenic steroid determinations,
    65
  to remove glucose interference in
    oestriol determination, 169
Brietal, 291
Bromide, 267, 309-310
  determination in serum, 310
  formed from carbromal, 309
  overdosage, serum values in, 310
  treatment of, 310
Budale, 279, 291
Buffer solutions, Tables of, 366-371
Buffy layer, ascorbic acid in, 256
Butanol-extractable iodine, 8
Butazolidine, displacing T_4 from binding
  to TBG, 39
Butobarbitone, 262, 275, 279, 290, 291,
  341
  extinction coefficients of, 296
  R_f value by TLC, 300

C_{18} steroids, 45
  determination, see Oestrogens
C_{19} steroids, 46
  colour reactions for, 62
  group reactions of, 55
  Zimmermann reaction for, 55
C_{21} steroids, 46
  group reactions for, 63
  oxidising agents for, 65
  reducing agent for, 65
Cafadol, 279
Caffeine, 264, 275, 279
CAH, congenital adrenal hyperplasia
Calcitonin, 2
Calcium sulphaloxalate, 348
Calomel, in teething powders, 332
Calorie, unit of energy, 26
Cannabis, 357
Carbamazepine, 284, 285
Carbimazole, inhibition of T_4 formation
  in the thyroid, 39
Carbon monoxide poisoning, 311
Carbrital, 262, 291, 309, 318
Carbromal, 262, 268, 291, 309, 318
  screening test for in gastric aspirate,
    318
Carbutamide, inhibition of T_4 formation
  in the thyroid, 39
Carotenaemia, 217
Carotenes, 215
  determination in serum, 217
  foods present in, 217
Carr-Price reagent, 216
Catecholamines, 193 *et seq.*
  conjugates of, 193
  determination in urine, 195, 196
    effect of drugs on, 200
    effect of MAO inhibitors on, 200
    fluorimetric method for, 196
    interpretation, 199
  formation and metabolism of,
    193, 194
  screening test for, 199
  secretion of, 193
  separation of, 196
  tumours containing, 193
Catechol-O-methyl transferase, 194
Celontin, 283
Cerebrospinal fluid, sulphonamides in,
  350
Chemicals, deaths from poisoning by, 265
Chloractil, 340
Chloral hydrate, 262, 319
  interference in determination of
    catecholamines, 200

Index 385

metabolism of, 319
simple screening test for in gastric
aspirate, 319
Chloramphenicol, 285
Chlorate, 267, 311-312
screening test for in gastric aspirate,
312
Chlordiazepoxide, 264, 268, 303, 304
absorption maxima of, 309
colour reaction for, 306
effect on determination of 17-OS, 61
fluorescence reaction for, 306
GLC for, 303
Chlormadinone, increasing plasma TBG,
39
Chlormethiazole, 264, 284
Chlormezanone, 279, 291
Chlorphentermine, 270, 274
absorption spectrum of, 273
Chlorpromazine, 340
absorption maxima of, 345
colour reactions for, 344
metabolism of, 342
Cholecalciferol (Vitamin D_3), 221
Chorionepithelioma (chorioncarcinoma),
143
HGC secreted by, 109
Chromosomes, abnormalities of, 112, 144
in gonadal dysgenesis, 144, 149
in primary testicular disorders, 144
Claudication, intermittent, tocopherol
for, 223
Clofibrate, interference in determination
of HMMA, 211
Clomiphene (Clomid), 116
as stimulus for the hypothalamus, 116
in gonadal function test, 140, 144
in induction of ovulation, 151
in infertility, 150, 153
Clomipramine, 263, 284, 304
absorption maxima of, 356
colour reactions for, 354
Clonazepam, 284, 304
absorption maxima of, 309
reaction for in urine, 306
Cloxacillin, effect on determination of
17-OS, 61
CNS-stimulant drugs, 270-271
deaths from poisoning by, 264
Cobalamins (Vitamin B_{12}), 243-249
coenzyme functions of, 243
deficiency, assessment of, 244
causes of, 243
consequence of, 244
determination in serum, 244

in folate deficiency, 245
in foods, 243
Cocarboxylase, coenzyme function of,
223
in thiamine deficiency, 226
Codeine, 264, 275, 279, 291
drug of abuse, 356
GLC for, 303
Codis, 275
Competitive protein binding (CPB)
technique for determining plasma
oestrogens, 118, 156
progesterone, 128
testosterone, 136
thyroxine, 14
Compound E, see Cortisone
Compound F, see Cortisol
Compound S, see 11-Deoxycortisol
Concordin, 353
Congenital adrenal hyperplasia (CAH),
91-94
amniotic fluid in, 188
due to 11-hydroxylase deficiency, 94
due to 21-hydroxylase deficiency, 91
infertility due to, 149
investigation of, 91-94
17-OS and 17-OGS excretion in, 91-94
oxygenation index in, 72, 92
pregnanetriol excretion in, 79, 93
salt-losing, 91
suppression tests in, 92-94
virilising, 92
Congestive heart failure
blood pyruvate in, 228
in aldosteronism, 91
Conn's syndrome, 91
Contraceptive pill
effect on excretion of 17-OS and
17-OGS, 60
on plasma transcortin, 77
in hirsutism, 147
increasing the amount of TBG, 45
of SHBG, 136
secondary amenorrhoea after taking,
149
Coproporphyrins, increased in urine in
lead poisoning, 324
Cornea, vascularisation of in riboflavin
deficiency, 229
Corpus luteum, during the menstrual
cycle and early pregnancy, 110-112
formation and control of, 105, 106,
110
secretion of oestrogen by, 105, 112
progesterone by, 112

386   *Index*

Corticosteroids, 46, 63
  excretion of oestrogens impaired by, 171
  reducing plasma TBG, 39
  17-side chains of, 64
Corticosterone, 49, 50, 63
  included in 11-hydroxycorticosteroids, 73
Corticotrophin-releasing hormone (CRH), 82
  in Addison's disease, 102
  secreted in response to hypoglycaemia, 85
  to fall in cortisol output, 102
Cortisol, 46, 49, 63, 84, 128
  binding globulin, 77
  drugs influencing the metabolism of, 71, 77
  inhibition of T_4 formation in the thyroid by, 39
  plasma, determination as an 11-OHCS, 73
    diurnal rhythm of, 96
    drugs influencing, 77
    in Addison's disease, 103
    in Cushing's syndrome, 96
    increase after taking certain substances, 77
  reducing plasma TBG, 39
  secretion rate, 77
    correlation with plasma cortisol, 77
Cortisone, 49, 63
  plasma cortisol increased after taking, 77
  reducing plasma TBG, 39
α-Cortol, 52, 63
α-Cortolone, 52, 63
CPB, competitive protein binding
Cremotresamine, 349
Cretinism, 40
CRH, corticotrophin releasing hormone
Cryptorchidism, 144-145
Cushing's syndrome, 95-102
  causes of, 95
  dexamethasone suppression test in, 99
  investigation of, 95-102
  metopirone stimulation test in, 100
  17-OS and 17-OGS excretion in, 96-98
  plasma cortisol in, 96, 102
  ratio of urine 17-OGS to 17-OS in, 102
  summary of findings in, 100
  symptoms of, 95
  TRH stimulation test in, 25
  urine, free cortisol in 98
    pregnanetriol in, 79

Cyclobarbitone, 262, 290
  extinction coefficients of, 296
  R_f value by TLC, 300
Cyanocobalamin, 243
Cyclizine, 264
Cyproheptadine, 353
  absorption maxima of, 356
  colour reactions for, 354
Cyst fluid, composition in polycystic ovary syndrome, 147
Cysteamine, in treatment of paracetamol overdosage, 270
Cystine aminopeptidase, 174
  determination in maternal serum, 174-176
Cytochrome-C reductase, 229

Dalmane, 304
Dalysep, 348
Daprisal, 275, 279, 291
Dartalan, 341
Deaths by poisoning in England and Wales 1973, 262-265
Dehydration, in aspirin poisoning, 276
9(11)-Dehydroaetiocholanolone, 56
  Zimmerman colour equivalent of, 56
Dehydroascorbic acid, 249
7-Dehydrocholesterol, 220
Dehydroepiandrosterone (DHA), 46, 49, 50, 84
  changes during the menstrual cycle, 137
  plasma at puberty, 142
    in females, 137
  sulphate, 83, 112-114, 137
  Zimmermann colour equivalent of, 56
Delimon, 279
11-Deoxycorticosterone (DOC) 49, 50
  inhibiting formation of T_4 in the thyroid, 39
11-Deoxycortisol (Compound S), 49
  excretion of metabolites in the metopirone test, 86
  in CAH due to 11-hydroxylase deficiency, 94
21-Deoxyketols, 63
  in CAH, 65
  reduced by borohydride, 65
11-Deoxy-17-oxogenic steroids
  determination in urine, 68
    effect of drugs on, 71
    of glucose on, 68
  in CAH, 68
  in the metopirone test, 87
  separation from 11-hydroxy-compounds, 72

Index

Deoxyribonucleic acid (DNA) disordered synthesis of, 244
Desipramine, 263, 351, 352
  absorption maxima of, 356
  colour reactions for, 354
Dexamed, 270
Dexamethasone, 82
  effect of plasma cortisol, 77
  suppression test, 89
Dexamphetamine, 270, 275, 279, 291, 341
  effect on diurnal rhythm of plasma cortisol, 77
Dexedrine, 270
Dexocodene, 275, 279
Dextrone, 337
Dextropropoxyphene, 275, 279, 291
  drug of abuse, 356
Dexuron, 337
DHA, dehydroepiandrosterone
Diabetes mellitus, amniotic fluid volume in, 187
  blood pyruvate in, 228
  carotenaemia in, 227
  HPL in pregnancy in, 173
  oestrogen excretion in, 171
Diamine oxidase, determination in maternal serum, 176
Diamox, inhibiting T_4 formation in the thyroid, 39
Diarrhoea, blood pyruvate in, 228
Diatriazoate, interference in metadrenaline determination, 207
Diazepam, 263, 303, 304
  absorption maxima of, 309
  colour reaction for, 306
  fluorescence reaction for, 308
  GLC of, 303, 309
Dibenzazepines, 350, 352
  colour reactions for, 356
  deaths from poisoning by, 263
Dibenzepin, 353
Dibenzocycloheptenes, 350, 352-353
  deaths from poisoning by, 263
  fluorescence reaction for, 356
Dibenzodiazepines, 350, 353
  colour reactions for, 356
  deaths from poisoning by, 263
Dibenzoxepin, 353
Dibenzthiepin, 353
Dichloralphenazone, 319
2,6-Dichlorophenolindophenol, 250
Diet, effect on basal metabolism, 35
  in carotenaemia, 217
Diethylbarbituric acid, see Barbitone
Diethylpropion, 271, 274.

Diethylstilboestrol, increasing plasma TBG, 39
Digoxin, effect on determination of 17-OGS, 72
Dihydrocodeine, 264, 275, 279
Dihydrotestosterone, 135, 142
Dihydroxyacetones, 63
3,4-Dihydroxymandelic acid, 194, 205
3,4-Dihydroxyphenylacetic acid (dopac), 194
3,4-Dihydroxyphenylalanine (dopa), 193, 194, 205
  effect on TRH stimulation test, 24
  formed in neuroblastomas and phaeochromocytomas, 205
  interference in determination of HMMA, 211
  plasma cortisol reduced by, 77
Diiodotyrosine (DIT), 2, 3
Diketo-L-gulonic acid, 249
Dilosyn, 341
Dimethodilazine, 340
  absorption maxima of, 345
  colour reactions for, 344
Dimipressin, 352
Dindevan, inhibiting T_4 formation in the thyroid, 39
Dipalmitoyl lecithin, in amniotic fluid, 182
Diphenhydramine, 322
Dipipanone, 263
Diquat, 336, 337
Distalgesic, 279
DIT, di-iodotyrosine
Diuron, 337
Diverticulitis, 245, 249
Dolalgin, 279, 294
Dolasan, 275
Doloxene, 275, 279
Doloxytal, 291
L-Dopa, see 3,4-Dihydroxyphenylalanine
Dopac, see 3,4-Dihydroxyphenylacetic acid
Dopamine (3-hydroxytyramine), 193 *et seq.*
  determination of as total catecholamines, 196
  excretion of, following ingestion of bananas, 199
  urinary excretion of, in neuroblastoma, 212, 213
Doriden, 320
Dothiepin, 263, 353
  absorption maxima of, 356
  colour reactions for, 354

388   *Index*

Doxepin, 263, 353
  absorption maxima of, 356
  colour reactions for, 354
  fluorescence reaction for, 356
Drinamyl, 291
Drugs, see also individual drugs
  deaths from poisoning by, 262-265
  general considerations, 260-261
  interfering in determination of plasma
      cortisol, 75
    serum thyroxine, 39
    urinary catecholamines, 200
      HMMA, 209, 211
      metadrenalines, 207
      oestrogens, 169
      17-OGS, 71, 72
      17-OS, 60
  interfering in TRH test, 24
  materials used in analysis of, 266
  methods for studying
    extraction procedures, 266-269,
      357
    chromatography, 269, 359
    spectroscopy, 269
  of abuse, 260, 356 *et seq.*
    list of common, 357
    TLC for, 359
Duanol, 337
Durenate, 349
Duromine, 270
Durophet, 270
Dysfunctional uterine haemorrhage
  (DUH), 115, 153

E1, oestrone
E2, oestradiol
E3, oestriol
Ectopic ACTH syndrome, 91, 102
Edrisal, 279
Emeside, 283
Energy, units of, 26
Enteramide, 348
Enterovioform, interference in
  determination of PBI, 8, 35
Epanutin, see Phenytoin
Epiandrosterone, 52
Epilim, 284
Epiphen, 283
Equagesic, 275
Equaprin, 275
Ergosterol, 221
Ergotamine, 264
Erythromycin, effect on determination of
  catecholamines, 200
  of 17-OS, 61

Esgram, 337
Ethanol, 313-317
  deaths from poisoning by, 264
  determination, 313-317
    by GLC, 316
    in postmortem material, 317
    using the Conway unit, 314
  fate in the body, 313, 317
  plasma cortisol increased by, 77
  rapid screening test for in urine, 314
  values in intoxication, 317
Ethchlorvynol, 262, 268, 319
  screening test for in blood, urine and
    gastric aspirate, 320
Ethinamate, 268, 318
Ethinyloestradiol, increasing plasma TBG,
  39
Ethipram, 352
Ethoheptazine, 275
Ethopropazine, 340
  absorption maxima of, 345
  colour reactions for, 344
Ethosuximide, 268, 283
Ethotoin, 268, 283
Evidorm, 291
Extraction methods for drug separation
  of basic drugs, 266-269
  of drugs of abuse, 357-359

FAD, flavin adenine dinucleotide
Fenfluramine, 270, 274
  absorption spectrum of, 273
Fentazin, 341
Fetal death, low oestrogen excretion
  following, 170
  use of plasma HPL as indicator of, 172
    urinary pregnanediol as indicator
    of, 172
Fetoplacental unit, 154
  function tests, 154 *et seq.*
    determination of maternal plasma
      oestrogens, 156
      progesterone, 171
      maternal urinary oestrogens,
        158-170
      pregnanediol, 171
      maternal serum HPL, 172-174
        urinary HCG, 174
      maternal serum cystine
        aminopeptidase, 174-176
      other maternal serum enzymes,
        176
    tests on amniotic fluid, 176-188
α-Fetoprotein, 188
Fetus, anencephalic, 157, 170

Index

"small for dates", maternal plasma
  oestrogens in, 157
    urine oestrogens in, 170
    maternal serum cystine
      aminopeptidase in, 175
  HPL in, 173
  respiratory distress syndrome in, 182
Fever, effect on basal metabolism, 35
FIGLU, formiminoglutamic acid
Filon, 271
Flame photometer, determination of
  lithium, 330
Flavin adenine dinucleotide (FAD), 229
Flavin mononucleotide (FMN), 229
Fludrocortisol (9α-fluorocortisol), 82
Fluorimetric techniques
  benzodiazepines, 306
  catecholamines, 196
  "cortisol", 77
  N^1-methylnicotinamide, 231
  11-OHCS, 73
  riboflavin, 229
  thiamine, 224
  total oestrogen, automated, 163, 168
    manual, 123, 161
  xanthurenic acid, 233
Fluphenazine, 264, 341
  absorption maximum of, 345
  colour reactions for, 344
Flurazepam, 304
FMN, flavin mononucleotide
Folate deficiency, causes of, 235
  consequences of, 237
  determination of serum folate in, 238
    urine FIGLU in, 239-243
  histidine loading test in, 239
  increased excretion of MMA in, 249
  red cell folate in, 239
Folate, in food, 236, 237
  metabolism of, 237
  reductase, 237
Folic acid, 235
Follicle stimulating hormone (FSH), 1,
  105
  at puberty, 142-145
  during normal menstrual cycle, 110,
    139
  in testicular disorders, 144
  menopausal and post-menopausal, 145
  releasing hormone for (LH/FSH-RH),
    109
Formaldehyde, interference in
  determination of catecholamines,
    200
Formaldehydogenic steroids, 65

Formiminoglutamic acid (FIGLU), 238
  determination in urine, 239
5-Formimino-THF synthetase, 237
Fortalgesic, 279
Fortral, effect on excretion of 17-OGS,
  71
Free thyroxine index (FTI), 20
FSH, follicle stimulating hormone
Fucidic acid, interference in
  determination of 11-OHCS, 75
Fujiwara's test for trichloro compounds,
  319
Fungicides containing mercury, 332

Ganglioneuroma, 193
  adrenaline and noradrenaline in, 205
Gantanol, 349
Gantrisin, 348
Gardenal, 284, 290
Gas-liquid chromatography (GLC) for
  amphetamines, 273
  anticonvulsants, 302
  barbiturates, 301
  basic drugs, 303
  benzodiazepines, 309
  ethanol, 316
  methylmalonic acid, 248
  pregnanediol, 130-132
  steroid profiles, 72, 130
  tricyclic antidepressants, 351
    (reference only)
Gastrectomy
  increased urine MMA following, 249
  low serum B^{12} after, 245
Gastric aspirate
  determination of barbiturates in, 295
  fluorimetric test for benzodiazepines
    in, 307
  in analysis for drugs, 267
  screening test on for carbromal, 318
    chloral, 319
    chlorate, 312
    ethchlorvynol, 320
    phenothiazines, 345
    tricyclic antidepressants, 351
Gerisom, 279, 291
Gevodin, 279
Girard reagent T, 57
GLC, gas-liquid chromatography
Glucocorticoids, 82
  control of secretion of, 82
  effect on TRH stimulation test, 24
  reducing plasma TBG, 39

390 *Index*

Glucose, interference in determination of
oestrogens, 168
of 17-OGS, 68
tolerance test in Addison's disease,
103
β-Glucuronidase, 55
γ-Glutamyl transpeptidase (γGT), as
indicator of liver damage, 283
Glutethimide, 262, 267, 268, 320-322
determination in serum, 320
drug of abuse, 357
interference in determination of
barbiturates, 297
of 17-OGS, 72
poisoning, symptoms in, 321
17,20-Glycols, 63
20,21-Glycols, 63
Goitre, 37
non-toxic, 42
Gonadal dysgenesis, 149
Gonadal function tests, 114 *et seq.*
clinical problems associated with, 114
determination of gonadotrophins, 138
oestrogens, 117
pregnanediol, 130
progesterone, 128
testosterone and metabolites, 134
dynamic methods using
clomiphene, 140
HCG, 141
LH/FSH RH, 139
interpretation of, 141-153
Gonadotrophins, 1, 108-111, 138
at puberty, 109, 142-145
at the menopause, 109
determination, RIA methods for,
138
during the menstrual cycle, 138-139
pregnancy, 109
human chorionic (HGC), 109
menopausal (HMG), 109
in amenorrhoea, 150
hypogonadism, 62
hypopituitarism, 103
testicular disorders, 144
post-menopausal, 145
Graafian follicle, 105
Gramonol, 337
Gramoxone, 337
Gramuron, 337
Grave's disease, 37, 40
Growth hormone, plasma, in the insulin
stimulation test, 86
in hypopituitarism, 103
γ-GT, γ-glutamyltranspeptidase

Guanethidine, interference in
determination of catecholamines,
200
of HMMA, 211
Gynaecomastia, 115, 144, 147

Haem, effect of lead on synthesis of, 324
Haemopoiesis, disordered, 244
Hallucinogens, drugs of abuse, 357
Haloperidol, 264
Hashimoto's disease, 41
HCG, human chorionic gonadotrophin
Heminevrin, 284
Heparin, impurities in, interfering in
determinations of 11-OHCS, 76
Heptabarbitone, 262, 290
R_f value by TLC, 300
Herbicides, 337
Heroin, 264, 356
Hexahydro compounds, 52, 63
Hexobarbitone, 262, 290, 291
R_f value by TLC, 300
5-HIAA, 5-hydroxyindole acetic acid
Hirsutism, in the female, 95
Histidine, effect of folate deficiency on
the metabolism of, 237-238
loading test, 239
metabolism of, 238
HMG, human menopausal gonadotrophin
HMMA, 4-hydroxy-3-methoxymandelic
acid
Homovanillic acid, 194
HPA, hypothalamic-pituitary-adrenal axis
HPL, human placental lactogen
Human chorionic gonadotrophin (HCG),
1, 109
for inducing ovulation, 151
in pregnancy, 111, 112
in tests of fetoplacental function, 174
of gonadal function, 141
secreting tumours, 143
Human menopausal gonadotrophin
(HMG), 109
for inducing ovulation, 151
Human placental lactogen (HPL) in
maternal serum, 172
Hydantoin, 283
Hydatidiform mole, HMG produced by,
109
Hydramnios, 187
Hydrocortisone, see Cortisol
11β-Hydroxyaetiocholanolone, 46, 52,
70

Index

391

effect of hot acid hydrolysis on, 56
Zimmermann colour equivalent of, 56
17β-Hydroxyandrogens, in simple
hirsutism, 146
11β-Hydroxyandrostenedione, 46, 47, 49
11β-Hydroxyandrosterone, 70, 71
3-Hydroxyanthranilic acid, 233
Hydroxycobalamin, 243
11-Hydroxycorticosteroids,
determination in plasma, 73
effect of drugs on, 75
determination in urine, 74
effect of acid hydrolysis on, 54
17-Hydroxycorticosteroids, 46
6-Hydroxycortisol, increased after taking
some drugs, 71
16α-Hydroxy DHA, 113-114
in plasma, in females, 137, 142
sulphate, 112-113, 142
5-Hydroxyindole acetic acid (5-HIAA),
increased in urine after eating
bananas, 199
11-Hydroxylase deficiency, 91
17α-Hydroxylase, 84
21-Hydroxylase deficiency, 91
3-Hydroxykynurenine, 232, 233
4-Hydroxy-3-methoxymandelic acid
(HMMA), 194, 205
determination in urine, 208
in neuroblastoma, 212, 213
in phaeochromocytoma, 211, 212
formation of, 194, 205
screening test for, 208
substances interfering with, 209
4-Hydroxy-3-methoxyphenylacetic acid,
205
4-Hydroxy-3-methoxyphenyllactic acid,
194, 205
4-Hydroxy-3-methoxyphenylpyruvic acid,
194, 205
16α-Hydroxyoestrone, 107
17-Hydroxypregnanolone, 49, 52, 70, 80
determination in urine, 79
increased in CAH, 94
reduction by borohydride, 79

3α-Hydroxy-5β-pregnan-20-one, 48, 84
17-Hydroxypregnenolone, 49, 50, 84
112
3β-Hydroxypregn-5-en-20-one, 48
20α-Hydroxyprogesterone, 128
8-Hydroxyquinaldic acid, 232, 233
17β-Hydroxysteroids, 138
3-Hydroxytyramine, see Dopamine
Hydroxyzine, 264

Hyperadrenocorticalism, see CAH, and
Cushing's syndrome
Hyperaldosteronism, 91
Hypercholesterolaemia, serum tocopherol
in, 223
Hyperpituitarism, TRH stimulation test
in, 25
Hyperthyroidism, 40
basal metabolism in, 40
plasma TSH in, 40
serum adenylate kinase in, 36
cholesterol in, 36
creatine kinase in, 36
PBI in, 40
T_4 in, 40
use of lithium salts in, 330
T_3 toxicosis as cause of, 40
T_3 uptake tests in, 17
Hyperventilation, in aspirin poisoning,
276
Hypnotics, 267
barbiturates as, 288
benzodiazepines as, 303
carbromal, 318
chloral hydrate, 319
deaths from poisoning by, 262
drugs of abuse, 357
ethchlorvynol, 319
glutethimide, 320
methaqualone, 322
Hypoglycaemia, in Addison's disease, 103
in aspirin poisoning, 276
stimulus for release of CRH, 85
for secretion of growth hormone,
85
Hypogonadism, due to pituitary failure,
62, 144
17-OS excretion in, 62
Hypokalaemia, in aspirin poisoning, 276
in hyperaldosteronism, 91
Hypon, 275
Hypopituitarism, ACTH stimulation test
in, 103
adrenocortical failure due to, 103
basal metabolism in, 35
determination of growth hormone in,
103
gonadal function tests in, 144
myxoedema due to, 41
secondary amenorrhoea due to, 103
testosterone in, 143
TRH stimulation test in, 25
TSH stimulation test in, 25
Hypothalamic-pituitary-adrenal axis
(HPA), 84 *et seq.*

392 — Index

Hypothalamus, control of glucocorticoid secretion, 82
  decreased activity at puberty, 143
  secretion of CRH by, 82
    LH/FSH RH by, 109
    TRH by, 1
  stimulation of, 85, 116, 139-141
  suppression of, 89
  tumours of, 143
Hypothyroidism, 40
  basal metabolism in, 35
  carotenaemia in, 217
  differentiation between primary and secondary, 41
  genetic defects as cause of, 41
  plasma TSH in, 23
  secondary amenorrhoea in, 149
  serum adenylate kinase in, 36
    cholesterol in, 36, 40
    creatine kinase in, 36
    PBI in, 40
    T_4 in, 40
  TRH stimulation test in, 24
  TSH stimulation test in, 24
  T_3 uptake test in, 17

Ileitis, regional, 245
Imidazolone propionic acid, 238
Imipramine, 263, 351, 352
  absorption maxima of, 356
  colour reactions for, 354
  interference in determination of catecholamines, 207
    HMMA, 211
Indicators, Lists of, 365-366
Infants, convulsions due to pyridoxine deficiency, 235
  low serum tocopherol in, 223
Infertility, in testicular feminisation syndrome, 148
  in the female, 115, 148
    anovular cycles in, 151
    in amenorrhoea, 148, 149
    in polycystic ovary syndrome, 147
  in the male, 115, 152
    testosterone in, 134
Insidon, 352
Insulin stimulation test, 85
  in Addison's disease, 104
Intraval, 291
Intrinsic factor, deficiency of, 243, 245
Iodide, in synthesis of thyroid hormones, 2
  increasing T_4 output by the thyroid, 39

Iodine, butanol-extractable, 8
  metabolism in the thyroid, 3
  protein-bound, 5
  radio active, ^{131}I or [132]I, use of, 4
Iodipamide, interference in determination of metadrenalines, 207
Ionamine, 270
Iothalamate, interference in determination of metadrenalines, 207
Iproniazid, 263
Isoniazid, inhibiting T_4 formation in the thyroid, 39
  inhibiting a hepatic hydroxylase, 285
Ittrich reagent, 122-125, 161, 164

Joule, unit of energy, 26

Kallman's syndrome, 144
Kelfizine, 348
Kethamid, 271
20,21-Ketols, 63
20-Ketones, 63
Kidneys, damage due to paraquat, 336
  to phenacetin, 278
  secretion of renin by, 83
Kits, Quantisorb T_4N, 21, 22
  Res-O-Mat 15, 17
  Res-O-Mat ETR, 21, 22
  Res-O-Mat T_3, 18
  Tetralute, 14, 17
  Tetrasorb, 14, 17
  Trilute, 18, 19, 20
  Trisorb Tm T_3, 18, 19, 20
  Thyopac 3, 18, 19
  Thyopac 4, 14, 17
  Thyopac 5, 21, 22
  Thyrolute, 21, 22
Klinefelter's syndrome, 144
Köber reagent, 122-125, 159-161, 163, 166
Kynurenic acid, 233
Kynureninase, 232
Kynurenine, 233

Lactation, basal metabolism in, 35
Largactil, 340
Laroxyl, 353
LATS, long-acting thyroid stimulator
Lead, 324-330
  biochemical findings in exposure to, 329
  determination in blood and urine, 325
    after EDTA, 330
    values in lead exposure, 329
  effect on haem synthesis, 324

Index
393

treatment of toxicity due to, 325

Lecithin, determination in amniotic fluid, 182

Lederkyn, 349

Lentizol, 353

LH, luteinising hormone

Librium, 304

Lithium, determination in serum, 330
salts, inhibiting T_4 formation in the thyroid, 39, 330
plasma cortisol reduced by, 77

Liver damage, due to chlorate, 311
to paracetamol, 279
to paraquat, 336
effect on rate of removal of ethanol from the blood, 317

Long acting thyroid stimulator (LATS), cause of thyrotoxicosis, 37

Lorazepam, 264, 303, 304, 309
colour reactions for, 306
fluorescence reaction for, 306

Lucidril, 271

Lucophen, 270

Luminal, 284, 290

Luteinising hormone, (LH), 1, 106
during pregnancy, 112
puberty, 142-145
the menopause and post-menopausally, 109, 145
the menstrual cycle, 109-111, 139
releasing hormone for (LH/FSH-RH), 109

Lysergic acid derivatives, increasing T_4 formation in the thyroid, 39

Lysergide, drug of abuse, 357

Lysivane, 340

M&B 693, 349

Madrinon, 348

Malabsorption syndrome, folate deficiency in, 237
retinol absorption test in, 220
serum carotenes in, 217
tocopherol in, 223
urine MMA increased in, 249

Mandelamine, interference in oestrogen determination, 169

Mandrax, 262, 322-323

MAO, monoamine oxidase

Mazindol, 271

Meclofenoxate, 271
absorption spectrum of, 273

Medazepam, 264, 303, 304, 309
absorption maxima of, 309
colour reactions for, 306
fluorescence reaction for, 306

Medicel, 349

Medocodene, 279

Medomin, 290

Megaloblastic anaemia, B_{12} deficiency in, 244
folate deficiency in, 242

Megimide, interference in determination of barbiturates, 297

Meglumine salts, in contrast media interference in determination of metadrenalines, 207
of 17-OGS, 72

Melleril, 341

Melsedin, 322

Menopause, androstenedione at, 146
FSH at, 145
gonadal function at, 145
gonadotrophins at, 109, 145
LH at, 145

Menstrual cycle, 109
anovular, 115, 142, 145, 148, 151
disorders of, 114, 115
gonadotrophins during, 138, 139
hormone changes during, 109
plasma androstenedione during, 137
17-hydroxyprogesterone during, 137
oestrogens during, 119
progesterone during, 129
urine oestrogens during, 126-127
pregnanediol during, 134
pregnanetriol during, 137

Mepacrine, interference in determination of 11-OHCS, 75

Mephenytoin, displacing T_4 from binding to TBG, 39

Meprobamate, 264, 268, 275
effect on determination of 17-OS, 61

Mercury, 332-336
compounds, interfering in determination of PBI, 39
daily excretion of, 335-336
determination in urine, 335
in vapours, 333

Mescaline, 357

Mesontoin, 283

Metadrenaline (metanephrine), 194
determination in urine, 205
drugs and dietary substances interfering in, 207
formation of, 194
urinary excretion of in phaeochromocytoma, 211, 212

Metaperiodate, oxidising agent in determination of HMMA, 209
of metanephrines, 206

394   *Index*

Metaperiodate—*cont.*
of steroids, 55, 65
Methadone, 263, 356
Methaemoglobin, in blood in chlorate
poisoning, 311-312
Methaqualone, 268, 322-323
determination in serum, 323
drug of abuse, 322, 357
GLC for, 303
symptoms of overdose, 323
UV spectrum of, 323
Methdilazine, 341
absorption maxima of, 345
colour reactions for, 344
Methedrine, 270
Methimazole, inhibition of T_4 formation
in the thyroid, 39
Methisul, 349
Methohexitone, 291
Methoin, 268, 283
Methotrimeprazine, 340
absorption maxima of, 345
colour reactions for, 344
3-Methoxytyramine, 194
Methsuximide, 268, 283
Methylamphetamine, 270, 274
absorption spectrum of, 273
effect on diurnal rhythm of plasma
cortisol, 77
spectroscopic identification of, 272
α-Methyldopa, interference in
determination of catecholamines,
200
β-Methyl-β-ethyl glutarimide, 297, see
Megimide
Methyl glucamine, see Meglumine
Methyl malonate (MMA), 245-249
determination in urine, 245-248
after valine loading, 248
in B_{12} deficiency, 248
Methyl malonyl CoA, 246
Methyl malonyl CoA mutase, 243, 246
N^1-Methylnicotinamide, 231
determination in urine, 231-232
Methyl phenidate, 271
absorption spectrum of, 273
Methylphenobarbitone, 284, 290
Methyl salicylate, 263
Methyl testosterone, not converted to
17-OS, 62
reducing plasma TBG, 39
5-Methyl THF, 237
5-Methyl THF methyl transferase, 237,
243

Methylthiouracil, inhibiting formation of
T_4 in the thyroid, 39
Methyprylone, 263, 268, 318
Metopirone (metyrapone) test, 86
in Addison's disease, 104
in Cushing's syndrome, 99
normal response, 87
Mineralocorticoids, 82
control of secretion of, 83
MIT, monoiodotyrosine
MMA, methyl malonic acid
Modecate, 341
Moditen, 341
Mogadon, 304
Monlinuron, 337
Monoamine oxidase (MAO) inhibitors
effect on catecholamine excretion,
200
HMMA excretion, 211
metadrenaline excretion, 207
Monoiodotyrosine (MIT), 2, 3
Morphine, 264
drug of abuse, 356
effect on 17-OGS excretion, 71
17-OS excretion, 60
Motival, 341, 353
Mouth, lesions of in riboflavin deficiency,
229
Mysoline, 284
Myxoedema, see Hypothyroidism

Nalidixic acid, effect on determination of
HMMA, 211
of 17-OS, 61
Napsalgesic, 275
Narcotics, drugs of abuse, 356
Nembutal, 290
Neomercazole, inhibiting T_4 formation in
the thyroid, 39
Nephritis, chronic, serum carotenes in,
217
Nephrosis, secondary aldosteronism in,
91
Neulactil, 341
Neural crest tumours, 193
Neuroblastoma, 193
comparison of tests for, 212
3,4-dihydroxyphenylalanine formed
in, 205
urinary adrenaline and noradrenaline
in, 205
catecholamines in, 211
dopamine in, 212
HMMA in, 211, 213
Neurodyne, 279

Index

Niacin, see Nicotinic acid
Nicotinamide, 231
  coenzymes containing, 231
Nicotine, 231, 264, 270, 274
  absorption spectrum of, 273
  excretion of, 274
Nicotinic acid, 231
  determination of, 231
  formed from tryptophan, 233
Nitrazepam, 262, 304, 305
  absorption maxima of, 309
  colour reactions for, 306
  GLC for, 303, 309
Nobrium, 304
Noctec, 319
Noradrenaline, 193, 194
  determination in tissue extracts, 203
    in urine, 200
  formation, 194
  metabolism of, 194
  oxidation of, 195
Noradrenochrome, 195
Noradrenolutine, 195
Norepinephrine, see Noradrenaline
Norethandrolone, reducing plasma TBG, 39
Norethynodrel, increasing plasma TBG, 39
Normetadrenaline (normetanephrine), 194
  determination in urine, 205
  effect of drugs on secretion of, 207
  formation of, 194
  urinary excretion of in phaeochromocytoma, 211, 212
Norpramine, 352
Nortriptyline, 263, 341, 351, 353
  absorption maximum of, 356
  colour reactions for, 354
Noveril, 353
Novobiocin, 349
Nydrane, 284

Oat-cell bronchial carcinoma, 102
p-Octopamine, interference in determination of metadrenalines, 207
Ocusol, 348
Oestradiol-17β (E$_2$), 45, 46, 49, 105
  in dysfunctional uterine haemorrhage, 153
  modifications of, in urine, 107
  plasma, during normal menstrual cycle, 110, 119

Oestrane, 45
Oestriol-16α, 17β (E3), 45, 46, 49, 105
  determination in maternal urine by automated method, 163-168
  glucosiduronate, 114
  modifications of, in urine, 107
  sulphate, 105, 114
  synthetic pathway during pregnancy, 112-113
Oestrogens, 105 et seq.
  conjugates of, 107
  determination in plasma, 117, 156
    normal range, 119
    values in pregnancy, 156
  determination in urine, 121, 158-168
    normal range, 126
    values in pregnancy, 169
  during normal menstrual cycle, 110
    pregnancy, 112, 169
    menopause and after, 145
    puberty, 142-143
  effect on determination of 17-OS and 17-OGS, 61, 71
    concentration of plasma transcortin, 77
    TRH stimulation test, 24
  increasing plasma TBG, 39
  metabolism of, 106-107
  modifications, present in urine, 107
  synthesis of, 105-106
Oestrone (E1), 45, 49, 105
  modifications of, in urine, 107
17-OGS, 17-oxogenic steroids
11-OHCS, 11-hydroxycorticosteroids
17-OHCS, 17-hydroxycorticosteroids
Oleandomycin, effect on determination of 17-OS, 61
Oligomenorrhoea, 115, 150
Oligospermia, 152-153
Onadox, 275
Opipramol, 263, 352
Opsolot, 284
Orisulf, 349
Orphenadrine, 265
17-OS, 17-oxosteroids
Ovary, steroid hormones of, 45, 105
Ovulation, induction of, 151
  biochemical tests in, 151
Oxazepam, 294, 303, 304, 309
  colour reactions for, 306
  fluorescence reaction for, 306
Oxazolidones, 284
11-Oxoaetiocholanolone, 52, 70
  Zimmermann colour equivalent of, 56
11-Oxoandrosterone, 71

Index

17-Oxogenic steroids (17-OGS), 65
  determination in urine, 66
    effect of drugs on, 71-72
      glucose on, 68
    in Addison's disease, 103
    in CAH, 68, 91-94
    in Cushing's syndrome, 96
    in the dexamethasone test, 89
    in the metopirone test, 87
    normal ranges for, 72
17-OGS/17-OS ratio, 97
  in Cushing's syndrome, 97
  in simple virilism, 95
17-Oxosteroids (17-OS), 46, 84
  determination in urine, 58
    at puberty, 142-143
    hydrolysis of conjugates for, 54
    in Addison's disease, 103
    in CAH, 91-94
    in hirsutism, 95, 147
    in hypogonadism, 62
    in the metopirone test, 87
    normal ranges for, 61
  Zimmermann colour equivalent of, 56
20-Oxosteroids, 60
  increased excretion in CAH, 92
    in pregnancy, 60
  Zimmermann colour equivalent of, 56
Oxygen, effect of thyroid hormones on
  consumption of, 1
Oxygenation index, in Cushing's
  syndrome, 98
  in CAH, 72, 92
Oxymethalone, reducing plasma TBG, 39
Oxyphenbutazone, inhibiting T_4
  formation in the thyroid, 39
Oxytocinase, see Cystine aminopeptidase,
  174

Pco_2, in aspirin poisoning, 276
Paedo-Sed, 319
pH, of blood in aspirin poisoning, 276
  in ectopic ACTH syndrome, 102
Panadeine, 279
Paracetamol (p-acetylaminophenol), 263,
  267, 268, 275, 278
  absorption maxima of, 281
  combinations with other drugs, 275,
    279, 291
  conjugates of, 279
  cysteamine in treatment of overdose,
    279, 283
  determination in serum, 281-283
  excretion of, 279

hepatic necrosis due to, 279, 283
  tests for assessing, 283
  other toxic effects, 283
  screening tests for in urine, 280
Paracodol, 279
Paradione, 284
Parahypon, 279
Parake, 279
Paraldehyde, 262
Paralgin, 279
Paramethadione, 268, 284
Paramol, 279
Paraquat, 267, 336-339
  determination in blood and urine, 337
  preparations containing, 337
  qualitative test for in urine, 337
  toxic symptoms due to, 336
    treatment of, 339
Para-Seltzer, 279
Pardale, 279
Pathclear, 337
PBI, protein-bound iodine
Peganone, 283
Pemoline, 271
  absorption spectrum of, 273
Penicillamine, in lead poisoning, 325
Penicillin, effect on determination of
  17-OS, 61
  interference with oestrogen
    production, 171
Pentobarbitone, 262, 290, 291
  extinction coefficient of, 296
  given with carbromal, 318
  Rf value by TLC, 300
Pentothal, 291
Perchlorate, inhibiting T_4 formation in
  the thyroid, 39
Pergonal, 116
  for induction of ovulation, 151
Periactin, 353
Pericyazine, 341
Pernicious anaemia, Schilling test for, 245
  serum B_{12} in, 245
  urine methyl malonate in, 249
Perphenazine, 264, 341
Pertofran, 352
Pethidine, 263, 270, 274
  absorption spectrum of, 273
  drug of abuse, 356
PGA, pteroylglutamic acid
Phaeochromocytoma, 193, 211
  3,4-dihydroxyphenylalanine found in,
    205
  tissue content of catecholamines in,
    205

Index

urinary catecholamines in, 199, 201
   HMMA in, 209-212
   normetadrenaline in, 208, 211, 212
Phanodorm, 290
Phasal, 332
Phenacetin, 268, 275, 278
  combinations with other drugs, 275, 279, 291
Phenazocine, 263, 279
  effect on excretion of 17-OGS, 71
Phenazone, 268, 319
Phenbutrazate, 271
Phenelzine, 263
Phenergan, 340
Pheneturide, 284, 285
Phenindione, inhibition of T_4 formation in the thyroid, 39
Pheniramine, 264
Phenmetrazine, 271
  absorption spectrum of, 273
Phenobarbitone, 262, 284, 290
  as anticonvulsant, 284-285, 288
  extinction coefficient of, 296
  GLC for, 303
  half-life of, 288
  R_f value by TLC, 300
Phenothiazines, 264, 339-346
  colour reactions for, 344
    interpretation of, 346
  drugs of abuse, 357
  effect on excretion of catecholamines, 200
    of metadrenaline, 207
    of 17-OGS, 71
    of 17-OS, 60
  inhibition of T_4 formation in the thyroid, 39
  metabolism of, 342
  mixed preparations of, 341
  screening tests for in urine, 343
  spectrophotometry of, 345
  therapeutic uses of, 342
Phensic, 275
Phensuximide, 268, 283
Phentermine, 270, 274
  absorption spectrum of, 273
Phenylbutazone, 263, 268
  displacing T_4 from binding to TBG, 39
  effect on cortisol metabolism, 71
    on determination of 17-OGS, 71
Phenytoin 264, 267, 283-287
  determination in serum or plasma, 285
  displacing T_4 from binding to TBG, 39
  effect on cortisol metabolism, 71
    on folate metabolism, 237

  on the metopirone test, 87
GLC for, 303
interference in the excretion of 17-OS, 60
metabolism of, 285
monitoring of, 288
Phospholipids, in amniotic fluid, 182
Phthalylsulphathiazole, 348
Pink disease, 332, 335
Pituitary tumours, 143
Placenta, formation in pregnancy, 111
  steroid hormones, of, 45
  substances studied in function tests of, 134
Placental insufficiency, congenital absence of sulphatase, 171
Plasma, determinations using, see individual substances
Poisoning by, see individual substances
Polycystic ovary syndrome, 146, 147
Polyglutamates, 236
Ponderax, 270
Porter-Silber reaction, 63
Post-menopausal period, 145
Potassium chlorazepate, 303, 304, 309
  absorption maxima of, 309
  colour reactions for, 306
  fluorescence reaction for, 306
Potassium, serum, in aspirin poisoning, 276
  in chlorate poisoning, 312
  in Cushing's syndrome, 95
  in ectopic ACTH syndrome, 102
  in hyperaldosteronism, 91
  in salt-losing CAH, 91
Praminal, 352
Prednis(ol)one, 82
  inhibiting steroid production, 94, 95, 147
  inhibiting T_4 formation in the thyroid, 39
Pregnancy, basal metabolism in, 35
  changes in plasma TBG during, 22, 37
  hormone changes during, 111
  in diabetics, 171, 173, 176, 187
  increased need for folate in, 237
  plasma gonadotrophins in, 109
    oestrogens in, 156-158
    progesterone in, 171
  serum alkaline phosphatase iso-enzymes in, 176
    cystine aminopeptidase in, 176
    HPL in, 173
    tocopherols in, 223
    toxaemia of, amniotic fluid volume in, 169

398

Index

Pregnancy—*cont.*
  urine oestrogens in, 171
    pregnanediol in, 172
  urine oestrogens in, 169
    17-OS in, 60
    pregnanediol in, 172
Pregnane, 45
5α-Pregnane, 47
5β-Pregnane, 47
Pregnanediol, 5β-pregnane-3α,20α-diol, 48, 52, 71, 108
  determination in urine, 131-134
    colorimetric method, 132
    GLC of, 131
  effect of acid hydrolysis on, 54
  urine, during menopause and after, 146
    normal menstrual cycle, 110
    puberty, 142
  normal values, 134
Pregnanetriol, 52, 63, 70, 84
  determination in urine, 78
  urine during menstrual cycle, 137
    in CAH, 79, 92-94
    normal values for, 79
5β-Pregnan-3α-ol-20-one, (pregnanolone), 48, 52, 71, 130
Δ5-Pregnenolone, 49, 84, 108
Prethyroglobulin, 2
Priadel, 332
Priglone, 337
Primidone, 264, 267, 284, 288
  GLC for, 303
  monitoring of, 288
Probenecid, reduced excretion of 17-OS due to, 60
Prochlorperazine, 263, 340
  absorption maxima of, 345
  as antiemetic, 342
  as antihistamine, 342
  effect on metadrenaline excretion, 207
Progesterone, 48, 105
  metabolites of, 50, 108, 130
    determination in urine, 130
  plasma, determination in, 128
    during menopause and after, 145
    menstrual cycle, 110
    pregnancy, 172
Progestogens, 46, 49, 63, 107
  increasing plasma TBG, 39
Prolactin, 1
Promazine, 340
  absorption maxima of, 345
  colour reactions for, 344
Promethazine, 264, 291, 340

absorption maxima of, 345
  as antiemetic, 342
  as antihistamine, 342
  colour reactions for, 344
Prominal, 284
Propionate, conversion to succinate, 246
Propylhexedrine, 270, 274
Propylthiouracil, inhibition of T_4 formation in the thyroid, 39
Protamyl, 291, 341
Protein-bound iodine (PBI) composition of, 5
  determination in serum, 5
    effect of iodine containing drugs and contrast media on, 8, 37
    normal range, 16
Prothiaden, 353
Prothipendyl, 339
  as antiemetic, 342
Protriptyline, 353
  absorption maxima of, 356
  colour reactions for, 354
  GLC for, 354
Pteroylglutamic acid (PGA), 236
Puberty, 114-115, 142 *et seq.*
  delayed, 114, 115, 143, 145
  gonadal function tests at, 142
  increased androgen excretion at, 61
  precocious, 114, 143
Pyridoxal phosphate, 232
  coenzymes containing, 232
Pyridoxine (Vitamin B_6), 232
  deficiency of, 232, 235
Pyruvate, determination in blood, 226
  after test dose of glucose, 228

Quantisorb T_4 N kit, 21
Quinalbarbitone, 262, 290, 291
  extinction coefficient of, 296
  R_f value by TLC, 300
Quinidine, effect on determination of 17-OGS, 72
    17-OS, 61
Quinine, 264

Radio immunoassay (RIA) techniques, discussion of, for
  maternal plasma HPL, 173
  plasma oestrogens, 118, 155
    progesterone, 128
    testosterone, 135
    T_3, 17
    TSH, 23
  urine gonadotrophins, 138
Rapidal, 290

Index

Reagents, properties of common
laboratory, 372
Red cell, diminished survival, 223
folate, 239
transketolase, 228
uptake tests for T_3, 18, 19
Renin, 83
Renin-angiotensin system, 83
Reserpine, causing low T_4 values, 39
effect on excretion of catecholamines,
200
of HMMA, 211
on Zimmermann reaction, 61
Res-O-Mat kits, 15-20
Respiratory quotient (RQ), 29
Retinol (Vitamin A), 215
absorption tests, 220
serum, determination in, 216
Revanol, 322
RH, releasing hormone
Rhesus isoimmunisation
amniotic fluid bilirubin in, 176
volume in, 187
plasma HPL in, 173
urine oestrogens in, 173
RIA, radio immunoassay
Riboflavin (Vitamin B_2), 229
coenzymes containing, 229
urine, determination in, 229
after standard dose, 230
Rickets, 220
Ritalin, 271
Rivotril, 284, 304
Ronyl, 271
RQ, respiratory quotient

Safapryn, 275, 279
Salazopyrin, 349
Salicylamide, 263, 268, 275
Salicylate, 275-278
serum, determination in, 277
Salicylic acid, 267, 275
Salt-losing CAH, 91
Salt loss in aspirin poisoning, 276
Saridone, 278
Saroten, 353
Schilling test, 245
Scurvy, 252, 253
SD, standard deviation
SE, standard error
Seconal, 290
Sedatives as drugs of abuse, 357
Septrin, 349
Serenesil, 319
Serenid, 304

Serum, determinations in, see individual
substances
Sex hormone binding globulin (SHBG),
117
Simazine, 337
Sinequan, 353
Skin lesions in riboflavin deficiency, 229
"Small for dates" fetus, see under Fetus
Sodium bromide, see under Bromide
valproate, 284
Solpadeine, 279
Solvents, properties of common, 373
Sonalgin, 291
Sonegran, 291, 341
Soneryl, 290
Sparine, 340
Spironolactone, effect on determination
of 11-OHCS, 75
17-OS, 61
Spray-Seed, 337
Sprue, tropical, 243, 245, 249
Standards for volumetric analysis, 366
Steatorrhoea, see Malabsorption
syndrome
Stein-Leventhal syndrome, 147
Steladex, 341
Stelazine, 340
Stemetil, 340
Steroids, chemistry of, 45
conjugates of, 53
hydrolysis of, 53
determination, general techniques for,
53
isomerism of, 47
nomenclature, 46
17β-Steroid reductase in gynaecomastia,
148
Strychnine, 264
Succinate dehydrogenase, 229
Succinimides, 283
Succinyl CoA, 246
Succinylsulphathiazole, 348
Sulfametopyrazine, 348
Sulfasuxidine, 348
Sulphacetamide, 346, 348
Sulphadiazine, 348, 349
Sulphadimethoxine, 348
Sulphadimidine, 348, 349
Sulphafurazole, 348
Sulphamerazine, 349
Sulphamethazine, 348
Sulphamethizole, 349
Sulphamethoxazole, 349
Sulphamethoxydiazine, 349
Sulphamethoxypyridazine, 349

400 *Index*

Sulphanilamide, 346
Sulphaphenazole, 349
Sulphapyridine (M & B 693), 349
Sulphasalazine, 346, 349
Sulphathiazole, 349
Sulphatriad, 349
Sulphonamides, 346-350
  determination in blood, 347
  inhibiting T_4 formation in the thyroid,
    39
Sulthiame, 284, 285
Surface area from height and weight, 34
Surmontil, 352
Synacthen, 83
  depot, 88
  in ACTH stimulation test, 88
  in Addison's disease, 103

T_3, Triiodothyronine
T_4, Thyroxine
Tanderil, inhibiting T_4 formation in the
    thyroid, 39
TBG, thyroxine binding globulin
TBPA thyroxine binding prealbumin
Tegretol, 284
Tenuate, 271
Tercin, 275, 291
Teronac, 271
Terraklene, 337
Testicular feminisation syndrome, 148
Testis, gonadal function tests in diseases
    of, 143
  primary disorders of, 45, 61, 105
  steroid hormones of, 45, 61, 105
  tumours of, effect on urine 17-OS, 62
Testosterone, 46, 49
  in infertility, 149
  in simple hirsutism, 146
  plasma, determination in, 63, 116, 135
    at menopause and after, 146
    at puberty, 142
    normal values for, 135
  reducing plasma TBG, 39
  synthesis of oestrogens from, 105
  urinary, 136
Tetracosactrin, see Synacthen
Tetracycline, interference in
    determination of catecholamines,
    200
Tetrahydro E, 52, 63, 70
Tetrahydro F, 52, 63, 70
Tetrahydro S, 52, 63, 70
Tetrahydrofolic acid (THF), 236
Tetraiodothyronine, see Thyroxine
Tetralute kit, 15, 17

Tetrasorb kit, 15, 17
Thalazole, 348
Theophylline, interference in
    catecholamine determination, 200
    in TRH stimulation test, 24
THF, tetrahydrofolic acid
Thiamine (Vitamin B_1), 223 *et seq.*
  coenzymes containing, 224
  deficiency, tests for, 224-229
  determination in urine, 224
    after test dose, 225
Thiazide diuretics, cause of low T_4
    values, 39
Thiethylperazine, 264, 340
  absorption maximum of, 345
  antiemetic, 342
  colour reactions for, 344
Thin layer chromatography (TLC) for
    barbiturates, 289-300
  for drugs of abuse, 359
Thiochrome reaction, 224
Thiopentone, 291
Thiopropazate, 341
  absorption maximum of, 345
  colour reactions for, 344
Thioridazine, 264, 341
  absorption maximum of, 345
  colour reactions for, 344
Thyopac-3 test kit, 18, 19, 20
Thyopac-4 test kit, 15, 17
Thyopac-5 test kit, 21, 22
Thyroglobulin, 2, 3
Thyroid function tests, 4 *et seq.*
  interpretation, 37-42
  choice of, 37
  combined T_4 CPB and T_3 uptake test,
    21
  comparison of normal values in, 16
  determination of basal metabolism, 28
    et seq.
    of serum adenylate kinase, 36
      butanol-extractable iodine, 8
      cholesterol, 36
      creatine kinase, 36
      iodinated hormones, 9-14
      normal values for, 16
    PBI, 5-8
      normal values for, 16
    thyroxine by CPB, 14-15
      normal values for, 17
    TSH, 23
  free thyroxine index, 20-22
    effect of change in TBG on, 20, 22
  interference by drugs, 39
  in vivo test of iodine uptake, 4

Index

401

RIA for T_3, 17
red cell uptake test, 18, 20
stimulation tests, 25
suppression tests, 23
T_3 uptake tests, 17-20
urine T_3 and T_4, 23
Thyroid gland, genetic defects involving, 41
  hormones of, 1, 2
    effect on rate of metabolism, 1, 25
  synthesis of T_3 and T_4 in, 2
  tumours of, 37
Thyroid stimulating hormone (TSH), 1
  determination in plasma, 23
    after suppression with T_4, 25
    in the TRH stimulation test, 24
    in thyroid disease, 23-24
Thyrolute kit, 21
Thyrotoxicosis, 37
  due to T_3, BMR useful in, 35
Thyrotrophin, see Thyroid stimulating hormone
Thyrotrophin releasing hormone (TRH), 1
  effect of drugs on, 24
  stimulation test using, 24
Thyroxine (T_4), 1, 2
  combination with proteins, 2
  drugs affecting, 39
  free thyroxine index (FTI), 20-22
  serum, determination in
    after suppression with TSH, 23
    by CPB, 14, 17
    by semiautomated method, 9, 16
    urine, 23
    increase in nephrosis, 39
Thyroxine binding globulin (TBG), 2
  drugs affecting, 39
  increase in pregnancy, 22, 37
  variations in, effect on T_4, 20, 39
Thyroxine binding prealbumin (TBPA), 2
Tinnitus, 276
TLC, Thin layer chromatography
Tocopherols (Vitamin E), 222-223
  determination in serum, 222
Tofranil, 352
Tolbutamide, inhibition of T_4 in the thyroid, 39
Tolnate, 339
Torecan, 340
Tota-Col, 337
Total 17-oxogenic steroids, 66
Toxaemia of pregnancy, amniotic fluid volume in, 187
  HPL in, 173

urine oestrogens in, 171
  pregnanediol in, 172
Tranquillisers, 268, 269
  barbiturates as, 288
  benzodiazepines as, 303
  deaths from poisoning by, 263
  phenothiazines as, 342
Transcortin, 77
  plasma, effect of drugs on, 17
  in pregnancy, 77
Tranxene, 304
Tranylcypromine, 263
TRH, thyrotrophin releasing hormone
Triazamide, 349
Trichlorethanol, 319
Triclofos (Trichloryl), 319
Tricyclic antidepressants, 269, 350-356
  metabolism of, 351
  screening test for in gastric aspirate and urine, 351
  symptoms due to, 351
  UV absorption spectra of, 356
Tridione, 284
Triiodothyronine (T_3), 1
  combination with protein, 2
  free, in plasma, 4
    determination of, 17
  thyrotoxicosis due to, 35
  uptake tests, 17, 19
  urine, 23
    increased in nephrosis, 39
Trilute kit, 18, 19, 20
Trimeprazine, 340
  antihistamine, 342
  colour reactions for, 344
Trimethoprim, 349
Trimipramine, 263, 352
  absorption maxima of, 356
  colour reactions for, 354
Trinuride, 284
Trisorb kit, 18, 19, 20
Trithioperazine, 264, 291, 340
  colour reactions for, 344
Tropium, 304
Troxidone, 268, 284
Tryptizol, 353
Tryptophan, loading test, 235
  metabolic pathway of, 233
TSH, thyroid stimulating hormone
Tuinal, 262, 291
Tumours adrenal, cortical, 143, 148, 149
  medullary, 193
  catecholamine-secreting, 193
    ganglioneuroma, 193, 211
    neuroblastoma, 193, 212

402 *Index*

Tumour—*cont.*
  phaeochromocytoma, 193
  hypothalamus, 143
  oestrogen-secreting, 148
  ovarian, 143, 149
  pituitary, 148
  testis, 62, 143, 148
  thyroid, 37
Turner's syndrome, 149
Tyrosine, formation of adrenaline from, 194
  thyroxine from, 3
  iodinase, 3

Urine, determinations on, see individual substances
  urobilinogen, increased in folate and B_{12} deficiency, 244
Urocanic acid, 238
Urolucosil, 349

Vallergan, 340
Vanillin, formation from metadrenalines, 206
  interference of dietary, in determination of HMMA, 211
Vasosulf, 348
Veganin, 275, 279
Vegetarianism, and B_{12} deficiency, 245

Vertigon, 340
Virilising CAH, 92
Vitamin A, see Retinol, 215
  B_1, see Thiamine, 223
  B_2, see Riboflavin, 229
  B_6, see Pyridoxine, 232
  B_{12}, see Cobalamins, 243
  C, see Ascorbic acid, 249
  D_3, see Cholecalciferol, 220
  E, see Tocopherols, 222
Volital, 271

Weed killers, chlorate in, 311
  diquat in, 336
  paraquat in, 336
  deaths from poisoning by, 265
Weedol, 337
Weedrite, 337
Weights, desirable, according to height and age, 374

Xanthine oxidase, 229
Xanthurenic acid, 232
  determination in urine, 232-235

Zactipar, 279
Zactirin, 275
Zimmermann reaction, 55
Zwitterionic biological buffers, 371